# Globalization, Water, & Health

The School of American Research gratefully acknowledges
the co-sponsorship of the Society for Applied Anthropology
in developing this volume.

Publication of the Advanced Seminar Series
is made possible by generous support from
The Brown Foundation, Inc., of Houston, Texas.

**School of American Research
Advanced Seminar Series**

George J. Gumerman
*General Editor*

# Globalization, Water, & Health

**Contributors**

Alfonso Cortez-Lara
*Dirección Regional de Mexicali, Colegio de la Frontera Norte*

William Derman
*Department of Anthropology, Michigan State University*

John Donahue
*Department of Anthropology, Trinity University*

Anne Ferguson
*Department of Anthropology, Michigan State University*

Tom Greaves
*Department of Anthropology, Bucknell University*

David Guillet
*Department of Anthropology, Catholic University*

Yixin Huang
*Jiangsu Institute of Parasitic Diseases*

Barbara Rose Johnston
*Center for Political Ecology*

Carl Kendall
*School of Public Health and Tropical Medicine and Department of International Health and Development, Tulane University*

Irene Klaver
*Department of Philosophy and Religion, University of North Texas*

Lenore Manderson
*Key Centre for Women's Health in Society, University of Melbourne*

Linda Whiteford
*Department of Anthropology, University of South Florida*

Scott Whiteford
*Department of Anthropology, Michigan State University*

# Globalization, Water, & Health
*Resource Management in Times of Scarcity*

*Edited by Linda Whiteford and Scott Whiteford*

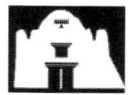

**School of American Research Press**
*Santa Fe*

## School of American Research Press
Post Office Box 2188
Santa Fe, New Mexico 87504-2188
www.sarpress.sarweb.org

Director: James F. Brooks
Executive Editor: Catherine Cocks
Manuscript Editor: Kate Talbot
Design and Production: Cynthia Dyer
Proofreader: Amanda A. Morgan
Indexer: Jan Wright

**Library of Congress Cataloging-in-Publication Data:**
Globalization, water, and health : resource management in times of scarcity / edited by Linda Whiteford and Scott Whiteford.– 1st ed.
    p. ; cm. — (School of American Research advanced seminar series)
  Includes bibliographical references and index.
  ISBN 1-930618-57-3 (cloth : alk. paper) – ISBN 1-930618-58-1 (pbk. : alk. paper)
  1. Water supply—Cross-cultural studies. 2. Globalization—Health aspects 3. World health. [DNLM: 1. Water Supply. 2. World Health. ] I. Whiteford, Linda M. II. Whiteford, Scott, 1942- III. Series.
  RA591.G57 2005
  363.6'1–DC22
                      2004030595

Copyright © 2005 by the School of American Research. All rights reserved.
Manufactured in the United States of America.
Library of Congress Catalog Card Number 2004030595
International Standard Book Number 978-1-930618-58-9 (paper).
First edition 2005. Second paperback printing 2011.

Cover illustration: Courtesy of WHO/TDR/Crump, image ID 9901821.

# Contents

|  | List of Figures and Tables | ix |
|---|---|---|
| 1. | Paradigm Change<br>*Linda Whiteford and Scott Whiteford* | 3 |
|  | SECTION I  Water-Linked Health Issues | 17 |
| 2. | Casualties in the Globalization of Water:<br>A Moral Economy of Health Perspective<br>*Linda Whiteford* | 25 |
| 3. | Water Reform, Gender, and HIV/AIDS:<br>Perspectives from Malawi<br>*Anne Ferguson* | 45 |
| 4. | Water, Vectorborne Disease, and Gender:<br>Schistosomiasis in Rural China<br>*Lenore Manderson and Yixin Huang* | 67 |
| 5. | Waste Not, Want Not: Grounded Globalization<br>and Global Lessons for Water Use from Lima, Peru<br>*Carl Kendall* | 85 |
| 6. | Whose Water Is It Anyway? Boundary Negotiations<br>on the Edwards Aquifer in Texas<br>*Irene Klaver and John Donahue* | 107 |

CONTENTS

| | SECTION II   Water Management and Health | 127 |
|---|---|---|
| 7. | The Commodification of Water and the Human Dimensions of Manufactured Scarcity<br>*Barbara Rose Johnston* | 133 |
| 8. | Water Struggles of Indigenous North America<br>*Tom Greaves* | 153 |
| 9. | Water Management Reforms, Farmer-Managed Irrigation Systems, and Food Security: The Spanish Experience<br>*David Guillet* | 185 |
| 10. | The Incredible Heaviness of Water: Water Policy and Reform in the New Millennium in Southern Africa<br>*William Derman* | 209 |
| 11. | Good to the Last Drop: The Political Ecology of Water and Health on the Border<br>*Scott Whiteford and Alfonso Cortez-Lara* | 231 |
| 12. | Concluding Comments: Future Challenges<br>*Scott Whiteford and Linda Whiteford* | 255 |
| | References | 267 |
| | Index | 303 |

# Figures

| | | |
|---|---|---|
| 2.1 | Map of Ecuador | 29 |
| 2.2 | Map of Bolivia | 39 |
| 3.1 | Map of Malawi | 47 |
| 4.1 | Boy with schistosomiasis | 77 |
| 4.2 | Woman washing clothes in a pond | 78 |
| 4.3 | Woman spraying vegetables with pond water | 79 |
| 5.1 | Map of Peru | 87 |
| 6.1 | Map of the Edwards Aquifer region | 112 |
| 6.2 | Cross-section of the Edwards Aquifer | 113 |
| 9.1 | Map of Spain | 186 |
| 10.1 | Map of Southern Africa | 210 |
| 11.1 | Map of United States/Mexico border region | 232 |

# Tables

| | | |
|---|---|---|
| 4.1 | Priorities of Yingjiang Villagers | 81 |
| 5.1 | Population of Metropolitan Lima | 94 |

*This book is dedicated to all those who suffer for water, with our hopes for a better future.*

# Globalization, Water, & Health

# 1

## Paradigm Change

**Linda Whiteford and Scott Whiteford**

This is a book about crimes and passions, about greed and global reach, illness and death, but also about the results of paradigmatic change—from the idea of health as a human right to one that elevates economics as the determinant of health. That change is played out through control of the very essence of life, water. In short, this is a book about the global contradictions in water use, ownership, and commodification, even in the very access to water. The crimes committed take the form of international contracts, corporate agreements, and local practices that divert water from small communities to larger cities and from households to agribusiness, that flood valleys to create dams, that shift resources from one state to another or from one country to another. This book is about the ongoing struggle for scarce resources among local communities, national governments, and international agencies such as the World Bank and the International Development Bank. In this struggle, even "virtual water" is commodified for future use, bought and sold in futures, and scarcity is manufactured to justify the diversion of water.

The anthropological contributions in this volume illuminate the cultural and political relations in a global arena where children die, adults sicken, and lives are cut short because of resource management techniques that privilege some over others. The authors combine their expertise in medical and ecological anthropology to challenge and deepen our understanding about water—its management, sale, and conceptualization—and its bearing on human health and well-being within the global nexus. The chapters are rich in ethnographic texture, history, and ironies as the authors offer in-depth insight into the cultures they discuss and the global political and economic processes they analyze.

It is no exaggeration to state that two major threats to world stability are the global disparities in health and in access to natural resources such as water—disparities that globalization only exacerbates. Drawing on anthropological studies and using social science theories, methods, concepts, and techniques, the authors explain the global processes affecting water management and health equity. The conclusions they draw should shape future policies and practices.

Most of the chapters in this book are based on long-term fieldwork, often carried out by teams of researchers. Increasingly, funders seek multidisciplinary teams because the problems under investigation are complex. The composition of each team reflects the subjects of inquiry. For example, research on resource management, health, and economic change frequently involves colleagues from disciplines such as medicine, geography, economics, and public health. This challenges many university-training paradigms that prepare anthropologists to work alone rather than in collaboration. Research on environmental and health issues, in particular, can be best accomplished by interdisciplinary teams of experts who can measure water quality, evaluate water structure delivery systems, define the economics of waste, understand the hydrology of a region or its ecosystems, draw blood samples, use field labs to diagnose samples, and analyze differential patterns of health system access and household use patterns, epidemiology, and political analysis.

Defining a study's boundaries is difficult, especially when examining health and social and environmental change in an era of globalization. Disease vectors such as mosquitoes, for instance, rarely if ever respect national or international boundaries unless these align with physical boundaries, such as mountains or lakes. The nature of the research problem defines the units of analysis. The chapters in this volume focus on individuals, households, watersheds, irrigation districts, and communities. Simultaneously, they examine vectors, hosts, and reservoirs of disease, as well as international discourses, power structures, and commodity chains. The authors creatively struggle with how to trace linkages in those chains, relating individuals to their larger, physical, social, and political surroundings. We want to point out that the units of study examined here differ drastically in size, but all fall within the purview of anthropological research and analysis. The authors take various theoretical perspectives—critical medical anthropology, economic anthropology, political economy, and political ecology—but all deal with the interplay between global and local forces and their effect on the environment and health.

Like many terms that have moved into the popular vernacular, *globalization* has multiple meanings. It has become important for anthropologists to examine the global network of cultural, economic, and political processes spurred by new technologies, and the consequences of these processes. Globalization is a theme and subject of inquiry in this volume for several reasons. First, world organizations such as the World Bank and the World Health Organization (WHO) have been disseminating an ideology of economic reform and waging global health campaigns, be they privatization or prevention campaigns, with worldwide effect. Greatly influenced by these ideologies, populations throughout the world have, in many cases, mobilized to resist, have reinterpreted, or have acquiesced to programs imposed by their nation-state governments. International nongovernmental organizations of many kinds have also engaged in global campaigns to stop HIV/AIDS, conserve virgin forests, or oppose modification of water. Transnational corporations such as General Motors, Upjohn, and Nestle have extended their markets and operate processing plants throughout the world with tremendous environmental and health consequences. These processes are occurring simultaneously in an era of neoliberal economic policies and global capitalism that characterized the decades (1980s and 1990s) before the eve of the new millennium.

This volume addresses changes occurring in response to global forces, translated into nation-state and regional agency policy or in local mobilization. As the chapters in this volume document, global processes transcend national borders, creating new, complex forms of organization. How social scientists, and anthropologists in particular, conceptualize the linkages between levels and forms of organizations as they trace meanings, power, and systems of power is one of the key issues for the future. We give different emphasis to global processes, even configuring them in diverse ways because of the diverse emphases of the questions they raise. The challenge we face is complicated by issues of scale, space, and time. As anthropologists, the authors' starting point is the local, defined in multiple ways; but in every case, their research methodology has extended beyond the local, to national and international policies or programs. This volume grapples with these challenges of scale and the complexity of interacting connections between levels and localities as the authors examine issues of poverty, illness, scarcity, power, local knowledge, resource degradation, and agency.

The authors used a wide range of research methods: surveys, life histories, discourse analysis, participant observation, epidemiological and clinical record reviews, water testing, soil testing, physical exams, focus groups, participatory research, cost-benefit analysis, archival research, spatial and institutional analysis, and clinical laboratory analysis. The diversity of methodological strategies attests to the complexity of the issues studied, the strength of forming interdisciplinary teams to tackle these highly complex issues, and the expansive and inclusive scope of anthropology.

Anthropology has a history of using local people as research assistants, and more recently as research partners. Structural and employment differences, however, often limit the equality of the partnership (Trostle 2000). Increasingly, community members of low-income neighborhoods are organizing to pressure the government for better water or health care or to address problems of contamination or failure of access. Participatory research is one way that scholarly inquiry can directly help local communities while also contributing to scholarly knowledge, enriched by the level of equality between the academic researcher and his or her research partner(s) from the community.

Most of the research in this volume not only stems from collaborative efforts but also is marked by an emphasis on historical analysis.

We agree with Farmer (2004:308) in his 2001 Sidney W. Mintz Lecture: "Erasing history is perhaps the most common explanatory sleight-of-hand relied upon by the architects of structural violence. Erasure or distortion of history is part of the process of desocialization necessary for the emergence of hegemonic accounts of what happened and why." We would like to underline the importance of historical research on patterns of water use, water access, and water conflicts. Relating water histories to health problems can provide an in-depth frame through which to connect issues that often appear disparate: resource management and health outcomes.

As mentioned earlier, whether in Africa, Latin America, or China, research almost always was conducted with colleagues from the country of study. This is increasingly important in anthropology, where both the Society for Applied Anthropology and the American Anthropological Association (among other professional associations) clearly identify in their ethical codes or guidelines the commitment to make one's research relevant to those with whom one works, that is, lending or service agencies, community members, and academics. This is particularly true in the fields of health and resource management because they so powerfully impact people's lives. Equally important is the commitment to publish or, in some other appropriate form, disseminate research results in the country where the research was carried out. Although this is a traditional component in anthropological discussions of methods and ethics, it is, unfortunately, frequently forgotten in the rush of academic or practitioner life.

Anthropology and the social sciences in general have an important role: to inform policy. The critical, structural approaches often employed in anthropology recognize that the social and political causes of structural violence against people based on gender, ethnicity, and economics require insertion into policy analysis. The policy issues addressed in this volume raise questions and issues such as whether water is a human right; how people should address the legitimacy of unequal access to safe drinking water within and among communities, regions, or nations; and what role public institutions, nongovernmental organizations, and the private sector should play in policy debates over decentralization, ethically based resource rights, and appropriate ways to price water to encourage equitable distribution and conservation.

These issues affect people in local communities all over the world; global influences are shaping policy and debate. Resolving disputes before they become violent is critical and requires interdisciplinary, international approaches using the watershed and community as units of management. Research needs to focus on how assumptions about the sustainable use of resources, growth, and environmental balance are similar or divergent and on the health implications of those assumptions. Research needs to expose the basis of assumptions and determine the forces leading to their creation and contributing to their maintenance. Research needs to be "ethnographically visible" and more, to expose the "materiality of the social" (Farmer 2004:305). Again quoting Farmer (2004:308), "I find it helpful to think of the 'materiality of the social,' a term that underlies my conviction that social in general and structural violence in particular will not be understood without a deeply materialist approach to whatever surfaces in the participant-observer's field of vision—the ethnographically visible."

Farmer's concept of "structural violence" provides the framework upon which this book rests. Whether the discussion centers on globalization processes, water use and misuse, or health and illness, we believe that the social, historical, economic, and political processes that underlie and are reified in social structures and organizations privilege some at the cost of others. Good health, like access to clean water, is never randomly distributed across sectors of society but rather advantages certain groups. Age, wealth, gender, ethnicity/race, and religion are examples of social categories often used to disenfranchise groups. We suggest that, in the study of globalization, resource management, and health, mechanisms of oppression must be made explicit, both as ethnographically visible and as the materialist conditions supporting that visibility.

Structural violence is a concept that makes explicit its focus on inequality and the mechanisms supporting it, and is therefore appropriate and necessary for our analysis. "The concept of structural violence is intended to inform the study of the social machinery of oppression. Oppression is a result of many conditions, not the least of which reside in consciousness" (Farmer 2004:307). The authors attempt to make explicit those cultural constraints whose sources lie in the invisible landscapes of history, politics, and dominance.

Why are we so interested in globalization, water, and health? To answer that question, we need to talk about people. The World Health Organization reports that 25,000 children die daily from illnesses associated with drinking water, that approximately four billion cases of diarrhea occur each year, killing more than 2.2 million people, and that some 1.7 billion people, more than a third of the world's population, live without access to a safe water supply (UNESCO 2003a). Water covers more than 70 percent of the earth's surface area, yet less than 1 percent of the world's water is available for human consumption. The extensive pumping of groundwater (Glennon 2002), increasing corporate purchase of water (Barlow with Clark 2002:130), and urban and agricultural divertissement of water (S. Whiteford and Melville, eds., 2003) are altering the world's water supply. The new millennium is seeing the intensification of the age-old robbery of water (and health) from the poor as global patterns of trade and consumption commodify water to increase capital generation.

One might ask, why do so many people suffer and die from diseases related to water? Not only is water an element essential for human survival, but it is also a medium for a wide range of diseases. Diseases related to water—such as cholera, some types of diarrhea, amoebic dysentery, schistosomiasis, and onchocerciasis—are usually discussed in terms of four conceptual disease categories: waterborne, water-washed, water-based, and water-related.

*Waterborne* diseases result from the ingestion of water containing pathogenic organisms: bacteria, viruses, or protozoa (cholera is a well-known example). Other waterborne diseases are typhoid, hepatitis, and giardiasis. All of these can be controlled through personal hygiene using safe water.

*Water-washed* diseases, also known as "water-scarce" diseases, occur when too little water is available for washing or personal hygiene. Water-washed diseases are often found when people who must conserve water do not have enough to wash their hands and face after defecating or when they endure common exposure to flies.

*Water insecurity* results when a history of water shortages causes people to adopt behaviors counter to hygiene practices recommended by public health standards, resulting in diseases such as scabies. Trachoma, pinworm, tinea, conjunctivitis, skin sepsis, and ulcers are also common outcomes of poor water quality, lack of access to soap, or failure of hygiene education.

*Water-based* diseases encompass a wide variety of illnesses linked by water. That is, humans are exposed to nonhuman hosts in which parasites live out part of their life cycle. Water in which people bathe, swim, or wash their clothing may be, for instance, contaminated by snails in which schistosomiasis or dracunculiasis (guinea worm) parasites and lung flukes live. The parasite is transferred as humans come into contact with the water in which the snails or flukes exist. Water access and management of black waters are critical to controlling the spread of water-based diseases.

The fourth category is *water-related* and includes diseases such as dengue and West Nile fevers, malaria, yellow fever, filariasis, and onchocerciasis (river blindness). The insect vector uses the water as a breeding ground, from which the vector emerges. Water is necessary, for instance, for the *aedes Egypti* mosquito to complete its life cycle. The mosquito is the vector (mode of transference) for diseases such as dengue fever that spread from one infected person to another by the blood meal process of the female mosquito. To reproduce, the female *aedes Egypti* mosquito must deposit her larvae in clear, still water, similar to the water often stored in and around homes.

Where sanitary systems are incomplete or absent, the disposal of water from households also is implicated in the spread of disease. Gray waters and black waters—waters containing household waste, including feces—may flow unchecked into streams and rivers, down gullies, and through peoples' yards and the ditches along roads. These water runoffs provide the breeding ground for other disease vectors, contaminate downstream water sources, and spread parasitic and vector-borne diseases.

Water quality, as well as water security, directly affects people's use of water to maintain their health through hydration and hygienic habits, to wash their foods, and even to keep their homes free of the vectors that carry disease. When water is scarce, unreliable, or of questionable quality, people reduce their use of it, often endangering their health. Thus, when water—the "blue gold," "human right," "liquid health," "fountain of youth and revival"—becomes commodified by trade agreements channeling it to some and excluding others, it becomes a mechanism that exacerbates already existing inequities and furthers the structural violence visited upon the poor and powerless.

Thirty years ago, Omran (1977) published an article describing a series of mutations in the interaction of humans, crops, and culture and the resultant health changes. What he referred to as "The Epidemiological Transition: A Theory of the Epidemiology of Population Change" was a sequence of complex interrelationships among increased population size, the domestication of grains and animals, and altered agricultural patterns and the effects of these on morbidity and mortality. Building on Omran's ideas and moving from the first epidemiological transition (occurring in prehistoric times, ten thousand years ago) through the second epidemiological transition (occurring in the late nineteenth and early twentieth centuries), Armelagos and others have identified what they refer to as the "Third Epidemiological Transition," occurring in the last third of the twentieth century. In the third epidemiological transition, societies have already conquered infectious and contagious diseases, and populations are faced with death and disability due not to infectious and contagious diseases, but rather to genetics and lifestyle.

The idea behind the epidemiological transition framework rests on the foundations of epidemiology (the population-based study of the determinants and distribution of disease) as applied to understanding emerging patterns of disease (Armelagos 1990). Human cultural changes producing new behavior and consumption patterns were analyzed to understand how population pressures, combined with access to newly domesticated foods or other resources, affect mortality and morbidity rates.

The second epidemiological transition was based, in part, on resource management of water and the capability of states to provide a reliable, potable supply of drinking water for their populace. Countries such as the United States emphasized the development of a public health infrastructure in the late nineteenth and early twentieth centuries, concomitant with the development of a Fordist workforce. As a result of adequate, publicly provided sanitation and potable water, reductions in the levels of infectious and contagious diseases transformed the US health profile, preparing for the third (and current) epidemiological transition. The development of vaccines to combat early-childhood diseases such as measles, mumps, and whooping cough, in combination with widespread access to potable water and sewerage disposal, created a health profile in which a larger number of children than ever before survived childhood.

Those who lived through childhood tended to succumb to diseases incurred through genetics, lifetime exposure, and lifestyle. In the early 1900s, the five leading causes of death in the United States were pneumonia, tuberculosis, diarrhea and enteritis, heart disease, and chronic nephritis. By 1990, the five leading causes of death in the United States were heart disease, cancer, stroke, injury, and lung disease. Cardiovascular diseases, malignant neoplasms, diabetes, and Alzheimer's disease replaced acute respiratory and diarrheal diseases as the primary killers of the population.

Understanding epidemiological transitions—for instance, from death and disability due to preventable diseases, to death and disability due to chronic and lifestyle diseases—is important because it provides the conceptual foundation for understanding potential health transitions generated by the globalization of commodities such as water. The second epidemiological transition occurred because public policies provided potable water and sanitary disposal of wastes as a public right. As world trade patterns increasingly determine access to water, basic health conditions and the assumptions about the role of the "public" in public health are changing. A brief recounting of the classic story of the Bank Street pump and its role in the history of protecting public health through supplying clean water and sanitation shows that those resources are necessary to achieving and sustaining the second health transition. Countries with little access to a reliable supply of clean water face almost insurmountable odds as they try to improve their health profile.

The second epidemiological transition was made possible because of informed, enlightened public policy and access to a reliable water supply. In the nineteenth century, cholera and other waterborne diseases were common killers. Cholera—the "blue death," that age-old and still current waterborne killer—was responsible for the first recorded documentation of disease transmission through water. During a cholera outbreak in London in the 1850s, thirty years before Robert Koch first identified the cholera vibrio, John Snow (1855

[1979]) identified and isolated water from a particular water pump as the source of the cholera infection. Snow, a physician and epidemiologist, mapped the topography of a cholera outbreak in a section of London by means of a door-to-door survey that enabled him to isolate the Broad Street pump as the source of contaminated water. After identifying the source, Snow removed the handle of the pump, thereby eliminating access to the contaminated water.

Not satisfied by merely eliminating access, Snow traced the way in which the Broad Street water supply became contaminated. He found that two water lines served a common neighborhood in London. One line, however, ran close to and was infected by a break in a sewage pipe. That water line provided water to those who used the Bank Street pump. Snow found that those who drank the water from the Bank Street pump (the most contaminated with sewerage) had a death rate nine times higher than neighbors who drank water drawn from a less polluted source.

In addition to tracing the mode of transmission, Snow identified the source of the infection and its consequences for the human gastrointestinal system. He conducted subsequent studies analyzing seasonal factors, gender differences in water-related behaviors, and occupational variables in the transmission of cholera. The scientific documentation from these early studies supported the national public-health policies aimed at public provision of clean water and safe waste disposal. The success of those initiatives made possible the second health transition, which dramatically improved the health profiles of countries such as the United Kingdom and the United States by the early part of the twentieth century.

WHO estimates that the quantity of water necessary for health varies not only with individuals' physical attributes (age, size, health status), but also with the climate in which they live. According to WHO, people living in temperate climates need 2 to 3 liters of water a day; those living in hot climates need between 6 and 10 liters of water a day. Although these amounts may be disputed, they give a rough idea of how much water is minimally required for sustainability. The UN High Commission for Refugees (UNHCR) suggests that a minimal amount of water is 10–11 liters during periods of high stress. In some countries, women expend up to kilocalories a day collecting water (see Ferguson, chapter 3 in this volume). Some estimates suggest that people can survive one month without food but only five to seven days without water. Those with limited access to water adapt their behaviors to accommodate water insecurity, often resulting in unhealthful patterns of water usage (L. Whiteford et al. 1999).

Now that we understand why water is critical to health, we may ask this question: why doesn't everyone agree that water and health are human rights and should be protected for everyone? The answer can be found in the paradigm shift. In this new era of globalization, health and water as human rights have been reconceptualized in an economically driven formula. Writing about this shift, Craig Janes describes a program called "New Century Scholar," which brought together thirty scholars from nineteen countries to discuss "Challenges of Health in a Borderless World." Janes (2004) writes that they were to "reflect on public health and health policy in a qualitatively new era of globalization. This era is marked in particular by the emergence of new, and powerful, non-state actors; shifts in health governance as the power of nation-states erodes; the ascendancy of the development banks as the drafters of health policy; the emergence of economics as the core social science of global health; and the dismantling of public health systems of health care and public health, increasingly replaced by private systems and NGOs."

Janes recounts his distress with the results of the WHO Commission on Macroeconomics and Health (Commission on Macroeconomics and Health 2001) and the Bill and Melinda Gates Foundation conceptualizations of global health challenges. Those challenges were constructed in terms of potential technological advances created by science and scientists and were measured by economics. Again quoting from Janes (2004), "the commission explained the relationship between poverty and disease, and their proposed solutions, illustrates the movement in global health policy from a focus on health as a human right to a utilitarian economics-based discourse, which, in this case, posits health as a determinant of global economic development." As the chapters in this volume clearly demonstrate, the shift in priorities from human welfare to economic development is not isolated to health but is a dominant theme in the commodification of water as well. Both the water and health discourses masquerade as means to reduce poverty and facilitate economic development but succeed best in continuing the structural violence visited on the least powerful.

In closing this first chapter, we find ourselves drawn to the eloquent writing of Vandana Shiva (2002; quoted in Hyatt 2004:x): "Paradigm wars over water are taking place in every society, East and West, North and South. In this sense, water wars are global wars, with diverse cultures and ecosystems, sharing the universal ethic of water as an ecological necessity, pitted against a corporate culture of privatization, greed, and the enclosures of the water commons." We hope that the following chapters will help students, colleagues, practitioners, and policy makers better understand the relationship between health and water and the necessity of restoring the human rights paradigm.

# Section I
# Water-Linked Health Issues

# Introduction

## Linda Whiteford and Scott Whiteford

In this volume, authors have tried to be attentive to the role scale plays in determining research questions and the methods appropriate to capturing global connections without losing sight of local applications. The chapters by Linda Whiteford (chapter 2) and Scott Whiteford and Alfonso Cortez-Lara (chapter 11), which begin and end the book, carefully document and describe how global trade agreements commodify, trade, and direct water rights. Those chapters powerfully trace how policies created by global agencies such as the World Bank and the International Development Bank directly and indirectly affect access to clean water, and human health, in communities in Mexico, Ecuador, and the Dominican Republic.

Chapters in Section I place their conceptual emphasis on health as they focus on the interstices between health outcomes and water access. Section II reverses the order of emphasis; authors focus on water and resource management, which they then relate to health. The authors address issues of scale in contemporary research, the cultural construction and interpretation of history, power, decision making, commodification, and the multiple, overlapping, often contradictory agendas being played out as global forces intersect with local realities.

In chapter 2, the opening chapter of this section, Linda Whiteford links the failure to bring health to the world-trade negotiating table specifically to the ascendancy of the "health as an economic outcome" paradigm. Developed by economists (Janes 2004), this paradigm has replaced the "health as a human right" model espoused by social justice advocates. Using the concept of structural violence, Whiteford argues that inequalities of power that disadvantage developing countries in global trade agreements manifest in higher levels of malnutrition, premature deaths due to waterborne and insectborne diseases, and prolonged disabilities disproportionately suffered by the poor, women, and the elderly. To illustrate these points, she draws on case materials from Ecuador and the Dominican Republic. Whiteford introduces the concept of the "moral economy of health," challenging us to ensure that discussions of health maintain equal footing with those of trade and commerce.

Questions of scale are also mediated by socially constructed concepts such as gender, as Anne Ferguson shows in chapter 3. She connects international water decisions with their gendered implications for the health of women in Malawi and the potential role of the HIV/AIDS epidemic. In many societies, gender plays a critical role in the allocation of activities and resources; in all societies, water and health are gendered concerns.

In chapter 3, Ferguson notes that in Southern Africa, where the rates of HIV/AIDS infection are the highest in the world, the disease is recognized as "both a health and a development crisis." New policies and laws on water, land, poverty alleviation, and natural resource management recently enacted in the region have, by and large, overlooked the implications of HIV/AIDS. Ferguson considers the gender and health implications of the neoliberal-inspired water reform being implemented in Malawi, one of the poorest countries in Southern Africa. While privatization of municipal water supplies has captured much international notice—and criticism—little attention has been given to the effects of "community-based" policies for rural water supply in the context of the HIV/AIDS epidemic. Here, too, enclosure is underway. Using research findings from southern Malawi, she suggests that the new water-reform policy may increase social and gender differentiation, creating greater inequality and causing more ill health.

Understanding the social construction of gender and its implications for health and water provides a critical link in the synthetic approach that is the aim of this book. In Ferguson's chapter 3, gender as a social construct is identified, in part, as a mediating variable between water reforms and health outcomes in Malawi. The same theme is also dominant in chapter 4, where Lenore Manderson and Yixin Huang highlight the disconnect between water management policies and disease prevention, demonstrated by the failure to control schistosomiasis in eastern China. They write that schistosomiasis is "the most important tropical disease of pubic health and socioeconomic importance" and the one vectorborne disease in which water is directly implicated. Manderson and Huang explore the epidemiology and social context of this disease, illustrating how social constructs such as gender and demographic, economic, and political factors influence exposure and rates of infection.

As a case study, Manderson and Huang focus on one small agricultural village on the Yangtze River in Anhui Province in eastern China. Schistosomiasis infections are endemic there, and the authors explore how water resource policies, the construction of large dams, and the wider processes of modernization and globalization affect the villagers' lives. Within the household, men and women share decision making about priorities and spend their limited discretionary cash on domestic buildings and marriage arrangements. At the level of village decision making, in which women have virtually no say, the priorities for expenditure are irrigation and roads, income-generating programs and small industries, and schistosomiasis control. The distribution of water resources, the maintenance of the irrigation system, and any new engineering works are village responsibilities. Although the villagers are well aware of various waterborne or water-washed diseases and diseases related to rudimentary hygiene and sanitation, few have the cash resources to improve their domestic facilities. None have the resources to prevent regular contact with water that is infested with snails and infected with schistosomes, other parasites, and viruses.

Carl Kendall's chapter 5 takes us to South America. Ethnographically set in Lima, Peru, Kendall situates his chapter in the anthropological concern with scale. Using Buroway's idea that imagination serves as a mediator between the local and the global, Kendall focuses on the management not of water, but of diarrhea, in a desert city where water consumption is low and diarrhea rates high. His chapter links Buroway's "grounded globalization" to traditional fieldwork in realist ethnography that interprets cultural constructs as a charter for social organization and material culture. The chapter discusses the global forces, connections, and imaginations creating the unusual situation in Lima, where daily water use per person is significantly less than the UN-reported minimum required for survival. As a result, the environment is contaminated, and the recorded levels of diarrheal disease in children are among the highest in the world. Limeños, in turn, have refigured these global forces into a liquid mirror, one that distorts globalizing forces and produces both a misguided "penny capitalist" response and a culture of controlled consumption to make those forces manageable. The analyses employed throughout the chapter provide alternative ways of conceptualizing global processes from both theoretical and practical viewpoints.

Chapter 6, the final chapter in section I, unites the two themes of health and resource management. Irene Klaver and John Donahue discuss public negotiations concerning water management of the Edwards Aquifer in southwest Texas. The topic of public health was not addressed in these negotiations, and the authors explain the meaning of this omission. Situating their analysis on the local political level of the Edwards Aquifer Authority, they contextualize their discussion with some of the global forces and agendas involved in drawing hydrological boundaries and setting resource rules. They show how one governing body, in particular, functions as a model-boundary object. Klaver and Donahue conclude that a broad partnership of citizens and professional, elected officials involved in planning, developing, and managing water resources enhances the success of integrated water-resource management. In detail, they also identify the potential conflict between the welfare of the ecosystem and the health of humans, a theme in many other chapters of the book.

The anthropological analyses in this section draw on ethnographically rich cases from Ecuador, Malawi, China, Peru, and the United States to demonstrate the continuing disenfranchisement of the world's most vulnerable populations. The cases exemplify how political and moral economy/ecology/medical anthropology perspectives identify key issues embedded in social, gender, and ethnic prejudices as they transform policies controlling access to the "public health commons."

# 2

## Casualties in the Globalization of Water

*A Moral Economy of Health Perspective*

**Linda Whiteford**

> Health should be seen as a global public good from which we can all benefit and to which we all should contribute.—*Kelley Lee*

The first casualty of the globalization of water may be a population of millions around the world. It has been more than one hundred fifty years since Snow discovered that contaminated water spreads cholera. It has been more than twenty years since the United Nations declared the International Drinking Water Supply and Sanitation Decade (1980–1990). The UN declaration was intended to bring attention to the plight of the world's population living without access to clean water and sanitation. Even with that decade of attention and the ten years between 1990 and 2000, population growth rendered those gains almost stagnant (UNICEF 2004). Every eight seconds, a child dies from drinking contaminated water (Children's Water Fund 2004). This chapter traces how failure to address health issues when water rights are traded and sold has contributed to declining health worldwide. Using several countries in Latin America and the Caribbean as examples, this chapter shows how neoliberal trade and lending regulations increase the structural violence and burden of waterborne diseases in the daily lives of the world's disadvantaged.

In the latter half of the twentieth century, national and international policies rejected the moral obligation to safeguard public health essentials (clean air, water, environment) in favor of protecting individual and corporate economic market interests. As a result, the valences of public policy also shifted, commodifying natural resources formerly considered a human right. As Barlow and Clarke note (Barlow with Clarke 2002:130), in the twenty-first century, corporate players such as the Global Water Corporation regard water not as a human right, but as "a rationed necessity that may be taken by force."

The "tragedy of the commons," traditionally referred to as the loss of shared productive land through uncontrolled overuse, now has new meaning. The new tragedy of the global commons is the loss of shared, publicly protected natural resources through their sale for economic gain. As clean water becomes more difficult to secure, the number of preventable deaths and disabilities due to unreliable and/or inadequate water supply increases exponentially.

As the Center for Policy Analysis on Trade and Health (CPATH 2004) notes, "health is both a universal aspiration of all peoples and governments and a mark of the egregious disparities that exist between the developed and developing worlds. In 2000, at the World Summit for Social Development in Geneva, leaders worldwide committed to attaining universal and equitable access to basic health care, sanitation and drinking water, to protect health, and to promoting preventive health programs. But too often health and a stable infrastructure of services are considered secondary to formulas for economic growth that may or may not succeed." The Free Trade Area of the Americas (FTAA) proposals, such as the North America Free Trade Agreement (NAFTA), are designed to liberalize trade by reducing tariffs and regulatory policies and thereby, according to some analysts, encourage trade. Their deregulatory stance, however, has negative implications in the areas of human rights and human health. The regulation of public health measures has been responsible for creating and assessing conditions that protect the public's health—clean water, safe housing, and a healthy environment. Again, according to CPATH (2004), "as under the foreign investment chapter (Chapter 11) of the North American Free Trade agreement (NAFTA), private companies can challenge laws and regulations adopted by democratically elected governments and officials. Any 'measure' is subject to elimination if it is shown that it is not 'necessary,' or is 'unduly burdensome to trade....FTAA could apply to public sectors.... No vital human service in the US would be exempted under these conditions, including health care, and water services would be subject to privatization and deregulation." The responsibility for protecting the public's health should not be for sale.

Lack of clean water and effective sanitation systems exposes between 2.4 and 3.5 billion people annually to preventable disease and death (Ahmed 2002). Parasites, such as cryptosporidiosis, are becoming common in many regions of the world, including the United States. *Cryptosporidium* has been found in drinking water, swimming pools, and streams accidentally contaminated by human feces.

An estimated two hundred million people worldwide are infected with schistosomiasis, and another two billion are at high risk of infection (WHO *World Water Day Report* 2001). Schistosomiasis, also known as "bilharziasis," is a debilitating waterborne disease most often infecting women who bathe or do the family wash in rivers where they come in contact with snails harboring the parasites (see Manderson and Huang's chapter 4 in this volume). Untreated schistosomiasis infects internal organs such as the liver, resulting in disability and ultimately death (Ahmed 2002).

Trachoma, another preventable hygiene-related disease, has blinded more than six million people, and perhaps as many as five hundred million people are at risk for blindness (World Bank 2002a; WHO 2000; WHO *World Water Day Report* 2001; Ahmed 2002). Trachoma is caused by *Chlamydia trachomatis*, a bacteria spread by physical contact and insect vectors. The World Health Organization (WHO) estimates that trachoma cases in some parts of Africa may reach as high as 40-percent prevalence in children (Ahmed 2002).

Intestinal worms infect nearly 10 percent of the population in the developing world (WHO 2000), causing malnutrition and anemia and, in the most severe cases, retarded growth. Bacterially caused diseases such as cholera, typhoid fever, and dysentery, even chronic diarrheas such as *Brainerd diarrhea*, are preventable with good hygiene, water, and sanitation. These interventions reduce diarrheal disease by 25 to 33 percent (WHO *World Water Day Report* 2001).

Even developed nations like the United States experience occasional and accidental exposures to waterborne bacteria and parasites. For less developed countries, the risks are higher and the exposures are constant. The 1990s cholera epidemic in South America is an example of the enduring health consequences when globalization diverts political will from investments in public water and sanitation. Privatization and decentralization in Ecuador have resulted in growing global investments, but often without global responsibilities for maintenance and sustainability. Water systems installed but never maintained and sanitary systems dumping wastes into the water of neighboring communities fail to protect community health.

Globalization exists in many forms and has many definitions. In this chapter, *globalization* means the "creation of new economic, financial, political, cultural, and personal relationships through which societies and nations come into closer and novel types of contact with one another" (Waters 2001:8). Much has been written about globalization, but this chapter is concerned with how trade practices—such as the "banana wars" in Europe in the 1990s, the continuing "coffee wars," or the current "water wars"—are decided by global trade organizations such as the World Trade Organization (WTO) and how those decisions impact community health. Health outcomes and health policies, practices and models, are intimately tied to economic and political decisions. Nowhere is that linkage more distinct than in the public health arena. The aim of this chapter is to promote cognizance of the unhealthy, unjust consequences of global neoliberal trade and to propose an approach that ties global trade to public health essentials. As the world adopts new covenants of global trade, those covenants must include the protection of public health commons: clean water and air.

The remarkable epidemiological shift that occurred in the United States and much of the developed world in the twentieth century was possible only because of an inexpensive, reliable, clean water supply and publicly underwritten sanitation. Using a political economy of health analysis, political decision makers of the late nineteenth century recognized that the maintenance of a stable, reliable workforce depended on the control of the communicable diseases ravaging large urban centers and decimating the populace. Fear of contagion was also a motivation. The burgeoning middle class, which could afford clean water and sanitary facilities, feared that it would lose its economic advantages if infected by others. The result was the creation of political and public health policies to deliver a dependable water supply and

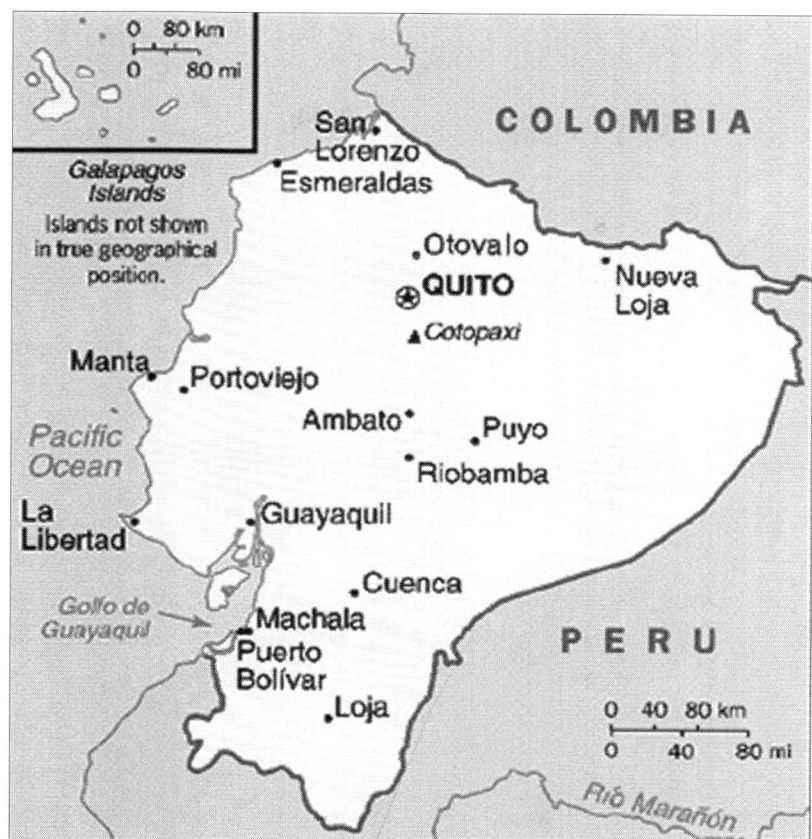

FIGURE 2.1
Map of Ecuador.

sanitation system not merely to those who could afford it, but to all members of the society.

By the 1930s, following prolonged and concerted efforts to provide water and sanitation to large urban centers, the incidence of communicable and contagious diseases—the early killers of children and the elderly, the wasting killers of those in their most productive years—dramatically decreased in many parts of the United States and Britain. Significant reductions in the disease rates among economically productive adults created the healthy, productive workforce critical to economic transformation.

In view of the social and economic gains realized by the first public-health transformation, this chapter suggests that it is now time to bring a *moral* economy of health perspective to the discussion of health costs incurred by globalization. A moral economy of health framework makes explicit a set of values that honor the obligation to protect common global resources, identify the underlying social and political structures of violence against disenfranchised populations, and defend health as a human right to be protected in global trade and lending agreements.

Most of the developed nations similarly reduced disease by offering essential basic services to protect public health. Today, however, much of the world remains without access to such basic services. In 1998 WHO, the United Nations' agency focusing on health, published a review of the first fifty years of its activities. In that report, the agency (WHO 1998) notes that even with the significant reduction of death and disease in many parts of the world, "21 million deaths—2 out of every 5 worldwide—will be among the under-50s, including those of 10 million small children who will never see their fifth birthday." By 1998 diarrhea and malaria (two water-related diseases) accounted for more than 5 million of those deaths, and more than 2.3 billion people still suffered from other diseases linked to water. To expose the structural violence of unequal access to clean water and sanitation, as well as the role played by globalization and neoliberal trade, the following case study applies a moral economy of health perspective to the Ecuadorian cholera epidemic of the 1990s.

## A CASE STUDY: CHOLERA IN ECUADOR

Many water-related pathogens have been identified since Dr. John Snow undertook his classic experiments in London with the Bank Street pump. But the distribution of disease—and its prevention—is a social and political activity as much as a biological one. The recent cholera epidemic in Ecuador demonstrates how a moral economy of health perspective identifies the local and global, social and political factors promoting the spread and continued reinfection of a marginalized, vulnerable population.

In March 1991 the El Tor strain of *cholera vibrio* hit Ecuador. Part of a widespread epidemic in northern South America, it would progress throughout the continent before being controlled. By the time this epidemic began to subside, in 1993, more than eighty-five thousand cases were clinically diagnosed in Ecuador, with more than one thousand fatalities. Although the epidemic hit the entire country, the majority of cases (80 percent) occurred in only twenty townships. To understand why this concentration occurred where it did, and its consequences, one must know about Ecuador's culture, history, and geography.

Ecuador is one of the smallest countries in South America, located in the northwest between its larger and more powerful neighbors, Colombia and Peru. Ecuador straddles the equator (hence, its name), situated in both the northern and southern hemispheres. Geographically limited (260,000 sq km), it encompasses both an extraordinary natural biodiversity of birds and plants and a rich cultural diversity. Indigenous cultures such as the Shuar, Chachis, and Achuar compose some of the more than fourteen distinctive ethnic groups (Perrottet 1993). Most travelers to Ecuador know the two primary cities—Quito, the Andean capital between the two cordilleras of volcanoes that create the "spine" running from the north to the south of Ecuador, and Guayaquil, the large coastal city on the Pacific side of the country. Other travelers know the Amazon in the south or the famous weaving center, Otovalo, in the north. While the cool, high mountains of the Andes attract many visitors, the lush and fascinating Amazon region draws others. Birders and hikers from around the world visit the Galapagos Islands with unlimited fascination.

As a secondary center of the Spanish Empire, Ecuador never experienced the degree of glory nor endured the hardships that Peru and Colombia did, but its customs and architecture reflect many cultural and physical inheritances from the Spanish occupation. Along with these, Ecuador adopted beliefs about European superiority, with the result that indigenous groups are among the most economically deprived in the country. They live in remote regions with limited access to resources, including water.

Cholera bacteria are transmitted through water, and cholera is a waterborne disease most commonly associated with fecal-oral contact. When the bacteria are introduced into the human system, they can cause severe constrictions in the human gut, resulting in excessive fluid discharges—extreme diarrheal crisis. That crisis can be reversed if treated in time; otherwise, dehydration causes other system failures, ending in death. One common consequence of extreme fecal discharge is contagion, through contact with water containing the *cholera vibrio* or with feces from infected persons.

After the *vibrio* is introduced into a water system, it can be stopped by practicing basic hygiene techniques—washing hands with soap and defecating away from water supplies—or by disinfecting the water supply. Both require access to water and sanitation infrastructures. During the cholera pandemic in Ecuador, the large urban areas of Quito and Guayaquil were able to control the outbreaks within eleven months. In the twenty townships in the rural Andes, however, it took almost three years.

To understand this unequal distribution of disease, we must ask why the spread of the disease was controlled first in the large urban areas and only much later in the rural, indigenous areas. We may also ask, what does the moral economy of health perspective tell us that helps illuminate the situation? How does a focus on the social, cultural, and political mechanisms underlying and reinforcing unequal patterns of disease provide insight into this case, and what are the moral concomitants of these mechanisms?

First, we must know something about the twenty townships where the epidemic continued to rage. They are in five states, two along the coast and three inland. The two coastal states or *provincias* (Esmeraldas and El Oro) were characterized as populated areas with inadequate access to water and sanitation, as well as continued ingress of international travelers. The three mountain states (Chimborazo, Cotopaxi, and Imbabura) have the largest concentration of Indians. These are states rich in traditions, festivals, rituals, and indigenous cultural beliefs and practices. All five states share high levels of poverty and the structural violence maintained by distance, both geographic and social, from power. The three mountainous states suffered also because their population was predominately indigenous, rendering them targets for prejudice and further isolating them from access to resources.

In 1994–1995, as the US medical anthropologist, I worked closely for twelve months with a team of two Ecuadorians—an epidemiologist/ physician and a community educator. We were brought together by the Ecuadorian government with the assistance of the US Agency for

International Development. The team, directed by the United States–based Environmental Health Project (EHP), was to conduct an in-depth investigation into why cholera persisted in the states of Chimborazo and Cotopaxi. In the third high-incidence state, Imbabura, the Harvard diarrhea project was conducting a study/intervention, so Imbabura was omitted from the EHP scope.

The EHP team was charged with (1) identifying cholera-related adult behaviors in high-risk communities, with the objective of isolating behaviors and beliefs associated with potential increased risk of cholera, (2) gathering and analyzing data on environmental and domestic health behaviors, (3) developing and implementing interventions to change high-risk behaviors, (4) setting up a monitoring system, and (5) training local people to continue the monitoring and to document activity results. We developed a health intervention model, the Community-Based Participatory Intervention (CPI). We trained fifty-five individuals in community education techniques and leadership skills, conducted ethnographic and epidemiological research, and designed and led community-based interventions (L. Whiteford with Laspina and Torres 1996). Following the intervention phase, a second project was conducted to evaluate the outcomes and the sustainability of the CPI model, documenting a successful and sustained change in behaviors that resulted in the control of the cholera epidemic in the study sites (L. Whiteford with Laspina and Torres 1996).

The project successfully identified detrimental beliefs and behaviors and brought about the sustained reduction of cholera in the two project states. Directly and indirectly implicated in the spread of cholera were several actions: defecation in fields or other areas close to living and eating activities; substandard hygiene related to water; food preparation by street vendors, as well as the conditions in which they served food; food preparation and distribution during religious and community festivals; and contact with migrants returning from endemically infected coastal areas. In addition, we identified contributing factors of environmental and political conditions, such as the disposal of hospital waste in open canals from which downstream residents drew their drinking water.

The behaviors contributing to the spread of cholera reflected information commonly available in the extant literature. What was too often neglected in the same literature, but is pertinent here, was the larger political arena that fostered the spread of waterborne diseases in some communities but not in others. In both Chimborazo and Cotopaxi, water is abundant, flowing from the slopes of numerous volcanoes throughout the area. But the conditions under which the water is transferred from source to ingestion are unprotected and easily contaminated by waste—human, animal, and hospital. Usually, the water is not piped into homes but is collected and stored by families. This means that water is a scarce commodity in the home, even though abundant at its source. Too often, piped water (in those communities where the infrastructure exists) is not chlorinated because the local community cannot pay water taxes necessary to buy disinfectants. Therefore, even if the water is piped, it may not be potable, a distinction typically unrecognized in local communities. We discovered that the provision of water was inadequate and often unsafe.

Like many other countries in South America in the early 1990s, Ecuador adopted neoliberal economic reforms that resulted in decentralization of economic responsibilities. In some cases, the central government promised economic resources to local agencies. That monetary transfer, however, was often inadequate or never occurred. The burden of paying for chlorination fell to the communities; they, in turn, levied a water tax. Members of those communities with piped water systems responded, "Why should we pay to buy chlorine for our water when we already have water that comes into our homes without paying?" Unfortunately, the water transported to their homes was unprotected from the wastes emptied into the system upstream. During the continuing economic crisis that Ecuador has experienced since the late 1990s, few families have had either the resources or the inclination to pay for something (chlorination) that appears to be unnecessary.

The globalization of trade further shifted the economic valences in the two states, increasing privation in the rural communities. Particularly hard hit were ethnic communities already marginalized from the global economy. In both Chimborazo and Cotopaxi, more men migrated to coastal communities where demand for temporary manual labor is constant and where cholera is endemic. Several times a year, the men returned to participate in communal rituals, sharing their food and drink. In several study communities, the incidence of cholera spiked following these migrants' participation in communal festivals. In this way, cholera continued to be re-introduced into the rural, indigenous communities.

As national governments turn their attention to global trade, they further exclude the marginalized, rural, indigenous communities from basic services. Placing the responsibility on local communities to provide the necessary resources for developing or maintaining infrastructure makes adequate water and sanitation—basic human rights, according to the moral economy of health perspective—impossible for the poor.

In the case of the cholera epidemic in Ecuador, the beliefs and behaviors of individuals in the most highly affected communities were relatively easy to identify. People recognized ways to change their own behaviors to reduce the likelihood of cholera, provided they could pay for soap, chlorine, and household water-storage tanks. With resources made available through project funds, five target communities were successful in controlling cholera and sustaining the reduction. But the larger problems remain: how to protect all the other communities at risk for waterborne, water-washed, and water-related diseases (see chapter 1) and how to encourage local, regional, national, and global powers to support basic water and sanitary systems for communities.

A moral economy of health analysis would propose that in order to achieve the second epidemiological transition—reduction of morbidity and mortality due to infectious disease—countries like Ecuador should obligate global trade partners in exchange for natural resources and labor. For instance, as part of trade agreements, Texaco and other companies would provide water and sanitation infrastructure to the communities where they extract resources. In such agreements, trade partners would commit to providing materials and technology to increase access to the public health "commons" in exchange for trade concessions. This argument is neither new nor novel and has most recently been articulated by Evelyne Hong (2000).

## GLOBALIZATION AND HEALTH DISPARITIES

Evelyne Hong, in her powerful indictment of global trade (Hong 2000), embeds her discussion in a historical framework starting with the colonial experience and slavery. She then moves to postcolonial development, free market reforms, the roles of the World Bank and the WTO, the Agreement on Technical Barriers to Trade (TBT), the Agreement on Trade-Related Aspects of Intellectual Property (TRIPS), and the General Agreement on Trade in Services (GATS). For the purpose of this chapter, the roles of the World Bank and the WTO are discussed as they affect health care reforms and health status in various countries.

In 1987 and in 1993, respectively, the World Bank published *Financing Health in Developing Countries: An Agenda for Reform* and *World Development Report: Investing in Health.* Both publications present agendas promoting the financing and delivery of health care by market forces but fail to address the economic disparity underlying poor health. "The Report recognizes that poverty is a threat to health but does not address the issue of economic inequality and poor health" (Hong 2000:27). In an attempt to quantify the effects of poor health on economic productivity, the report calculates the impact of the burden of disease on a population through the Disability Adjusted Life Years (DALYS)—a formula for measuring how many days of an economically productive life are potentially lost because of morbidity (illness). Using such a calibration, the World Bank recommended the following three actions: (1) initiation of clinic user fees, (2) decreased national spending on health services and a transition of health care programs from a model of universal access to primary health care to a model of selected primary health care, and (3) the privatization of health services through the market system. The neoliberal reforms espoused in the last twenty years of the twentieth century resulted in many health-care systems abandoning policies of free or low-cost care and the central government turning over essential functions, such as the purchase of vaccines, to local government.

One example of the high price of cost reduction comes from Colombia. In the 1990s, privatization and decentralization of health care resulted in fewer immunizations against childhood diseases. The vaccines were too costly for local governments, and the national community-health infrastructure that supported local communities had been devastated through neoliberal reforms. Since then, the Colombian government has returned to centralized purchasing and distribution of drugs essential to protect the population (Duque 2002).

In 1999, however, an outbreak of measles—a disease easily preventable by immunization—had a much greater epidemiological potential to sicken and kill than it otherwise would have, because many children along the Colombian-Venezuelan and the Colombian-Ecuadorian borders were not immunized.

In conjunction with the push to decentralize and privatize health services, the World Bank instituted structural adjustment policies (SAPs) to reduce the likelihood of countries defaulting on loans. Many developing countries negotiated loans with the World Bank during the more economically lush periods of the 1970s and early 1980s, only to find themselves unable to repay the interest, let alone the principal. In 1982, when Mexico defaulted on its loans, the World Bank instituted SAPs to discourage other countries from following Mexico's lead. The World Bank used SAPs to encourage countries to generate money for paying off their loan debts by cutting state subsidies from their internal markets. But the institution of SAPs provoked heated discussions, antigovernment backlash, and riots. In 1985, for instance, SAPs resulted in food riots in the Dominican Republic, where state subsidies for beans and rice were removed and prices rose beyond what many could afford (L. Whiteford 1997, 1998, 2000). People burned tires in the streets of Santo Domingo to block the police and ransacked stores in protest. At least one protestor was killed when the police arrived to quell the disturbance.

Countries like the Dominican Republic were encouraged to seek international markets in order to obtain foreign currency and to develop products for export rather than develop local, domestic economies. For many countries, SAPs meant the removal of price controls and basic food subsidies, the reduction of social services such as health care and education, and the devaluation of their currencies—in some cases, even the loss of their national currency, as occurred in Ecuador in 2000 when the US dollar became the national currency. These measures eventually led to inflation; price hikes for food, consumer durables, gasoline, fuel, and farm equipment; curtailed government spending; decreased real wages; civil service job layoffs; closure of schools, hospitals, and clinics; and a collapse in public investments and domestic manufacturing (L. Whiteford with Laspina and Torres 1996:14–15). These measures undermined the government's ability to support the public health infrastructure, provide low-cost medical care, and create and maintain potable water and sanitation systems.

Decentralization and privatization of government services—two basic tenets of neoliberal reform—have intensified disparities and inequities experienced by the poor as their access to affordable health care diminishes (see S. Whiteford and Cortez's chapter 11, Johnston's chapter 7, and Guillet's chapter 9 in this volume). In Bolivia, particularly in the rural areas, decentralization translated into a loss of services. In 1997 externally mandated and internally executed decentralization plans meant that local communities had greater decision-making opportunities. Community groups met to discuss and identify local health needs. To compensate for the loss of services from the central government, they designed local, low-cost health care strategies to reduce water-related diseases. But rural communities often did not receive enough financial support from the national government in La Paz to carry out their plans. Decentralization, for them, became responsibility without resources (L. Whiteford et al. 1999).

The privatization of health care has had similar disastrous consequences. While the government concentrates on creating a health care system designed to recover costs, the poor are turned away because they cannot pay user fees. Because government health services must attract paying clients, the system has to aim at serving the upper and middle classes. In South America, it is not uncommon to have multiple health systems, each servicing a specific social group. The Dominican Republic, for instance, has four health systems: a publicly funded, low-cost public system serving the poor, a private health-care system serving the middle and upper classes, a social security health-care system funded jointly by the government and employers, and a health-care delivery system for the military and their families (L. Whiteford 1997, 1998, 2000). The public health delivery system, always underfunded and overutilized, received even less state funding when the World Bank encouraged the Dominican Republic to develop a free-market public health system through the use of SAPs. In this free-market model, health is no longer considered an inalienable right: it is a private good (L. Whiteford with Laspina and Torres 1996:29). As health care becomes a commodity, state welfare systems are disintegrating.

As the public infrastructure deteriorates, governments give less

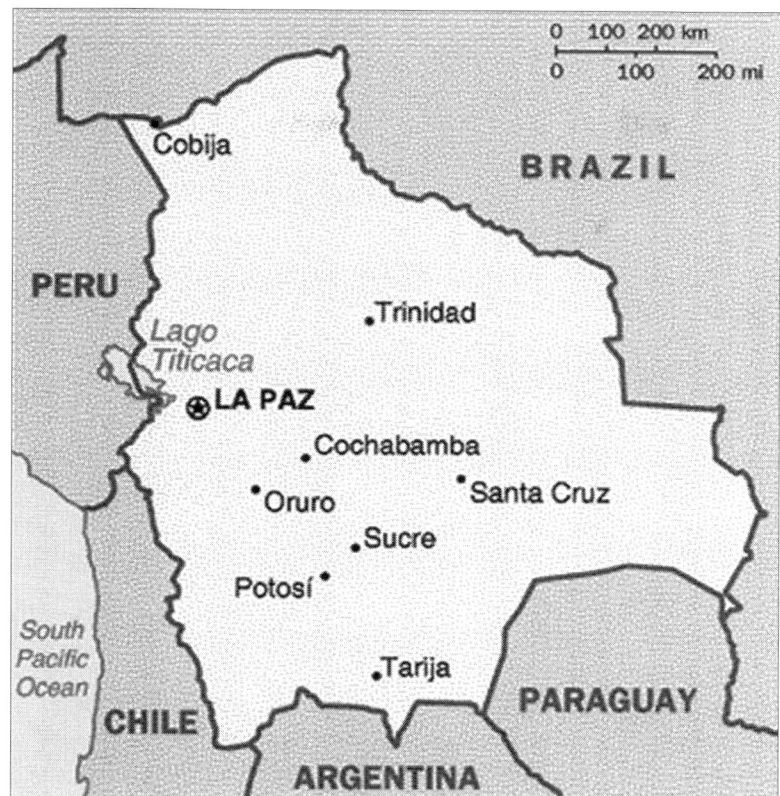

**FIGURE 2.2**
*Map of Bolivia.*

attention and funding to the provision of water and sanitation systems. SAPs, and other mechanisms used to protect global lending systems, are penalizing the poor (Kawachi and Kennedy 2002). Middle- and upper-class families can afford private systems. The poor, such as families in Guayaquil, Ecuador, may be forced to pay more than their monthly wage to have potable water delivered in tank trucks (Hong 2000; L. Whiteford with Laspina and Torres 1996).

Fully a third of the world's population lives without a safe water supply, exposed to dangerous bacteria, viruses, protozoa, and helminths (R. Reid 1998); the most vulnerable are children. In the years between 1965 and 1990, almost five million children under the age of five in Latin America and the Caribbean died of diarrheal diseases, and uncounted millions suffer continued morbidity from water-related diseases (UNEP 1997:23). According to the UN "Global State of the Environment Report," in the early 1990s some sixty thousand children under five years of age in Latin America and the Caribbean died of preventable diarrheal diseases. And that number may well be underrepresented by 20–40 percent. Even then, that represents a loss due to preventable mortality of perhaps 15 percent of that age cohort (UNEP 1997).

Debt servicing and the structural adjustment policies that often accompany it impact the middle class negatively as well. In September 1999 Ecuador announced its inability to make its interest payments on international loans (Lane 2003:122). In the years immediately preceding this announcement, more than 41 percent of government expenditures had gone to servicing the foreign debt, reducing the money the Ecuadorian government spent on health by 50 percent in the three years between 1995 and 1998. In an attempt to stabilize the government and reduce inflation and as part of a two-billion-dollar loan package negotiated with the International Monetary Fund, the World Bank, and the Andean Development Corporation, in 2000 Ecuador was allowed to reschedule its debts with foreign lenders (Lane 2003:126). This arrangement, however, carried with it mandated structural adjustments such as increased privatization (that is, privatizing the national petroleum industry). This involved sales to international companies, the elimination of subsidies for many essential services, higher taxes, and the loss of the *sucre*, the national currency, which was replaced by the US dollar.

Rather than immediately reduce inflation, the move to the US dollar led to a continued increase in prices as people unaccustomed to US coins rounded prices up to the next dollar value. In 2000 the average increase in the consumer price index was 90 percent, with food costs increasing by 107 percent and health costs by 102 percent (Lane 2003:132). At the same time, salaries for government employees remained unchanged. By the new millennium, health care was beyond the reach of the poor, and food was barely attainable. The middle class also felt the sting, particularly because its bank accounts and savings accounts had been frozen by the government the year before and were still unavailable.

## CASUALTIES IN THE GLOBALIZATION OF WATER

As a result, middle-class families lost the resources to pay private physicians, and poor families became even more dependent on the ever-dwindling, state-provided health services. Health programs designed to provide households with potable water through home chlorination were discontinued, and the cost of bottled water rose.

Water shortages not only result in high rates of waterborne and water-washed diseases, but also are directly implicated in the spread of vectorborne diseases such as dengue fever and malaria (Gubler with Kund 1997; L. Whiteford 1997). Dengue fever has been endemic in Southeast Asia for many years, but its more recent spread into the Americas and the Caribbean is linked with lack of reliable water systems. Household water storage creates a breeding ground for the mosquito vectors. Families store water for future use, use less water for basic hygiene, reuse water, and repeatedly expose themselves to infections. Without basic sanitation systems, people defecate in streams, fields, and household areas, exposing their family and neighbors to diseases.

Globalization has eviscerated public health infrastructures by emphasizing export industries, reduced state subsidies by adopting structural adjustment policies, and commodified basic human necessities. It is time to reintroduce health into the global discussion.

## CONCLUSION: WATER AND THE MORAL ECONOMY OF HEALTH

As the process of globalization has empowered multinational banks and trade partners, the force and effectiveness of the World Health Organization has dwindled. In 1978 WHO presented the Alma Ata Declaration, with its slogan "Health for All." The slogan came to epitomize the world's concern with health, particularly that of the most vulnerable—the poor, the very young, and the very old. Along with the ideal of health for all came the primary health-care (PHC) model and later the selective primary health-care (SPHC) initiatives. In 1978 WHO introduced the Action Programs on Essential Drugs, in 1981 the WHO Assembly passed the International Code of Marketing Breast Milk Substitute, and in 1988 WHO approved a list of ethical criteria for medicinal drug promotion. The purpose of each initiative was to protect vulnerable populations from intrusions aimed at creating or controlling markets. The International Code of Marketing Breast Milk Substitute, for instance, was a response to the increase of infant mortality when women switched from breastfeeding to using powdered milk formulas requiring the addition of water. Lacking a secure and safe water supply, women were forced to put contaminated water in the powdered milk for their babies, many of whom became sick and died. Since the development of the WTO in 1995, many protections of the world's most vulnerable populations have vanished. Health is no longer a basic human right (Hong 2000:30).

WTO agreements not only guide trade but also determine, directly and indirectly, quality of health. The Agreement on the Application of Sanitary and Phytosanitary Measures (SPS), for instance, claims to protect the rights of humans, plants, and animals if adequate, conclusive, scientific evidence of risk exists (Hong 2000:34). The WTO, however, has not recognized any specific standard or code describing what should be considered risk, thereby emasculating any potentially protective measures. The result is ambiguity that favors the commercial interests of the developed world at the cost of health for the underprivileged (Hong 2000:34). "Given that the overarching aim of the WTO is to facilitate trade, the guiding principles for food safety measures [are] towards 'downward harmonization' of health and environmental standards, risks assessments supported by scientific evidence and equivalence" (Hong 2000:35). That is, health and other social issues become secondary to trade interests. As Hong points out, the contradiction in the WTO aims to facilitate trade but also develop health and food safety standards pits powerful commercial interests (for example, tobacco producers and manufacturers) against a small, dispersed group of public health advocates.

Another WTO agreement, the Agreement on Technical Barriers to Trade (mentioned earlier), addresses elements associated with food and product labeling and "with claims relating to health and nutrition, which are made for food products" (Hong 2000:36). The WTO Agreement of Trade Related Aspects of Intellectual Property (TRIPS) affects patents, copyrights, and trademarks, among other elements. In terms of health, this agreement has direct implications for "knowledge-based" property and "intellectual property" affecting indigenous groups and third world countries where little time and effort has traditionally been given to formally legitimating ownership claims to ideas (through patents or copyrights) and/or products such as pharmaceuticals or transgenic crops (Hong 2000:36). The power differential cannot be ignored and should be brought forward and addressed.

The moral economy of health perspective argues that health must be on the agenda of any discussion concerning global trade. Just as protection of human health and the environment should be a factor in water agreements, it should also be part of debt-restructuring negotiations. High-tech medical innovations, the medicalization of health, and the diminution of the global public health "commons" conspire to silence the discussion of health at the trade table.

The moral economy of health perspective identifies immunizations, secure and reliable water, and sanitation as basic human rights that governments should work together to ensure for all. To counteract the "globalization of disease" and enhance the "globalization of health," health for all—public health—must become a priority in the consideration of multilateral trade negotiations and structural adjustment policies, setting structural conditions for global trade and linking them explicitly to improvements in basic human health conditions (K. Lee 2000; Hong 2000; Farmer 2003).

How can the moral economy of health perspective gain the support necessary to change global health conditions? First, the decision to bring health to the negotiating table must be made. WHO must be strengthened; it needs to approach the bargaining table with policies to protect the environment, health, social well-being, and vulnerable populations. WTO can monitor inequities by reviewing trade agreements and their impacts on social, environmental, and health policies and pinpoint those issues affecting basic human rights, public health, and welfare (Hong 2000).

In the past twenty years, much of medical anthropology, particularly what has come to be called "critical medical anthropology" or the "political economy of health," has focused on the social and political conditions underlying health disparities (Baer with Singer and Susser 1997; Baer and Singer 1995; Farmer 1992, 2003; Kim et al. 2000). Much has been written using epidemiological patterns to describe the determinants and distribution of disease. Those numbers paint only part of the picture, however. Power, prejudice, racism, and what Paul

Farmer (2003:231) refers to as "pernicious moral relativism" complete the picture. This is not a hopeful picture, but rather one where the most vulnerable are ravaged. It is time to change the models of engagement, the paradigms of provision, and to require accountability in the global distribution of basic human resources. It is immoral to block approved loans for clean water, education, and health care to countries such as Haiti in order to make a political point, inflicting suffering on those least able to effect change. It is ethically unjustifiable to permit the pollution of drinking water by allowing pesticides from nearby fields to contaminate a community's streams and rivers.

Protecting the most vulnerable requires a global approach to eliminating the resource inequities that result in billions of deaths each year. Working together, the World Health Organization and the World Trade Organization can globally foster the civil and economic well-being of an informed, healthy populace in which the burden of disease does not rest on the least advantaged. Physicians, anthropologists, economists, public health officials, politicians, and policy makers have the data necessary for world trade negotiators to make informed decisions about health issues. As Farmer (2003:238) reminds us, it is time to "make health and healing the symbolic core of the agenda." To do less is to fail the future.

# 3

## Water Reform, Gender, and HIV/AIDS

*Perspectives from Malawi*

**Anne Ferguson**

At the World Summit on Sustainable Development in Johannesburg in September 2002, water emerged as a powerful symbol of what President Mbeki and others called "global water apartheid"—a world divided between those who have access to safe water and those who do not. In many ways, those of us who study the water resource policies of the World Bank and other multilateral lending institutions were surprised at the attention clean drinking water and sanitation received at the summit. The paradigm shift in water management over the past decade has directed attention away from supply-side concerns with potable water and sanitation to demand-oriented approaches focused on watershed and river basin management, use of water for productive purposes, pricing, and stakeholder participation. The demand management–based strategies adopted by major lenders and many governments place emphasis on cost recovery and water as an economic good.

At the same time, however, this approach is being challenged. Organizations, scholars, and activists who advocate the moral economy of health perspective (see L. Whiteford, chapter 2 in this volume) point to structural violence in the health sector (Farmer 2003) and call for recognition of water as a social good and a human right. In 2002, for example, the United Nations moved to recognize the human right to water as part of the International Covenant on Economic, Social and Cultural Rights. Water now is at the center of contestations that surround sustainable and just development policies and practices.

To explore the links among the processes of globalization, water resource management, and health, we must challenge the boundaries separating disciplines such as medical anthropology, gender studies, and political ecology, as well as those in the real world separating ministries of health from those of agriculture, environment, and water. In particular, I concentrate on the shift in international water-management paradigms within the context of the HIV/AIDS epidemic afflicting Malawi, a poor country located in Southern Africa. The research reported here was interdisciplinary and collaborative, involving a sociologist, an environmental historian, and a hydrologist at the University of Malawi.[1]

While privatization of municipal water supplies has captured much international notice—and criticism (see Johnston, chapter 7 in this volume)—the effects of new, demand-driven, community-based policies for rural water supply have been overlooked. Here, too, *enclosure*—processes restricting access to resources that were once considered a common good—is underway (*The Ecologist* 1993). The new rural water-services paradigm in Malawi and other countries of Southern Africa calls for community and user-group ownership of boreholes, wells, and other sources of water, with very little oversight by local or national government. This, I argue, is not in the best interest of public health. In the context of the HIV/AIDS epidemic, it may limit the most vulnerable households' access to clean water. As a solution to diminished state resources and responsibilities, user-group and community ownership of rural water supplies may increase class and gender differentiation, inequality, and ill health.

## PARADIGM SHIFTS

Current approaches to water resource management are reflected in international statements from the Johannesburg Summit, the Dublin Principles, the Rio Summit's Agenda 21, and most donor and

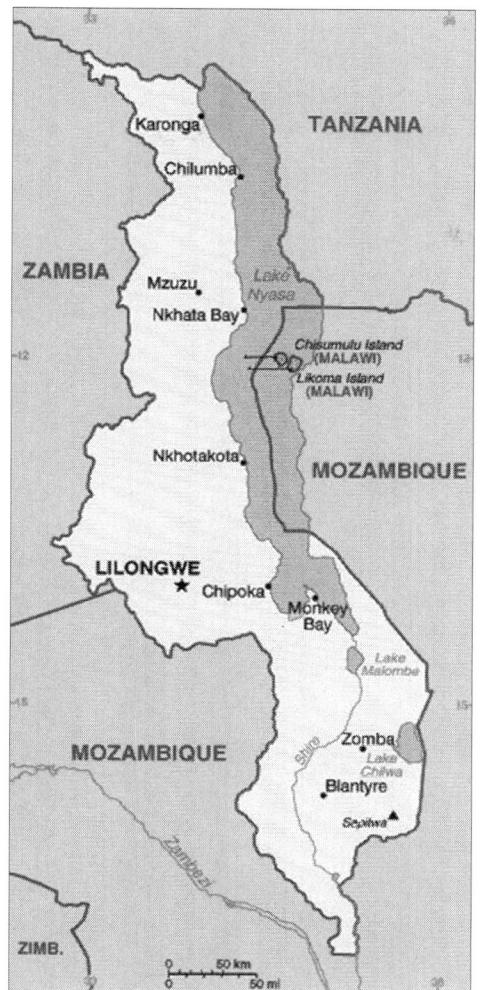

FIGURE 3.1
*Map of Malawi.*

international lending organization policies. Five general trends can be identified in this literature. First is the removal of subsidies, accompanied by pricing and other regulatory measures to limit the demand for water and channel its use to the most productive economic sectors (see Guillet, chapter 9 in this volume). Second is the development of decentralized management institutions incorporating stakeholder participation and responsibilities. Third is an integrated approach to water management, promoted through a focus on river basins and cross-sectoral collaboration among ministries. Fourth is recognition of the rights of the environment itself to water, and fifth is increased gender, class, and racial equity in access to water and voice in water-related institutions.

These trends mirror broader transformations associated with globalization and pervasive neoliberal economic and political reforms espoused especially by the World Bank: reduction in the size and functions of the state, decentralization, privatization, free trade. They mark a significant alteration in direction from policies followed in the 1970s and 1980s. A demand-side orientation has largely replaced supply- side dynamics—particularly state provision of infrastructure such as dams, irrigation schemes, potable water, and sanitation facilities. Comprehensive river-basin management strategies involving stakeholder participation and emphasizing markets, pricing, and technology are being implemented to promote water use efficiency, recover costs, and conserve the resource. Many of these policies constitute loan conditionalities imposed by the World Bank and other international lenders in very poor countries like Malawi, which are dependent on donor funds to function.

The literature on women, gender, and water now spans more than two decades and reflects more general trends in gender and feminist studies. The 1980–1990 United Nations International Drinking Water and Sanitation Decade did much to bring women's roles in water management at the household and community levels to the attention of policy makers (PROWWESS/UNDP 1991). As a result, women gained visibility, but the way this was achieved was problematic. The goal was to identify women's roles and document their workloads in isolation from those of men and from changes in the wider economy and society. A static picture emerged, which failed to differentiate women by class, race, age, or other social attributes or to examine how their roles were mediated by their relationships with men and with broader social, economic, and political institutions. Women-centered projects and projects in which women provided labor but had little say in decision making were often the outcome.

This approach, found in much of the women-in-development (WID) and ecofeminist literature, fed popular stereotypes depicting women as natural caretakers of water and other environmental resources ostensibly because of their close contact with nature and their familial responsibilities. Further, the focus on the private or domestic sphere of water and sanitation ignored women's use of water for farming and other enterprises. This orientation has proven conceptually inadequate for studying gender relations and environmental change, frequently resulting in facile policy recommendations and programs that have increased women's work burdens or otherwise contributed to project failure.

As a counterpoint to WID and ecofeminism, scholars such as C. Jackson (1993), Cleaver and Elson (1995), Cleaver (1998a, 2003), and Agarwal (2000) propose an analytical framework that is contextualized and centers on gender divisions of rights and responsibilities in the productive and reproductive spheres related to land, water, and other natural resources. These authors demonstrate that there is nothing inherent about women that makes them better resource managers or more caring of the environment than men. Indeed, in some situations, women's "closeness" to the environment may derive from their subordinate positions and lack of power relative to men ( C. Jackson 1993).

Researchers have begun to scrutinize the implications for gender equity in the recent paradigm shift that has taken place in water resources management. Studies examining what this change means for women's access to water and their part in the new water-management institutions began to emerge in the mid-1990s (Cleaver and Elson 1995; Green and Baden 1994; Zwarteveen 1997). Researchers are divided on the potential impacts. Some argue that these reforms lead to greater recognition of the economic value of women's work in water collection and management. They also contend that the decentralized, participatory approach and the creation of new management institutions associated with the reforms may give women more voice in decision making than in the past. Others point to the possibility that women's use rights to water may be marginalized and that new, decentralized, formal decision-making structures may not be any more open to them than earlier ones, nor as effective as older, informal institutions (Cleaver 2003).

As an alternative approach, the conceptualization of water as a human right has recently gained momentum. Gleick (1999) argues that, with growing global water scarcity, a right to water is necessary to protect the poor and vulnerable from having an essential ingredient of life priced beyond their means. His rationale is similar to that used by those who endorse a human right to food. In an earlier paper, we also proposed a human rights–based approach to water reform (Ferguson and Derman 1999). Using the framework of the Convention on the Elimination of All Forms of Discrimination against Women, Hellum (2001) suggests ways for water planners to legally recognize women's rights to water and to include them in planning and policy making. With the growing importance of a human rights approach to development, a rights-based approach to water is beginning to rival the commodity-focused one. The United Nations' recent (2002) recognition of a human right to water illustrates this shift as it conceptually transforms water from a welfarist social need or a commodity into a basic right of all citizens.

The gender and health implications of changes in water policies and laws can be understood only by considering these reforms in the context of the broader processes of political, economic, and social globalization of which they are a part. Because Southern African governments have reduced their size and functions as a result of structural adjustment policies (SAPs), government funding of services previously provided to citizens, albeit often poorly, has decreased. In rural areas, responsibilities for supplying and maintaining potable water and sanitation facilities are being delegated to donors, nongovernmental organizations (NGOs), churches, communities, and user groups, often under the guise of an ostensible stakeholder, community management, or a participatory empowerment strategy. Many of these new decentralization policies have not adequately taken into account the impacts of the neoliberal reforms instituted over the past two decades, which have increased, rather than reduced, inequality and poverty. Nor, in most cases, have the effects of HIV/AIDS been considered. The case study presented below examines these processes in Malawi.

## WATER REFORM, POVERTY, AND HIV/AIDS: MAKING THE LINKS IN MALAWI

More than 85 percent of Malawi's population lives in rural areas. Ninety-three percent of women live in these areas, and approximately 85 percent of them earn their living primarily from agriculture (Mbaya

## WATER REFORM, GENDER, AND HIV/AIDS

2002). The economy is dependent on the export of primary agricultural products—particularly tobacco—for which the terms of trade declined in the 1990s. Per capita incomes have decreased significantly since the imposition of SAPs in the 1980s. Approximately 45 percent of the population presently lives below an absolute poverty line of $40 per capita per annum, and 65 percent is considered poor by more conventional standards (Devereux 2002a:3). The number of poor is projected to grow unless a GDP growth rate of 6 percent per annum is realized, an unlikely figure, given that growth has averaged only 2.9 percent over the past twenty years (Devereux 2002a:3; World Bank 1999b:1).

Researchers point to the role of Washington Consensus neoliberal economic policies in explaining this growing impoverishment (Devereux 2002a; Owusu and Ng'ambi 2002). These authors highlight Malawi's high debt burden and its consequent financial dependence on and lack of autonomy in negotiating with the International Monetary Fund (IMF), the World Bank, and other powerful donors. Beginning in the late 1980s, new government policies promoted by the World Bank and the IMF restricted state intervention in the economy. Institutional arrangements that had provided basic subsidies for fertilizers and for staple food (maize) at affordable costs were dismantled, and social services were curtailed, including support to health, water, and sanitation. The Ministry of Water Development is among the lowest-funded government ministries. Projected private-enterprise development, economic growth, and poverty reduction have been slow to occur.

As in other sub-Saharan African countries, poor women bear the brunt of these structural reforms as their work burdens increase and formal sector support declines (Bakker, ed., 1994; Sparr, ed., 1994). Provision of affordable basic food (maize), potable water, and sanitation, as well as other services, has devolved to the private sector, donor projects, NGOs, churches, communities, and district assemblies. Increasingly, national government's role is limited to policy making, monitoring, and evaluating. In his analysis of social safety-net policies in Malawi, Devereux (2002a:11) describes this process of substituting discrete, donor-designed and funded, noninstitutionalized projects for institutionalized government programs as the "projectization" of social protection. He argues that it represents a breakdown of the social contract between the government and its citizens.

In the mid-1990s, Malawi had one of the worst nutritional, health, and poverty statistics of any nonconflict country in the world, with no significant improvement in sight (Devereux 2002a:6). In 2002 the country experienced its worst famine in recent history (Devereux 2002b). Deepening poverty and chronic food shortages point to fundamental failures in development and poverty alleviation strategies. In particular, many policies and strategies have not considered the implications of the HIV/AIDS epidemic (DeWaal 2002; Drimie 2002).

In Southern Africa, HIV/AIDS is now widely recognized as both a health and a development crisis. The eight highest rates of HIV/AIDS infection in the world are in the Southern African Development Community countries. Malawi ranks eighth in the world, with an overall adult rate estimated at 16 percent (UNAIDS 2000). Considerable variation in prevalence exists, with the Southern Region, where our research is located, showing a prevalence rate of 24 percent (Mbaya 2002). Most infections occur within the 15–24 age group, and AIDS is now the leading cause of death in the 15–49 age group. The World Health Organization (WHO) reports that Malawians aged 15–59 have more than a 60 percent risk of dying of AIDS (reported in Devereux 2002a:12). By 2010, if the epidemic continues unabated, life expectancy in Malawi is projected to fall to 34.8 years and population growth to .7 percent (Drimie 2002:6).

Unlike other infectious processes, which kill the very young or old, HIV/AIDS strikes people in their most economically productive years. Because those infected are responsible for supporting families, this characteristic of the disease is particularly devastating. Through its demographic and socioeconomic impacts, HIV/AIDS is changing the nature and dynamics of poverty.[2] The implications of the disease for development are beginning to be documented in Southern and Eastern Africa (Drimie 2002:8; du Guerny 2001). Recent studies on the implications of AIDS for agricultural production in the Central Region (Shah et al. 2002) and for land use and tenure in the Southern Region of Malawi (Mbaya 2002) point to a number of changes occurring. The age structure and composition of the poor are altering as the young adult population is decimated and children and the elderly become increasingly impoverished. Intergenerational poverty is on the rise as households dissolve and the fragile asset base of the poor is eroded. Surviving children, especially girls, are likely to receive less schooling because girls are more likely than boys to be taken out of school when labor is needed in households and on farms (Mbaya 2002). Loss of labor results in irreversible livelihood shocks, including not only lower agricultural productivity but also switching to less labor- and input-intensive crops that may be less nutritious. The erosion of the poor's household asset base may be permanent and may result in destitution. This is especially the case when more than one household member is affected and when the household loses access to land. Asset distribution in the form of land, livestock, and labor is becoming more unequal. Poorer households, especially those with the smallest land holdings, are less able to cope with the effects of HIV/AIDS than are the wealthier ones. Better-off households and those with few or no ill members may benefit from the sale of assets by their relatives and neighbors.

In Malawi and elsewhere in the region, women tend to be more vulnerable than men to the infection and its social and economic consequences. The infection rate of girls in Malawi, for example, is four times higher than that among boys of the same age. Walker (2001), Drimie (2002), and Shah et al. (2002) attribute this to women's lack of power to negotiate their sexual relationships, especially in marriage, and to the gendered nature of poverty. Overall, the number of poor female-headed households, especially those composed of young widows with small children and grandmothers looking after grandchildren, has increased as a result of the epidemic (Drimie 2002:8). In particular, as noted above, the stresses on poor women as a result of SAPs and downturns in the economy over the past two decades have placed them in a precarious position. To their workloads, HIV/AIDS has added caregiving for dying relatives and orphans and escalating responsibilities for generating cash and supplying food for the household through agricultural production and labor. In some areas, women have become more susceptible to sexual exploitation and trading of sexual services to secure income for household needs (Loewenson and Whiteside 1997; Shah et al. 2002). Given the dependency on women for caregiving and household food provisioning, the death of a woman is particularly devastating for a household.

Mbaya (2002:10–11) and Shah et al. (2002:64) note that, because of the rising mortality rate, it is becoming more common for widows and orphans to lose access to property, including land. This is especially the case for widows living under patrilineal systems of inheritance, as well as those who follow patrilocal residence in the matrilineal inheritance systems of southern and central Malawi.[3]

Development strategies in Malawi and elsewhere in the region have not yet fully factored in the implications of the epidemic. While mention is made of HIV/AIDS in Malawi's new land and poverty alleviation policies, the disease's social, economic, and political dimensions are not integral to the analysis presented in these documents (Mbaya 2002). In the remainder of this chapter, I draw on results from an ongoing research project in southern Malawi to explore some of the gender and health implications of the Water Resources Management Policy and Strategies (GOM 2000) passed by Parliament in 2000.

### Malawi's New Water Policy

Malawi has an extensive network of rivers and lakes that covers more than 21 percent of the territory. *The Country Situation Report on Water Resources in Malawi* (Kaluwa, Mtambo, and Fachi 1997:x) indicates that there are renewable freshwater resources of about 3,000 cu m per capita per year but that the distribution across the country is irregular and varies by season and year. Ninety percent of the runoff in rivers and streams occurs between December and June, and only an estimated 0.1 percent of this is captured for later use. Access to potable water remains very limited. *Water Resources Management Policy and Strategies* (GOM 2000:4) reports that the existing urban and rural water-supply schemes and systems provide potable water for nearly 54 percent of the population. This figure, however, dwindles to 32 percent at any one time because of breakdowns, sources drying up, and other operational and maintenance problems.

Only three of Malawi's cities—Blantyre, Lilongwe, and Zomba—have central sewage systems. *The Country Situation Report on Water Resources in Malawi* (Kaluwa, Mtambo, and Fachi 1997:43) notes that only 5.5 percent of the population has adequate sanitation and 30 percent has no sanitation at all. In urban areas, coverage is greatest, with approximately 30 percent of the population having access to adequate sanitation. In Zomba District, our research site, 88 percent of the population has access to "some form of sanitation," but only 5.5 percent has "access to adequate sanitation" (Kaluwa, Mtambo, and Fachi 1997:45). Indeed, at the time of our study, the sewage treatment plant in Malawi's fourth largest city, Zomba, was nonfunctional.

HIV/AIDS-positive people with impaired immune systems are more susceptible to common illnesses such as influenza and gastroenteritis, as well as to more serious yet still common diseases such as tuberculosis, malaria, and schistosomiasis (Ashton and Ramasar 2002; World Bank 1999a; UNAIDS 2000). Poor drinking-water quality due to inadequate water treatment increases health risks (Ashton and Ramasar 2002). Release of untreated sewage directly into rivers and streams is a major cause of water pollution in our research site and in Malawi in general. The population is beset by a wide range of conditions. There are annual outbreaks of waterborne disease, including cholera, typhoid, giardiasis, and dysenteries. In the dry season, water-scarce diseases are prevalent, including scabies, conjunctivitis, skin sepsis, and ulcers. Water-based and water-related diseases, particularly malaria and schistosomiasis, are endemic. The high prevalence rates of these conditions contribute to shortening the lives of many Malawians, especially those with impaired immune systems. In these circumstances, water supply and quality issues should be integral components of, not add-ons to, national water, health, poverty alleviation, and development policies.

The water policy passed by Parliament in 2000 represents a step backward in this regard. The 1994 water policy, which it replaced, gave priority to provision of potable water supplies, as reflected in the National Water Development Project. In 2000 the new direction became decentralization, institutional reorganization, and capacity building in urban water supply and, to a lesser extent, waterborne sanitation services. The Lilongwe and Blantyre Water Boards were reorganized, a water board was created for each of the country's three regions, and, although they remained government-owned, all were mandated to operate on a commercial basis emphasizing cost recovery.

By the late 1990s the Malawi government and its donors, particularly the World Bank, had identified shortcomings in the 1994 document: It was not in line with the new trends in international water management. It did not address development and management of water for productive purposes, conservation, or poverty reduction. It also did not recognize international and regional conventions and agreements on water resources to which Malawi was a signatory. Further, it made no real provisions for monitoring, assessment, or developments related to watershed management, conservation, or the mitigation of floods and droughts.

The new policy (GOM 2000) and draft law reflect the international trends in water resource management outlined above and bring the water sector in line with other new legislation and development trends in Malawi: poverty alleviation through market liberalization; promotion of private enterprise, demand management, and cost recovery; decentralization and greater stakeholder involvement; and sustainable and efficient use of resources. Water is considered a social and economic good, with special emphasis placed on the economic dimension of cost recovery and transfer of ownership of boreholes, wells, and piped gravity systems to communities and user groups.

The 1994 policy recognized women's roles in the provision of water for domestic purposes, and it contained stipulations for their participation in community-based organizations. Neither women nor gendered interests in water are featured in the new policy.[4] Instead, the primary strategy for alleviating poverty is the promotion of a business culture, with equitable access to water by "individuals and entrepreneurs." Similar to other new policy documents in the natural resource sector, the term *community* is used unproblematically throughout the document, overlooking power relations and differing interests in water by gender, age, and class within communities.

The policy document is divided into five sections: policy principles and institutional provisions; water-resource management policies and strategies; water services policies and strategies; institutional roles and arrangements; and capacity building. Here, my focus is on the water services policies and strategies.[5] The document identifies the central government as the custodian of the nation's water resources; the government's powers are to be exercised as a public trust. Highest priority is given to water for domestic use and environmental sustainability: "The protection and use of water resources for domestic water supplies will be accorded the highest priority over other uses, with water for basic human needs and maintaining environmental sustainability being equally guaranteed as a right" (GOM 1999a:sec.6.4.3). "Domestic purposes" is defined as the provision of water for household and sanitary purposes and for the watering and dipping of stock (GOM 1999a:Part I:1).

At the same time, the policy makes no mention of the HIV/AIDS epidemic or the necessity of potable water to mitigate illness. Given the minimal government funding the ministry receives and the continued restructuring and downsizing of the civil service, the policy stresses demand management strategies, promoting commercialization of water for domestic and other purposes to control its use. Users must undertake cost, maintenance, and ownership responsibilities. In urban areas, the five water boards have been further opened to private sector participation and investment. The policy also broadens water board responsibilities for sanitation and pollution control, stressing cost recovery, pricing, and creation of a positive environment for private sector investment.

In rural areas, the policy calls for enhanced community participation and empowerment. As the government withdraws from its responsibilities, people have to initiate demand for services and progressively assume the costs of installation, maintenance, and repair of boreholes, wells, and gravity-fed piped water systems. In other words, at the same time that many rural people find themselves increasingly impoverished by the combined effects of HIV/AIDS and failed economic policies, they are left with nearly sole responsibility for water supply. Nowhere in the policy document are the contradictions between the recognized right to water reconciled with the commodity and cost recovery focus.

The Ministry of Water Development has a long-standing engagement with community-based management, having trained rural people in shallow well, borehole, and piped water maintenance and sanitation since the 1980s. Many boreholes and gravity-fed piped water systems built under these older programs, however, are no longer functional (Kleemeier 2000, 2001; Schroeder 2000). The ministry attributes this to lack of local ownership. Consequently, the new policy is designed to "empower" communities (GOM 1999a, 1999b, 2001), calling for "the empowerment of the community or beneficiaries to own, operate, maintain, and manage their own water facilities and services, with the involvement of the public and private sectors, NGOs, and donors" (GOM 2000:sec.5.2.6).

The central government's role has been redefined to minimize expenditures for construction and maintenance. Instead of providing these services, the policy calls for it to regulate and monitor those offered by NGOs, communities, and "beneficiary user associations." The 2000 policy envisions partnerships among communities, NGOs, and the private sector to supply rural water, based on in-kind or cash contributions from communities and/or the levying of fees and rates for water. In this respect, it is not clear what the right to water for domestic purposes, recognized in the policy, means if rural users must pay the cost.

In actuality, the rural water-supply provisions of the 2000 policy are a continuation of practices initiated over the preceding decade as government funding diminished and NGOs, churches, and other organizations instituted rural water-supply projects of their own. How do these affect rural people's access to water in the context of the deepening poverty and HIV/AIDS crises? What, in particular, are the gender dimensions of the conjunction of poverty, HIV/AIDS, and neoliberal water reform? The final section of this chapter explores these issues, drawing on research results from Zomba District in southern Malawi.

### Water Reform, Gender, and HIV/AIDS in Zomba District

A major goal of our study was to examine whether the new water policy and practices were broadening people's access to water and to the new institutions established for water management. It involved study of water use practices among four clusters of users living along the Likangala River in Zomba District: peri-urban residents of Zomba Municipality, estate owners and workers, irrigation scheme farmers, and farmer/fishers near Lake Chilwa. As part of this investigation, we carried out household-level water use surveys, focus groups, and mapping of existing water points (boreholes, wells, streams, and rivers) in the research sites. We also interviewed key district and national actors, including representatives of donor organizations in water-related institutions. Although, as noted above, approximately 24 percent of the regional population is estimated to be HIV/AIDS-positive, we did not focus on households affected by AIDS, because this is a sensitive subject.

In rural areas, the provision of boreholes has become a highly politicized development activity. The pace of borehole construction quickened substantially before the last general elections, when the government announced a program to construct three thousand boreholes nationally. The Ministry of Water Development was to manage the program, but the boreholes were allocated on the basis of political constituencies. Because the ministry lacked the capacity to carry out construction, it engaged unregulated private contractors. This program presented ample opportunity for graft and corruption. It is estimated that fewer than 50 percent of the boreholes were drilled; of these, no more than 30 percent are functional (DeGabriele personal communication 2001).

Zomba District has experienced many of these problems. Here, too, private drilling companies, often lacking the necessary technical expertise, have sprung up to meet the demand for borehole drilling. Focus groups and interviews with water users indicated that the flow of many new boreholes was inadequate to meet expected needs. Overall, twenty-two of the forty water sources identified in our study area were nonfunctional during the dry season (Chilima et al. 2001).

The breakdown of the social contract described above by Devereux (2002a) is well advanced with regard to rural water supply in Zomba District. The newly enacted environmental policies in Malawi and the region mirror the transfer of responsibility from the state to communities and user groups through participatory strategies (Ferguson and Mulwafu 2001). An emerging literature critically assesses the equity impacts of these policies (Cooke and Kothari, eds. 2001; Ferguson 2002). As currently executed, they may be particularly inappropriate when applied to a resource essential for life, such as clean drinking water in the context of the HIV/AIDS epidemic. Considered here are three ways that this approach does not serve the interests of public health and disadvantages poor women and households affected by HIV/AIDS.

First, the proliferation of rural water programs has resulted in confusion, lack of coordination, and collapsed facilities. In the research clusters, boreholes and protected wells are being constructed by the Water Department, NGOs, churches, and donor-sponsored programs such as the World Bank–funded Malawi Social Action Fund. All stipulate that villagers organize themselves and contribute. Sometimes two or more projects, sponsored by different organizations and demanding different forms of participation, coexist in the same locale, creating confusion among community members.[6] Organizations sponsoring construction of boreholes and wells require the formation of one to three committees (construction, maintenance, and health and sanitation) for each borehole or protected well. Not surprisingly, we found that many of these village-level committees were nonfunctional. This does not indicate a lack of interest in water sources, but rather the time- and labor-consuming nature of the requirements as households struggle with deepening poverty and HIV/AIDS.

Malawi's 1998 Local Government Act stipulates that NGO, church, and donor water projects coordinate their work with area development committees, district assemblies, and district development committees. We found that many NGOs and churches were reluctant to have their autonomy restricted, preferring to work directly with village headmen rather than through newly established local government structures.[7] As a consequence, no central records exist indicating where boreholes and wells have been constructed: Some villages are well served, but others have few improved water sources. This makes rural water-supply planning—a vital public-health function in the midst of the HIV/AIDS epidemic—virtually impossible to carry out.

The maintenance committees required by NGO, church, and other programs frequently experience difficulties raising funds for repairs, locating spare parts, and identifying help for repairs that are beyond local capacities. Only one NGO in the area offered maintenance assistance for a year after construction was completed. The district-level Ministry of Water Development water monitoring assistants, formerly tasked with this responsibility, no longer have the financial and other support needed to perform these functions. Spare parts are not readily available in local stores. Consequently, many new water sources, even if properly constructed, cease to function within a year.

A second consequence is that the community-based approach promoted by government, donors, and NGOs may undermine the health of poor households, especially those afflicted with HIV/AIDS. Although the term *community* suggests that water sources are available to all villagers, many water programs run by NGOs work with user groups—members within the community who donate labor and building materials and/or make cash contributions to the construction of

## WATER REFORM, GENDER, AND HIV/AIDS

the water source (DeGabriele 2002). Boreholes and shallow wells constructed by one of the most active NGOs in the area, for example, belong to the households that contributed to construction. Lists of approved users may be posted, and the borehole handle may be removed during off hours to prevent noncontributors from using the facility. Field assistants observed that households unable to contribute labor or money often turn to highly polluted sources of water—unprotected shallow wells, the Likangala River, and irrigation canals—for drinking and bathing purposes.

Third, critical water-quality issues remain unaddressed by the community-based strategy. The Ministry of Water Development does not have sufficient funding to monitor water quality on a regular basis and, for that matter, does not know the location of many rural waterworks constructed by NGOs or churches. Few, if any, NGOs or donor projects carry out regular water-quality monitoring. The result is a potentially serious health risk, especially for those with impaired immune systems.

In 2000 we engaged two Ministry of Water Development technicians to collect water samples from thirteen widely used water sources in our research area. The fecal coliform counts at all sites, with only one exception, were considered too high for safe human consumption.[8] Readings were particularly high (fecal coliform count of 8,000 per 100 ml) at the Likangala Health Center, the source of primary medical care for many of the Lake Chilwa Basin's residents. Cholera, typhoid, and schistosomiasis are persistent health problems reported at this clinic during the rainy season.

Further, many of the most acute water problems experienced by study sites were not local in origin and cannot be solved by community-based participatory strategies alone. These include pollution of river water and degradation of the watershed. The Zomba municipal sewage system was designed in the 1950s for what was then a city of approximately thirty-five thousand but now numbers more than eighty-five thousand people. The treatment plant has collapsed. Untreated sewage from the hospital, the army barracks, and numerous other large institutions flows directly into the Likangala River, producing high levels of fecal contamination in the river and nearby boreholes and shallow wells. For years, rural dwellers living downstream and using the river for drinking and bathing have suffered from dysentery, cholera, typhoid, and scabies. They can do little about the situation at the village level because the problem originates elsewhere.

Community-based strategies such as promotion of sanitary practices around village wells and boreholes, advocated by the Ministry of Water Development and many NGOs, help control contamination but do not address the pollution of rivers, groundwater, and shallow aquifers caused by the city's faulty sewage treatment plant. Strong antipollution regulations and penalties for noncompliance are needed. Existing legislation and fines are inadequate and are seldom levied. For example, in early 2000 Zomba Municipality received only a small fine from the Water Resources Board for dumping sewage into the Likangala River. More effective than the fine itself was the negative publicity in the press, which sped identification of a donor loan to upgrade the sewage treatment plant.

Poor households affected by HIV/AIDS are particularly vulnerable to the weaknesses identified in the community-based management strategy. First, they lack the time, labor, and money to contribute to water programs or serve on committees, making them ineligible to use the improved water facilities. This enclosure, far from constituting a right to water, represents a form of privatization. More study is necessary to determine how widespread this practice is and what its consequences are. Second, in such cases, some women turn to other, more polluted water sources (often located farther from home), which pose a significant health threat to those with impaired immune systems and increases women's work burdens. Third, even where access to boreholes and protected wells is open to all, facilities fail to provide steady supplies of clean water because of shoddy construction practices, as well as lack of water-quality monitoring and means of repair.

## CONCLUSIONS

This review of Malawi's new water policy and strategies raises several critical issues regarding the "moral economy" of states and donors in Southern Africa in the face of worsening poverty and the HIV/AIDS epidemic. The shift in Malawi's water policies over the past decade is similar to changes instituted in other countries in the region. Despite recognition of a right to "primary" water in the new policies, concerns with health and gender equity frequently have been sidelined in practice.

While devolution of authority does hold the potential to empower people, complex processes involved in this transfer can ultimately serve local elites rather than promote broad-based democracy (Cleaver 2001; Cornwall 2003). Communities are usually hierarchically structured, so some individuals, often men and women who are better-off economically, are positioned to benefit over others from these devolution processes. HIV/AIDS has created new levels and kinds of vulnerability, expressed in differential and often gendered access to and participation in user groups and other new local-level institutions of water management. In addition, local-level empowerment by itself is insufficient to remedy many problems related to water quality and quantity, because their origins are not local.

The concept of structural violence (Farmer 2003) is helpful in our understanding the changes described above. In the context of the HIV/AIDS epidemic, neoliberal development policies in the water sector and other sectors have brought about new political, economic, and social structures that disproportionally threaten the health of poor households, particularly the women.

What might realistically be done to address these concerns? Our research suggests, first, that consideration of HIV/AIDS and its gendered dimensions should be made integral to the drafting and implementation of the new water, land, and poverty alleviation policies in Southern Africa. Malawi's new land policy, for example, may disadvantage poor women and households affected by HIV/AIDS. It advocates that customary land be privatized in the form of "customary estates" registered in one family member's name and that those most able to use land for productive purposes be favored.

Second, states must recognize a right to potable or primary water and reconcile this right with the prevailing demand-management, user-pays, commodity focus of the new water policies. Means need to be developed to ensure access to clean water for the poor in rural and urban areas, especially those who, because of HIV/AIDS, cannot contribute to rural water-supply programs or pay the escalating cost of water in urban areas. User-group or community ownership of water sources in rural areas must not exclude these households, which otherwise may fall prey to high-priced local water vendors or, more commonly, turn to unprotected water sources.

Third, strong institutions, standards, laws, and enforcement procedures at the national and international levels are needed to backstop the transfer of responsibility for rural water supply from the state to local governments, the private sector, and communities. The present focus on community empowerment must be coupled with support at the national level for the development of standards, monitoring processes, and other means to hold these new private-sector and local-level actors accountable. In the context of the vulnerabilities created by the HIV/AIDS epidemic, effective monitoring and enforcement of national standards and other regulations guaranteeing a right to potable water are essential. For the most part, these are not now in place in Malawi, nor are sufficient funds available to support these critical functions. In many instances, what is now being termed "community empowerment" amounts to little more than the government's efforts to reduce its responsibilities and expenditures.

Finally, as advocated at the Johannesburg Summit, potable water and sanitation must be brought back into the equation in developing an integrated, cross-sectoral approach to water management in the Southern African region. The neoliberal water-management paradigm widely promoted at international conferences and by donor organizations usually stresses integration across the "productive" sectors of the economy, such as water use in agriculture, forestry, fisheries, transport, and tourism. The 2000 water-reform policy in Malawi has de-emphasized potable water and sanitation concerns in favor of water uses for productive purposes, even though the country faces its most severe health crisis in recent history. If present trends continue, the new water-management policies in Malawi and elsewhere in the region are likely to amplify, rather than resolve, global water and health inequalities.

### Notes

1. This collaborative research on the impacts of water reform in Malawi was funded by the Broadening Access and Strengthening Input Market Systems (BASIS) Collaborative Research Support Program (CRSP). The principal investigator at Chancellor College, University of Malawi, was W. O. Mulwafu, an environmental historian. Dr. Stanley Khaila, a sociologist and past director of the Centre for Social Research at Chancellor College, was the first principal investigator with the project. Geoffrey Chavula, a hydrologist at the Polytechnic campus of the

University of Malawi, also participated in the study. US researchers in addition to me include Pauline Peters, anthropologist, Kennedy School of Government, Harvard, and John Kerr, resource economist, Department of Resource Development, Michigan State University. Graduate students supported by the project at Chancellor College—Ms. Grace Chilima, Mr. Bryson Nkhoma, and Mr. Diamon Kambewa—are to be thanked for collecting some of the data on which this chapter is based.

2. HIV/AIDS is not only a disease of poverty in Southern Africa. Countries with the highest GDPs in the region—Botswana, South Africa, and Zimbabwe—have the highest prevalence rates. The high prevalence rate among the middle and upper classes has implications for the functioning of institutions at the community, district, and national levels. In Malawi, it is estimated that nearly 50 percent of professionals will die from AIDS by 2005 (Mbaya 2002:5). Governments, NGOs, and private enterprises face losing their trained personnel. Also, absenteeism due to illness, caretaking, and attendance at funerals undermines the effectiveness of institutions and raises recruitment and training costs. Focusing on South Africa, Ashton and Ramasar (2002) identify many of these same trends in the water sector.

3. There is some evidence that men in matrilineal and matrilocal areas of Malawi may also lose access to land and property upon the death of their spouse.

4 *The Community Based Rural Water Supply, Sanitation and Hygiene Education Implementation Manual* (GOM 1999b:6), however, does make mention of women and gender. It calls for a gender-sensitive, democratically elected committee to manage water in communities and for women especially to take charge of all stages of the water project implementation cycle.

5. For an analysis of other sections of the policy, see Ferguson and Mulwafu 2001.

6. For example, water programs typically vary along many dimensions. They require participation at different stages of the construction process, different types and amounts of contributions from the user group, and different committee structures and rules concerning access to and use of the borehole. Villagers often do not understand why these requirements vary.

7. The government has produced the *Community Based Rural Water Supply, Sanitation and Hygiene Education Implementation Manual* (GOM 1999b), which stipulates procedures to be followed in rural water supply by all participating parties. Because of the severe budgetary constraints it faces, however, the Ministry of Water Development lacks the capacity to monitor or enforce these provisions.

8. Sites included the Likangala River, boreholes, shallow wells, the Likangala irrigation scheme and health clinic, and Kachulu Harbor on Lake Chilwa. BASIS paid for the transport of the technicians and for the chemical analysis at the ministry laboratory (because the ministry lacks funds to carry out such surveys). According to the Malawi Ministry of Water Development standards, the fecal coliform count should not exceed 50 per 100 ml of water. WHO standards are set at 0 per 100 ml (Chavula and Mulwafu 2001).

# 4

# Water, Vectorborne Disease, and Gender

## *Schistosomiasis in Rural China*

### Lenore Manderson and Yixin Huang

Water is vital: for drinking, cooking, bathing, cleaning, for raising animals and growing crops. Yet, perhaps more than any other element, it is also the source of death and disease, as all authors illustrate in this volume. Extreme shortage and surfeit of water—drought and inundation—dramatically affect people's health and well-being by changing the local ecology, disrupting disease-control measures, and creating new pathogenic environments. As both Linda Whiteford and Carl Kendall explain, water is the media of life-threatening viruses, bacteria, and parasites. Many, such as *cholera vibrio*, can be benign in minute quantities with sufficient hygiene and sanitation, but they are lethal when dense. The vectors and parasites with which we are concerned in this chapter have largely disappeared from high- and middle-income countries, but where prevalent, these continue to have a devastating effect on human health.

Water is also a deeply political resource, as shown throughout this volume. War is often fought over access to fresh water for productive purposes, domestic needs, and transport. Many nation states and regions are divided by rivers—the river being the shared and often disputed resource, the two banks delineating territorial borders.

The vector is often a critical part of the equation in the epidemiology of the most prevalent and dangerous diseases in the world. Mosquitoes, flies, and snails provide the safe havens of their own bodies to parasites and viruses that reproduce and then transmit to humans. These organisms thrive in or around water sources. Most target diseases of the WHO/TDR (Special Programme for Research and Training in Tropical Disease) are vectorborne and water-related.[1] Per annum, the TDR target diseases account for 1.3 million deaths. While geographic distribution is wide, they predominantly affect the poor. Those who have the fewest resources personally, and whose countries have the least capacity to prevent disease and deliver timely diagnosis and treatment, are at greatest risk of infection and are most likely to die or be severely incapacitated.

Despite major efforts by control programs, these vectorborne, water-related diseases have continued to be prevalent as a result of new land being opened up, forestry and mining projects, irrigation schemes, new dams, and, increasingly, rapid urbanization. Ecological and demographic changes affect the epidemiology of such diseases by creating ideal breeding places for mosquitoes, flies, and snails. With both urban and rural development, the movement of nonimmune populations to endemic areas and infected populations into areas where the vector is present has led to increased infection rates.

With globalization, water's commodity value has expanded. One of the most audacious examples of planning for future water dominance is China—a country already controlling the water resources for 50 percent of the world's population. The Three Gorges Dam, as well as the projected Upper Mekong/Lancang and Zipingqu Dams, will give China dominance over its poorer downstream neighbors—Thailand, Laos, Cambodia, Myanmar, and Vietnam—in a manner unparalleled by other economic or political mechanisms. The impetus for building these dams includes enhanced irrigation, hydroelectricity, and urban water supply, but those most enthusiastic for the dams claim that the benefits will include flood control, environmental protection, and tourism. Others, in their efforts to prevent the dam, raise the risks of environmental damage, increased flooding, and continued transmission of water-related disease (Jackson and Sleigh 2000). One of these diseases is schistosomiasis, of which the endemic form, *S. japonicum*, has resulted in serious morbidity and mortality in China.

These oppositional arguments have had no effect: the final step for the Three Gorges Dam—the closing of the Yangtze River's sluice gates—took place on May 31, 2003. By mid-2003 approximately 700,000 people in China had been relocated. An estimated 1.3 to 1.9 million people will be directly affected by 2009, but as many as 200 to 300 million people could be affected if the damming produces silting that inhibits flood control. The dams foreshadowed for the Upper Mekong will affect the livelihood of 60 million people in neighboring countries, as well as the ecology of these countries.

In this chapter, we explore the epidemiology and social contexts of water-related, vectorborne diseases, illustrating how social constructs such as gender influence exposure to disease and rates of infection. We concentrate on schistosomiasis, which has been particularly implicated in the context of water resource management and the construction of large dams. As a case study, we focus on one small village on the Yangtze, downstream from the Three Gorges Dam, to illustrate the ways in which the lives of those with the least power over and the least benefits from water resource management are vulnerable to its exigencies.

## SOCIAL ASPECTS OF SCHISTOSOMIASIS

Schistosomiasis (bilharziasis, or snail fever) is, after malaria, the most important tropical disease of public health and socioeconomic importance. The disease is caused by a species of waterborne flatworm, or blood flukes, named *schistosomes*, which enter the human body as people swim, wash, collect water for domestic purposes, fish, and farm. *S. haematobium* (causing urinary schistosomiasis) is found in fifty-three countries in the Middle East and Africa and, to a limited degree, in India. *S. mansoni* (causing intestinal schistosomiasis) is found in fifty-four countries, including the Arabian peninsula, north and sub-Saharan Africa, Brazil, and parts of the Caribbean islands. *S. intercalatum* (also intestinal) occurs in the rain forest belt of central Africa. *S. japonicum*, including *S. mekongi*, is endemic in China and both mainland and island Southeast Asia, causing "Asiatic" intestinal schistosomiasis.

The vector of schistosomiasis is a snail: *Bulinus* snails are the primary vector for *S. haematobium*, *Biomphalaria* for *S. mansoni*, and *Oncomelania* snails for *S. japonicum*. Infection occurs when intermediate snail hosts release larval forms of the parasites (cercariae), and these penetrate the skin of people in the water. The snails themselves become infected by another larval stage of the parasite (miracidium), which develops from eggs passed out in the urine or feces of infected people or other hosts, such as cattle or buffalo. Peak cercarial shedding occurs around the middle of the day, when humans use water for leisure, domestic, and personal purposes, agriculture, and fishing. These activities are gendered, a point we return to later.

According to WHO/TDR estimates, schistosomiasis affects more than two hundred million people, of whom one hundred twenty million are symptomatic and twenty million have a severe form of the disease. Direct mortality is low, but the disease burden is high in terms of chronic pathology and disability. In *S. haematobium*, bloody urine indicates damage to the urinary tract; untreated schistosomiasis causes further damage to the bladder, ureters, and kidneys, and bladder cancer in advanced cases. Intestinal schistosomiasis is identified symptomatically by blood in stools; the disease is slower to develop but includes enlargement of the liver and spleen, intestinal damage, and hypertension of the abdominal blood vessels. Death is mostly due to bleeding from varicose veins in the esophagus. In addition to urinary and intestinal damage, extensive morbidity is experienced by women, with eggs for both *S. haemotobium* and *S. mansoni* (but not *S. japonicum*) found in cervical, vaginal, and vulva tissue (Helling-Giese, Kjetland, et al. 1996; Helling-Giese, Sjaastad, et al. 1996; Kjetland et al. 1996; Feldmeier et al. 1998; Liu et al. 2000). Children are especially vulnerable to infection and develop chronic disease if not treated.

The global distribution of schistosomiasis has changed significantly in the past fifty years. The interruption of transmission through control of the vector has been achieved in much of Asia, the Americas, North Africa, and the Middle East. An estimated 80 percent of all cases, and the most severely affected, are now concentrated in Africa. Its continued endemicity is related particularly to large-scale water development and associated environmental changes, but also to increasing population size, density, and movement that spreads the disease to areas in sub-Saharan Africa that previously had low or no endemicity. Local variations in the level and intensity of infection, the seasonality of transmission, the presence of intermediate hosts, and the effect of different treatment schedules with praziquantel influence the overall infection levels and reinfection rates. Also, limitations in hygiene and sanitation infrastructure contribute to continued transmission.

The relationship between large-scale water development and schistosomiasis infection has long been known, illustrated in some of the earliest studies conducted in Egypt following the construction of the Aswan Dam (Farooq 1973). As Lerer and Scudder (1999) show, communities living near large dams do not necessarily benefit from water transfer or electricity generation. Changes in the management of water, including its diversion to supply urban areas with piped water and its use for hydroelectricity and irrigation, can increase the incidence of communicable diseases such as schistosomiasis and other parasitic infections. As discussed in this volume, changes in access to water, food insecurity, and the social disruption caused by construction, labor migration, and involuntary resettlement also compromise health. The Diama Dam on the Senegal River, for example, was built to block seawater intrusion and to control river flow in order to extend irrigation for agriculture, improve river navigation, and produce hydroelectricity. Completed in 1986, the dam disrupted the ecosystem, with negative impact on both animals and humans. Excess stagnant water upstream of the reservoir, in particular, led to an increase in urinary schistosomiasis and introduced intestinal schistosomiasis to Mauritania and Senegal (Southgate 1997; Southgate et al. 2001; Sow et al. 2002).

Similar changes in the incidence of schistosomiasis occurred after the construction of two large hydroelectric dams in central Cote d'Ivoire (N'Goran et al. 1997). Schistosome parasites and their snail hosts have also been introduced through land reclamation projects and land settlement programs in areas lacking water and sanitation infrastructure, health services, or access to health care. In Egypt (Mehanna et al. 1994) and in northeastern Brazil (Barbosa, da Silva, and Barbosa 1996), mobile populations with no previous exposure to the disease and without any immunity became infected. Schistosomiasis is also spread through forced population movement: refugee movements and population displacements in the Horn of Africa have introduced or extended the distribution of intestinal schistosomiasis in Ethiopia, Somalia, and Djibouti (Birrie et al. 1993).

In urban areas, as Mott and colleagues (Mott et al. 1990) noted more than a decade ago, the increasing incidence of schistosomiasis results from the migration of infected persons to nonendemic urban areas, introducing transmission in environments where the vector was present, and from the migration of infected and noninfected persons to urban areas that are already endemic. Patterns of domestic water usage, and the hygiene and sanitation behavior of migrants to urban areas, potentially increase the risk of disease transmission. The conditions under which people migrate and live—without piped water or safe sanitation facilities—inhibit their choices regarding where to wash clothes and dishes, urinate, defecate, and bathe.

Many studies of urban schistosomiasis, in very different locations and contexts, question the association between water-supply and toilet facilities and infection. Rather, these illustrate that, even with a safe water supply and sanitation, people may not avoid other water sources, whether or not they know those sources to be infested. In urban as in rural areas, social and demographic variables and water contact are most likely to predict infection. A study conducted in Cameroon, for example, showed that despite the availability of clean water from safe (schistosomiasis-free) sources, for reasons including habit and convenience, the population still used the river and streams for most bathing, laundry, and swimming. Knowledge about schistosomiasis infection did not result in reduced contact with infested water (Sama and Ratard 1994). In urban Niger, recreational use of water was the primary means of infection (Ernould et al. 2000). Firmo et al. (1996), on the basis of research conducted in Belo Horizonte, Brazil, similarly identified age, gender, and frequency of water contact as predictive, with adolescent males swimming or playing in water at greatest risk of infection.

## GENDER AND DISEASE

Any disease or infection is influenced by gender for various reasons: because risk of infection varies according to the ways in which women and men, girls and boys, differentially use the environment and are exposed to pathogens and vectors, because biological differences influence the pathogenesis of disease, and because the relative status of men and women determines access to health services and treatment. Gender influences the prevalence, distribution, determinants, and social consequences of infectious disease (L. Whiteford, chapter 2 this volume; Vlassoff and Manderson 1998). For schistosomiasis, the difference in disease morbidity and mortality globally suggests that men are at greater risk. As recent research on female genital schistosomiasis illustrates, though, the clinical manifestation and biological consequences of disease have been largely underestimated until recently (Poggensee et al. 2001; Remoue et al. 2001). In general, men appear to be at great risk of infection because of their work in agriculture, fishing, and other productive activities. This pattern varies, however, depending on the role of women in domestic and productive work, and defies any easy formula for identifying risk and developing interventions (Huang and Manderson 1992).

Because water use for recreational, domestic, and productive purposes varies by sex, infection rates and the intensity of infection vary also. Watts et al. (1998) have illustrated in Morocco that, in rural areas especially, at the many scattered water-contact sites, activities vary according to the rhythms of household and productive activities. Those involved in activities around the middle of the day during the period of peak cercarial shedding—women doing their washing, for instance—are at a much higher risk of infection than those who bathe in the river or pond at the end of the day. Older boys and young men often have high levels of infection because they are mobile and free to play in water. Studies of water contact in seven similar communities in Kenya, by Fulford et al. (1996), drew attention to the particular vulnerability of young women who spend more time at the water than males because of work activities. In Brazil, too, women engaged in domestic activities are at greater risk of infection because of longer periods of water contact than men (Almeda et al. 1994). As men are drawn into global labor markets and leave their natal communities for extended periods to earn wages, women take on more agricultural, as well as domestic, work that increases their exposure to infested water and their risk of infection.

Age and gender interact, influenced by patterns and sites of water use. Young children are at risk of infection because of their lack of immunity and hygiene training, as well as their intense exposure playing by and in water while their mothers work. One recent study in Nigeria (Mafiana et al. 2003) documented an infection rate of 72 percent among preschool children, whose exposure and infection are due to accompanying their mothers as the women perform domestic and occupational (fishing) activities. While sex differences are usually low or absent among preschool children, boys continue to have a high incidence of disease because they recreate in the water more than girls. By adulthood, there is some acquired immunity. Heavy infection, though, results in continued morbidity. The infection cycles, if not interrupted, result in further infection and continued morbidity.

In China, as discussed below, sex differences often vary in even small localities. Infection is sustained because people have economic and domestic reasons to continue using water sources, regardless of snail infestation and potential risk of infection. Cycles of infection are ongoing also because of inequalities in access to care and treatment. Resources and choices for men differ from those for women, in terms of their own health and the health of others within the household and in terms of village access to resources and participation in measures to reduce transmission of infection. In addition, men are most likely to move to areas of heavy industry and construction, leaving women to maintain family farms.

## SCHISTOSOMIASIS IN CHINA

In China during the early decades of the communist government, impressive steps were taken to control schistosomiasis: focal mollusciciding, environmental management, and the manual removal of millions of snails through the efforts of village work teams. The Patriotic Health Campaign, established in the 1950s, proved both successful and well accepted at its outset, with local leaders motivating program staff and village volunteers to eliminate the snails and eradicate the disease. In Guanxi, for instance, schistosomiasis was successfully eradicated through tenacious case finding and treatment, the killing of snails, and alteration of their habitat to prevent snail reinfestation (Sleigh, Jackson, et al. 1998; Sleigh, Li, et al. 1998). The program was multisectoral, with central policy development and strong local involvement. By the end of 1980, through the periodic treatment of humans and domestic animals, health education to encourage screening and early diagnosis and treatment, environmental modification, and focal snail control (Li et al. 1997; Li et al. 2000; Chen 2002), schistosomiasis had been successfully circumscribed in much of the country, in particular, the east coast provinces. Success was only partial in a number of poor provinces and areas, however, with continued transmission especially in the middle reaches of the Yangtze River, the Dongting and Poyang Lakes in central China, and Sichuan and Yunnan.

In 1992 the World Bank loaned US$71 million, with better-than-matching funds from the Government of China and the governments of endemic provinces, for schistosomiasis control through mass chemotherapy in areas of high prevalence, selective chemotherapy in other areas, and focal mollusciciding. This approach reduced morbidity in intervention areas but did not prevent the reinfection of human inhabitants or livestock. Research conducted during this period, mostly funded with a small portion of the loan (Yuan et al. 2000), showed marked local variations in infection by age and gender. A small comparative study conducted in Sichuan and Yunnan Provinces (Zheng et al. 1997) demonstrated that women were more likely than men to be infected in endemic areas with plateau canyons because the rice fields where women worked were heavily infested with snails. Infection was transmitted through the feces of wild animals and domesticated cattle, so chemotherapy alone would do little to disrupt the transmission cycle (Jiang et al. 2002). In the plateau basins, in contrast, the pollution source was human feces, and the infection rate in men was higher than that in women. The men were infected through production and daily activities along canals and ditches full of infectious snails.

In the Dongting Lake region, one study indicated that as much as 98 percent of water exposure was due to economic activity and only 2 percent to swimming or bathing, washing, and other necessities of daily life, suggesting that household water supplies and sanitation would do little to interrupt transmission. In this region, men had significantly greater exposure and infection than women, with fisher folk also significantly at greater risk than farmers (Li et al. 1997; Li et al. 2000). Similarly, Booth et al. (1996) noted that infection and morbidity varied by age, sex, and occupation, the former variables determining the latter. Men having higher levels of infection were more likely to suffer morbidity, but they were also more likely than women to have been treated for schistosomiasis.

**Priorities and Power: A Village Tale**

In this section, we draw on an ethnographic study conducted in an agricultural village, Yingjiang Village, in Anhui Province, eastern

China. Huang Yixin was resident in the village for twelve months, from 1993 to 1994. During this period, in addition to routine participant observation, he collected data formally through interviews with ninety-five villagers, gathered information on water use and exposure (through water contact observation), held focus group discussions, made a household survey of 303 households regarding patterns of water use, health status, and health and other priorities, and conducted document analysis. He used the Kato-Katz technique to collect data on the status of schistosome infection (Huang and Manderson 1999, 2003).

The village, like others in the area, is situated by the backwaters of the Yangtze River, the stagnant ponds and dense reeds of which provide an ideal environment for snails. Both animals (domesticated and wild) and people transmit schistosomiasis, limiting the value of control through case identification and treatment; animals are critical to the village economy. Intermittently, people are encouraged to force-feed praziquantel to water buffalo and cattle, but the numbers of animals theoretically host to schistosomiasis make this impractical, and more drastic measures against the animal population to reduce disease transmission are neither economically viable nor acceptable.

Similarly, the ecology of the backwaters, and changes in environment throughout the year with the rise and fall of the water, makes focal mollusciciding unfeasible and uneconomic. In other provinces, attempts have been made to irrigate ditches and seal river embankments with concrete to prevent habitation of Oncomelania snails, consequently preventing rice fields and vegetable gardens in areas adjacent to rivers from becoming transmission sites. But, again, this is not feasible for extensive areas because of time and cost: it can take three years to seal roughly 60 sq. km. Neither running water nor modern sanitary facilities are available in the village, despite its relative proximity to the regional capital and the highly industrialized and urban provinces of Jiangsu and Shanghai. People in the village cannot afford the luxury of such facilities.

Epidemiological data are not available, but village and town health officials maintain that schistosomiasis and hepatitis A are the most prevalent diseases; these are regarded as the most important by villagers. Their awareness of schistosomiasis stems from their experience

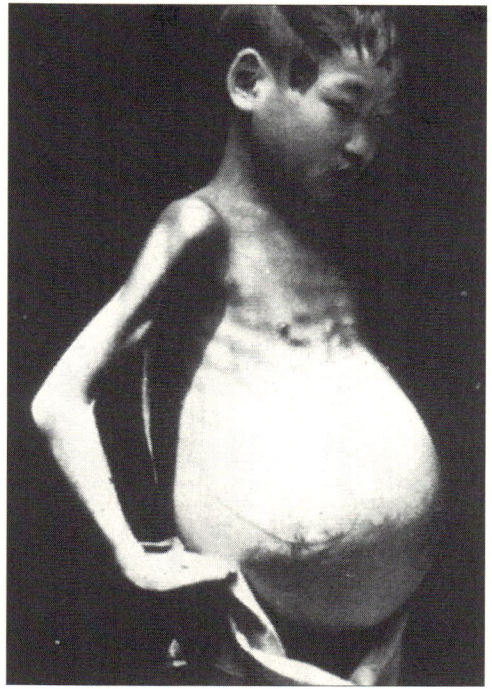

**FIGURE 4.1**
*A thirteen-year-old boy with schistosomiasis, including hepatosplenomegaly, ascites, muscle atrophy, pyrexia, anemia, and hemorrhage from the gastrointestinal tract (China, 1989). (Courtesy of WHO/TDR/Vogel, Image ID 9101068)*

with *S. japonicum* and the sustained propaganda from the health workers of the national schistosomiasis control program set up in the 1950s. Pictures of stunted children and adults, with hepatosplenomegaly, were commonly used for public health purposes, and cases of people with growth retardation and hepatosplenomegaly characteristic of extreme infection still exist (figure 4.1). People also identified the following as serious health concerns: ascariasis, hemorrhagic fever, skin infections, tuberculosis, diarrhea, and hookworm—all being hygiene and sanitation problems.

Changes in land tenure and distribution—combined with an increasing need of cash for household purposes, including food and medicine, and a growing desire for certain prestige consumables—

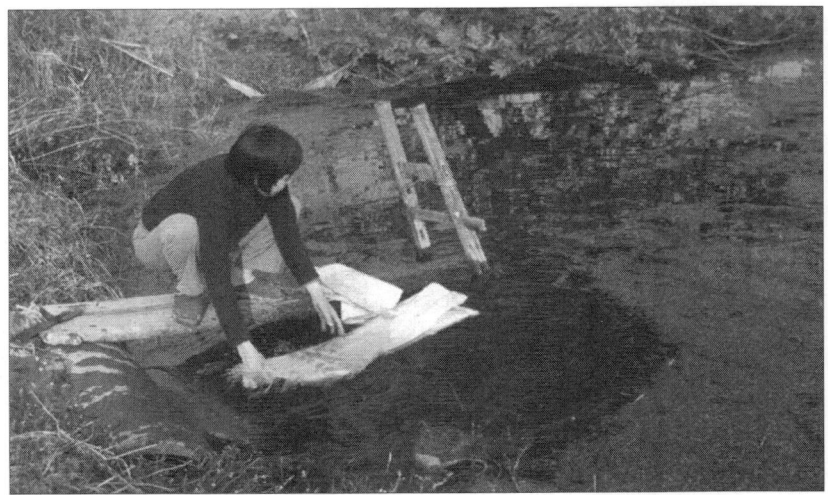

**FIGURE 4.2**
*A woman washes a knife and some cloth in a pond near her house and, in so doing, is exposed to infection from the water (China, 1999). (Courtesy of WHO/TDR/Crump, Image ID 9901821)*

have placed intense economic pressure on families. In the face of growing poverty and widening income gaps between rich and poor, there is more concern about income generation. Most villagers were farmers; those who had another occupation—clerical, service, or sales—supplemented their income with farm activities. Further, although parents largely valued education and hoped that their children would do well in order to gain good employment, increasing numbers of children were not completing school but were withdrawn after a couple of years to do farm labor. Girls, especially, left school early to help their mothers maintain vegetable gardens and orchards and care for domestic animals. Older male youths and adult men went to the provincial capital and other industrial centers (such as Shanghai) for wage work.

Women and girls are at particularly high risk for schistosomiasis and hepatitis A because of their economic and domestic activities (figure 4.2). The division of labor between men and women in the village is relatively strict. Almost all water-contact work is undertaken by women: the collection of pig feed and other by-products of the Yangtze's backwaters used for the village, the collection of water, washing of clothes, and watering of domestic animals. Rice planting is also

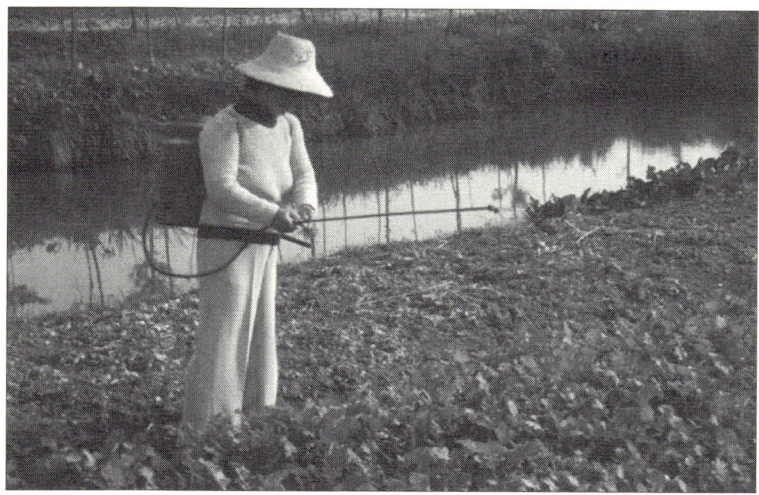

**FIGURE 4.3**
*A young woman uses a backpack spray to water the vegetables she is growing in her fields. She is exposed to infection when she fills the sprayer with water from the nearby pond (China, 1999). (Courtesy of WHO/TDR/Crump, Image ID 9901827)*

woman's work, so women are particularly vulnerable to infection from schistosomes as they stand for long periods through the day planting rice, watering plants, or gathering vegetables in infested fields or using water from infested ponds and streams (figure 4.3).

Women's involvement in productive and reproductive (domestic) work—in many cases, their role is essential while their husbands are away—suggests a relatively egalitarian environment, but this is not the case. In Yingjiang, the social status of women is low, so they have little political influence. Mobility among women is restricted. Many older women said that they had never been to the city in their county, let alone farther away.

Children, both male and female, have more advantages than their parent's generation because the economy has improved, but also because the birth control program means fewer children than in former generations. When children reach about nine years of age, they usually begin to help their parents in the fields when not in school. Twice a year, the school allows a "harvest vacation" for both students and teachers, two weeks in late spring and in middle autumn. Almost all children attend primary school from the age of six or seven, but in recent years some of them have been unable to finish. Since around 1990, children from the age of approximately thirteen have been able to go to middle school in the nearest town, but to do so, they must stay in boarding school and come home on weekends only. The expenses are much higher than for primary school (about 1,000 yuan per year—US$120.80 for each student), so this is even less affordable. In general, girls have less opportunity for education; they attend school for fewer years than their brothers. More adult women are illiterate than men.

Sexual division of labor is marked in the village. As villagers describe it, men work in the fields and rest at home, but women work both in the fields and in the home. Women "get up when early birds cry, go to bed when the ghosts cry" (*niao jiao zuo dao gui jiao*). Men's work includes ploughing fields, carrying heavy things (human porterage is still common in the area), purchasing chemical fertilizers and pesticides, and selling crops. Both men and women carry and apply fertilizer to the fields and may spray pesticides. Women's work includes transplanting rice seedlings, planting cotton and weeding, raising livestock, and going to marshland to collect pig feed. Their housework comprises cooking, washing, cleaning, looking after children, the old, or the ill, mending, making shoes and simple clothes, and fetching water. Men sometimes also fetch water, but men avoid doing "women's work" and say that "the more a man does woman's work, the poorer the family is."

Within households, men and women tend to share priorities and spend any discretionary cash on domestic buildings, marriage arrangements, and health care. Villagewide priorities for expenditure are, in order of priority, irrigation and roads, developing income-generating programs and small industries, and schistosomiasis control (table 4.1). The former People's Commune built and maintained a relatively complete irrigation system from 1958 into the 1970s. Under the private production system, however, the distribution of water resources, the maintenance of the irrigation system, and any new engineering works are village responsibilities. This leads to regular difficulties in maintaining canals and irrigation ditches, village pathways and embankments. Quarrels over water use occur between adjacent landowners, particularly in planting seasons.

Other priorities include improving sanitation, building biogas-

**TABLE 4.1**
*Priorities of Yingjiang Villagers*

| Priorities | Number of Persons | Percentage |
|---|---|---|
| Building irrigation works | 16 | 18.8 |
| Building roads | 16 | 18.8 |
| Developing enterprises | 15 | 17.7 |
| Controlling schistosomiasis | 14 | 16.5 |
| Building village clinic | 8 | 9.4 |
| Improving safe water supply | 7 | 8.2 |
| Other | 9 | 10.6 |
| Total | 85 | 100.0 |

generating pits to dispose of waste, improving education, building a home for destitute old people, improving agricultural technology, and improving communication.

Only men attend important village and town meetings to discuss issues such as the redistribution of land or the repair of irrigation ditches. Accordingly, officials from the town council and other government officers hear only men's views, not women's. Health, education, and the care for the frail and destitute are rarely brought up in public arenas, despite concern about such issues at a household level. People are well aware of various waterborne or water-washed diseases, or diseases related to rudimentary hygiene and sanitation, but few have the cash resources to improve their own domestic facilities. None have the means to undertake activities that might reduce regular contact with water infested with snails and infected with schistosomes and other parasites and viruses. Consequently, the transmission of schistosomiasis is sustained.

### Village Priorities and Gender Inequities

Yingjiang is not atypical of rural villages elsewhere in Anhui or in neighboring provinces in eastern and central China. In recent years, there has been substantial migration of men from the village (and from their agricultural and fishing activities) to work for wages in towns and rural industries such as manufacturing, heavy industry, and construction. Most town centers and peri-urban areas of provincial capital cities have some industry, and there are substantial changes throughout China towards "de-collectivization" and "de-agriculturalization" (Song 1999; Wang 2000). This involves a shift towards a market economy—for men, an increased move from mixed farming to monocropping, construction, forestry, and heavy industry, and for women, the major responsibility for maintaining family land interests, sustaining the household economy and agricultural production, and ensuring intergenerational rights.

Rural reform not only changed peasants' occupations but also provided opportunities for men to work in cities while women stayed in villages. Men find employment away from the village, particularly in manufacturing industries that are expanding to meet export markets. As a result, to some extent they can take advantage of local material changes (the introduction of cable television even in remote counties, for example). Education has changed to meet the technical needs of nonagricultural work, but this has particularly privileged young boys. As both Song (1999) and Wang (2000) note for Zhejiang and Yunnan provinces also, girls are often withdrawn from school to contribute to the domestic economy. Women's incomes play an increasingly important part in the household economy, but this has not been matched by increasing authority within the household or in the community. When men are at home, women do not determine the disposal of income, and there is rarely discretionary income. Economic change has not expanded women's opportunities for work or education, nor has it improved the material conditions of their everyday lives.

Health care is available to Yingjiang villagers at clinics in three adjacent villages or at larger health facilities in the nearest townships. Villagers feel that even the local village clinics are too far away for regular visits and that the quality of the services, both diagnostic and therapeutic, is variable and the charges are not standardized. If villagers have a complicated illness, they have to go to the County City Hospital more than 30 km away. Because of transport difficulties, the long distance from these hospitals, and the high charges, ordinary villagers tend to seek symptomatic relief for conditions. They use herbs and massage provided by fellow villagers. They seek treatment from visiting antischistosomiasis workers and family-planning motivators. (For a while, they took advantage of the medical anthropologist's medical expertise.) Men who work elsewhere in Anhui province, in Shanghai, or further afield often have access to better quality medical services. Even though globalization has heightened awareness of modern technologies, facilities, and treatments, the affordable reality for village women is decidedly local.

## CONCLUSION

Gender differences in priorities may have many outcomes, but inequalities in distribution of power and decision making influence the direction of choices. Health education, improved sanitation, and safe water supply can improve the health of rural people, but in villages such as Yingjiang there are few resources to improve infrastructure, limited cash for facilities such as toilets, and no economic or efficient way to prevent transmission of schistosomiasis. People depend on water for general living purposes and for their livelihood, and because the disease is transmitted through animal as much as human feces, it is particularly difficult to eradicate.

The irony is that schistosomiasis and other waterborne infections persist in Yingjiang and other villages along the Mekong in a relatively well-developed and industrialized province, illustrating that development is uneven throughout China at local and national levels. While China has had remarkable success nationwide in interrupting the transmission of schistosomiasis and reducing the incidence of other water-related, vectorborne diseases (malaria and filariasis, in particular), the control of disease is problematic in areas where environmental and epidemiological patterns favor continued transmission. The conventional approaches to eradicate schistosomiasis in the past—focal mollusciciding, the manual removal of snail hosts, and mass treatment in areas of high prevalence—are not feasible in areas with persistent endemicity.

As we suggest here, under conditions of rapid social change, men have found outside employment and are now at lower risk of infection than women or children. Women, however, live on the income they are able to generate from their own rice fields, vegetable gardens, and animals. They have few resources to seek treatment and are least able to influence village or county decision making to improve village infrastructure or extend health care.

Moreover, water management policies and disease prevention are not necessarily complementary. While the villagers of Yingjiang struggle simply to meet their everyday needs, those further west—in the provinces of Sichuan and Hunan, for example—are faced with larger problems associated with the construction of the Three Gorges Dam. Although the intent of the World Bank loan project was to increase schistosomiasis control, the dam is implicated in its continued transmission. By the turn of this century, China had commenced major works to build the world's largest dam by impounding the Yangtze River at the Three Gorges, providing work opportunities for men in the short term but displacing 1.3 million people in the process. The economic aim of this venture is to use the hydropower and improve navigation and flood control to develop the economy. This highlights the contradictory development goals of the health and agricultural departments (Jackson and Sleigh 2000). In the scope of things, the economic and health status of a few thousand villagers is of little account. But that is the point: it is all too easy to overlook the well-being of those without a voice while the waterways of nations are reshaped with economic growth as the goal.

### Notes

1. With the exception of schistosomiasis, all these diseases are transmitted by mosquitoes or flies. Malaria, lymphatic filariasis, and dengue fever are parasitic infections transmitted by mosquitoes (*anopheles*, *culex*, and *aedes*, respectively), which breed in water. Each species has its preferred feeding patterns, resting places, and breeding grounds, leaving larvae in the edges of streams, on the gentle surfaces of river backwaters or irrigation ditches, or in still pools on a broad leaf, in the husk of a coconut, or in a discarded can or tire. Sandflies and blackflies also thrive in the microenvironments of different waterways. Trypanosomiasis (sleeping sickness) is transmitted primarily by tsetse flies living in areas near human habitats, cultivated land, and small rivers or pools of water frequented by people. Onchocerciasis (river blindness) is transmitted by *Simulium* flies (black flies) that bite by day and are found near rapidly flowing rivers and streams.

# 5

## Waste Not, Want Not

*Grounded Globalization and Global Lessons for Water Use from Lima, Peru*

**Carl Kendall**

el idioma del agua fue enterrado, las claves se perdieron
o se inundaron de silencio o sangre.

*Pablo Neruda, "Amor América"*

This chapter explores what water use may be like in many communities in the future by examining water scarcity—and adaptations to it—in Lima, Peru. It demonstrates the continuing power of local histories to illustrate global dilemmas and to model solutions. To make the link between this local case study and global concerns, the chapter adapts Burawoy's theoretical approach and case study methodology, called "grounded globalization" (Burawoy et al. 2000). I link grounded globalization, in turn, to earlier traditions in ecology and structural-functional ethnography, such as C. Daryll Forde's *Habitat, Economy and Society* (first published in 1934), which interpret local culture as both a charter for social and symbolic organization and a material solution to problems of survival. Following Forde, this chapter focuses on water scarcity and adaptations in Lima, Peru, a city where daily water use per person in many parts of the city is significantly less than the United Nations–reported minimum required for survival in refugee camps and local adaptations to it. Following Burawoy, this chapter begins with a discussion of the global forces, connections, and imagination that play out in this local response to scarcity. The interaction between cultural constructs and material circumstances has the unanticipated effect of creating a contaminated environment and one of the highest recorded levels of diarrheal disease in children in the world. With respect to water, Limeños have reconfigured global forces into a liquid mirror, one that distorts globalizing forces and creates a culture of controlled consumption to make them manageable. Lessons for the rest of the world are apposite.

Burawoy and his students created a project to resurrect ethnography. They carried with them a commitment to "hermeneutic sociology: participant observation, open-ended interviewing, ethnography" (Burawoy et al. 2000:ix). But they found that the case studies they generated in this way "were caught up by that great mishmash of migrations, capital flows, hostilities, and opportunities jostling within the hot signifier of globalization" (Burawoy et al. 2000:ix). Globalization studies, as portrayed in the work of Clifford, Appadurai, Grewal and Kaplan, and others, seemed inimical to traditional ethnography (see Appadurai 1996; Clifford 1989; Grewal and Kaplan 1994). As Teresa Gowan and Sián Ó Riain, students in the seminar and two of Burawoy's co-authors, put it: "Whether derived from post-colonialism, political economy, cultural studies, or feminist theory, what our sources held in common was not so much their diverse definitions of globalization as their high degree of abstraction" (Burawoy et al. 2000:x). Their volume, *Global Ethnography* (Burawoy et al. 2000), was the rejoinder.

Global ethnography builds on the traditional strengths of ethnography: the extension of the observer into the world of the participant and sensitivity to issues of domination, objectification, and normalization. It also adds to the traditional by emphasizing the extension of observations over time and space and the extension from micro processes to macro forces. As Burawoy and his students conducted fieldwork and considered global effects, they came to see globalization as composed of three axes: "All our studies accomplished three things: first, they delved into external forces; second, they explored connections between sites; and third, they discovered and distilled imaginations from daily life. Forces, connections and imaginations became the three essential components" (Burawoy et al. 2000:5).

The cases presented in Burawoy's volume demonstrate the power of this approach. By utilizing local accounts of the lived experience of

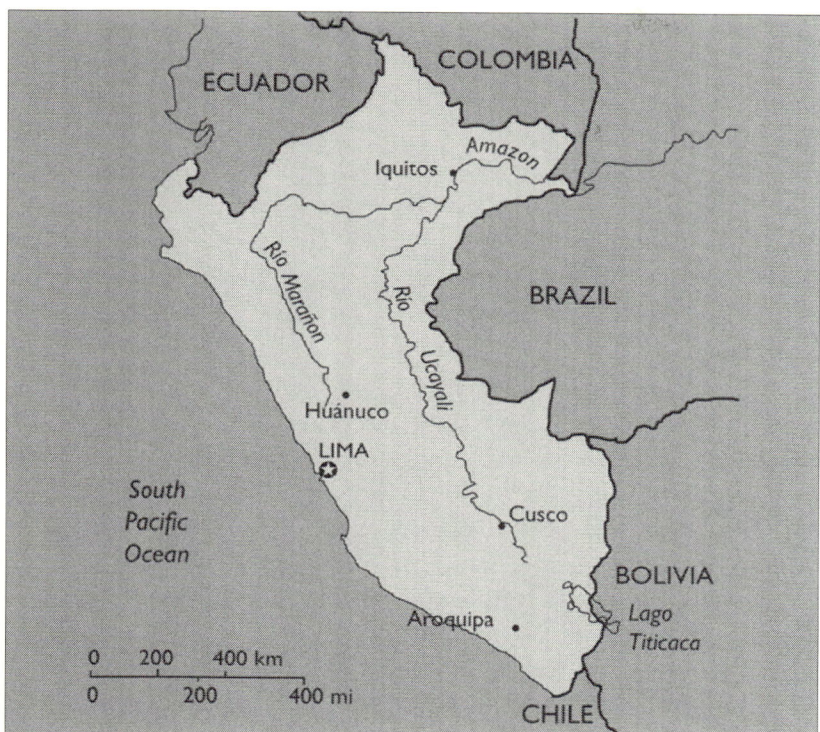

**FIGURE 5.1**
*Map of Peru.*

events to discuss exploitation, deindustrialization, deinstitutionalization, migration, "traveling theories" of feminism (see Clifford 1992), and other ideologies, they demonstrate the impact of globalization and the simultaneous self-reflexive interaction that creates this experience of globalization. Several case studies present the positive ways in which the local has appropriated and reconstituted these global forces to serve local needs, but, overwhelmingly, the case studies serve to document the manifold and negative impact of global changes on local life.

Burawoy derives his three axes—forces, connections, and imaginations—not only from the globalization literature but also from a review of anthropology that he documents in his introduction. By *global forces*, Burawoy means the global economy and polity as composed of extralocal forces that are manifested widely.

Global forces are felt through mediators—agents, institutions, and ideas—that work within a globally normalized framework of values and knowledge that they both constitute and transmit. Global forces are resisted, avoided, and negotiated at the local level. Although much is made of the stateless quality of transnational mechanisms, global forces are facilitated through the contractual and legal mechanisms developed among states and among individuals represented by those states. To make the link to structural functionalism, global forces represent the economic, political, or jural domain (see Fortes 1969) of globalization.

*Global connection* in Burawoy's scheme refers both to the links and to the underlying grid of interpersonal connections. Connection addresses migration and population flows, extensive networks of kinship, friendship, and patron-client relations. It defines new local and extralocal peers. Our new, connected world order offers fresh opportunities, the expansion of geographical boundaries, and occasional escape—for individuals and families—from oppressive environments. Global connections represent globalization as the social, interpersonal, domestic domain of globalization (Fortes 1969).

The third dimension, *global imagination,* addresses the diffusion and adoption of values, images, and memes transmitted around the world. This process constructs new "globalized" identities (modern and "traditional"), disembedding local identities and authorities. Global imagination addresses symbolic culture but also participates in the creation of new goals and values—global secular religion, if you will. Imagination is culture, in some application of this polysemic term. To continue the explicit association between grounded globalization and structural-functional anthropology of the 1930s and 1940s, this third dimension is the religious or spiritual domain (Fortes 1969).

These three axes, or domains, shape the stage on which local responses are mounted. They interpenetrate the local through accommodation and resistance and create new ideologies and material adaptations. The case study of Lima's water use illustrates these accommodations and this resistance.

This chapter examines grounded globalization in a case study of water and water use in Lima. The findings reported here are the product of a project titled "Health Behavior Interventions to Reduce the

Incidence of Diarrhea in Lima, Peru (HBIRID)," which ran from July 1, 1987, to December 31, 1991, funded by the Thrasher Foundation and the World Health Organization. The project was a collaboration of the Center for International Community-Based Health Research, the Department of International Health, The Johns Hopkins University (JHU), the Instituto de Investigación Nacional, Lima, Peru (IIN), and the World Health Organization's Diarrheal Diseases Control Program (CDD). The project took place in the peri-urban slums surrounding Lima.

The goal of the project was to isolate the risk behaviors associated with high rates of diarrheal disease infection. To identify protective hygiene behaviors, the project used a positive deviance methodology to compare mother and infant pairs having high diarrheal disease rates with those living in the same environment and having low diarrheal disease rates (our deviants). During phase 1 of the project, ethnographic research was conducted; during phase 2, epidemiological surveillance and structured direct observations were used to identify behaviors associated with transmission. From September 1987 through December 1988, the author, the late Peruvian anthropologist Dr. Mary Fukumoto and her students, and Dr. Duncan Pedersen conducted ethnography in a community in Canto Grande, a *pueblo joven* ("young town," a suburban community expanded mostly through extralegal land invasions) of about ten thousand inhabitants in the District of San Juan de Lurigancho, Lima. Initial site visits and participant observation research in the first year of the project was conducted by the author in San Juan de Lurigancho and in a distant pueblo joven with similar conditions (see Kendall and Gittelsohn 1994).

## FORCES AND LOCAL (DIS)CONNECTIONS: THE PROBLEM OF WATER

The linking of an ecological approach that recognizes human needs, finite resources, and population pressure to grounded globalization, as is done in this chapter, is necessitated because it is missing from Burawoy's presentation of global forces, and from many social scientists' accounts of the impact of globalization (for example, J. Ferguson 1999). The terrific forces unleashed by global economic and population growth are contested phenomena, often analyzed solely within disciplinary frameworks, with disputed data or timelines, from diverse ideological points of view, and with different ontological and epistemological premises. The problem this creates is a debate about these premises that is abstracted too far from the lived reality of the global changes. For example, there is debate about the causes of climate change and whether the observed changes reflect a new trend or are normal and periodic, rather than how populations cope with these changes. Notwithstanding these methodological concerns, there can be little dispute that the environment is changing. Water is an excellent example of this change.

A series of reports (Clarke 1993; Gleick, ed., 1993; UNFPA 1993; World Commission on Health and the Environment 1992; Engelman and Leroy 1993) document the growing challenge of freshwater availability and quality. One third of the world's population—all in the developing world—lives in countries with documented water stress (defined as 10 percent more water use than renewable resources permit), and that number could rise to two thirds in the next thirty years. In 2000 one-sixth (1.1 billion people) of the world's population lacked access to an improved water supply, and two-fifths (2.4 billion people) lacked access to improved sanitation (WHO 2000). Linda Whiteford's chapter 2 in this volume provides a framework for understanding these health problems and details the complaints.

This problem is magnified by rapid urban growth. In 1950 fewer than one hundred cities had populations greater than one million, and none exceeded ten million. Chilton (1998:1) predicted, "By the year 2000, some 23 cities—18 of them in the developing world—will have populations exceeding 10 million. On a global scale, half of the world's people will live in urban areas." The United Nations Population Fund (UNPFA 1993) predicted that these cities would be home to 90 percent of the poorest populations in Latin America and the Caribbean, 45 percent in Asia, and 40 percent in Africa. By 2003, 48 percent of the world's population lived in urban areas. The UNFPA estimated that the world's urban population will grow at double the rate of the world as a whole from 2000 to 2030. Urban areas in developing countries will grow even faster, averaging 2.3 percent per year during 2000–2030 (UNEP 1999b). Urban infrastructures can take years to develop, however. Today that development is failing to keep pace with urbanization and population growth.

Although urbanization and population growth contribute to the problem, they do not account for the increased water demand. The World Resource Institute documents that water use grew sixfold between 1900 and 1995, more than twice the rate of population growth (Ravenga et al. 2000:4). Greater water usage is associated with rising standards of living, including potentially unsustainable levels of irrigated agriculture. This is just one of the ways in which the causes of scarcity can have both a physical and social component.

Water quality is deteriorating in many areas of the developing world because of factors as varied as population growth and salinity caused by industrial farming and as overextraction rises. About 95 percent of the world's cities still dump raw sewage into their waters. In many developing countries, river pollution from raw sewage reaches levels thousands of times higher than the recommended safe limits for drinking and bathing (Clarke 1993). Polluted water has pushed 20 percent of freshwater fish species to the edge of extinction. Industrial and agricultural runoff threatens water quality with high levels of heavy metals and arsenic in the wastewater stream (UNEP 1999b).

Chilton notes other impacts in areas of rapid urbanization: increased costs for water, with competition between wealthy developed areas and periurban slums; seawater intrusion; mixing of industrial and human waste flows with drinking water, and the need to collect water from distant sources; and subsidence (Chilton 1998).

Drinking and bathing in polluted water supplies are among the most common routes for the spread of infectious disease. Clarke (1993) claims that nearly half the world's population suffers from water-related (both waterborne and water-washed) diseases. Such diseases are the second most important causes of death for infants in developing countries—diarrhea alone was estimated in the 1980s and early 1990s to cause four million deaths a year (Gleick, ed. 1993)—and access to safe water correlates strongly with the survival of children under five years old. Every eight seconds, the UNEP estimates, a child dies from a water-related disease (UNEP 1999a).

Chapter 2 details the impact of cholera in Ecuador. That epidemic began in Lima, Peru, in 1991, when nearly three thousand deaths were attributed to cholera. A disproportionate number of these deaths occurred in disadvantaged communities like Canto Grande, the site discussed in this chapter.

Repeated calls to respond to the water crisis have not been answered. The inaction of governments to the 2002 World Summit on Sustainable Development in Johannesburg, South Africa, is an example. Global meetings manifest the political, economic, and cultural values of the contestants: the United States promotes privatization and national solutions, while much of the rest of the world encourages collectivism and collaboration. The resulting compromises leave few benefited.

Current environmental trends expose the vulnerabilities of our global system but yield little insight into solutions. A global response to environmental concerns will take decades to be realized. In the meantime, populations must adapt to these threats. A few government and donor-sponsored programs have been tried, but most, like the World Bank's attempted privatization of Lima's water system (Alcázar, Xu, and Zuluaga 2002), have ended in spectacular failure.

National, not rational, values are played out in the congresses concerning water crises, and much symbolic, instead of financial, capital is spent. Approaches from economics and engineering abound, but the world seems to be moving away from these solutions. Missing from the discussions is what people are doing about problems. Exploration of the local, clearly linked to the consequences of water use, provides a better clue as to what water use will be like in the future. This chapter deals with these issues in describing water use in Canto Grande; conditions in Lima throw global issues into high relief.

## THE PROBLEM OF WATER IN LIMA

The population of Lima is difficult to count, for many of the reasons discussed in this chapter, but is somewhat more than 8 million, a large proportion of the total Peruvian population of 27.5 million. Lima also accounts for approximately 80 percent of the national industrial production. The urbanized area of the city is constrained by the Andes mountain chain, which runs parallel to the coast, and future growth is likely to be along this strip of desert and in three adjacent river valleys: Chillon, Rimac, and Lurin. One consequence of this is that Lima is very spread out, covering 2,800 sq. km.

In the past forty years, Lima has grown rapidly, in part because of immigration from other regions. Since 1971 the population is estimated to have more than doubled, from 3.3 million to 8.9 million people, almost a third of the entire country (*World Gazetteer* 2004; see also table 5.1). The increase in population has led to greater numbers of people living in nonplanned settlements, or "invasions," such as Canto Grande, many of which are not served by water, sanitation, or the electric power grid.

Lima is situated just 12 degrees below the equator, but its temperatures, modified by the Humboldt Current, average 21.0 C in January and 15.0 C in July. It has an arid climate with low precipitation (the average annual precipitation is 26 mm), with sea mists and occasional light drizzles and fog supplying moisture during the winter (*Britannica* 1998). Lima's location on the coast was necessitated by trade, and repeated hostilities postconquest made it the seat of government. Today global trade, food insecurity in the highlands, and the availability of services in Lima drive people to the city.

Lima's sources of raw water are scarce and variable. Located in the coastal region of Peru, Lima receives less than 15 mm of rainfall a year. The river flow through this region is strongly seasonal: twenty-five of the fifty-three main rivers dry up entirely during the dry season, from May to December. As a result, the average availability of surface water in the coastal area was estimated at 2,885 cu m per capita in 1996, compared with an estimated world average of 8,500 cu m (Macroconsult 1996). Engelman and Leroy have much lower estimates: 1900 cu m in 1990, falling to 1500 cu m in 2000. Engelman and Leroy project water scarcity (defined as 1,000 cu m per person) as early as 2025 (Engelman and Leroy 1993).

Pollution aggravates the scarcity problem. The major source of Lima's water supply is the Rimac River, which is contaminated by heavy metals from nearby mines, high levels of nitrates and other organic compounds, and untreated sewerage. About a third of Lima's water comes from wells, which depend on a shrinking supply of groundwater. When the water table near the ocean drops because of increased pumping in the dry season, salinity pollutes the aquifer (World Bank 1994). Peru represents a special case of waste as well. In the developed urban areas with piped water supplies, distribution losses (and the possibility of mixing with effluent) are eighteen times greater than average annual rainfall (360 mm versus 20 mm) (Chilton 1998).

Because of Lima's rapid population growth and urbanization,

**TABLE 5.1**
*Metropolitan Lima: Total Population (x 1,000)*

|            | 1961  | 1972  | 1981  | 1993  | 1998  | 2002  |
|------------|-------|-------|-------|-------|-------|-------|
| Total Pop. | 1,837 | 3,297 | 4,700 | 6,343 | 7,060 | 7,691 |

*Source: Instituto Nacional de Estadística e Informática.*

the increase in demand for water is substantial. Lima was growing by an average of about 2.7 percent a year from 1981 to 1992 as terrorism and economic factors drove rural populations into low-income communities such as Canto Grande. In 1991 pueblos jovenes accounted for 58 percent of Lima's population of 6.5 million. The result is an overextraction of groundwater that is unsustainable because the water table drops 1–2 m every year (Rojas, Howard, and Bastram 1994). Thus, both surface and groundwater resources are shrinking.

Fecal contamination of the Lima aquifer is significant, which adds to the public health risk. For those fortunate to be on a water distribution network, many of the groundwater sources are chlorinated to disinfect the water. Studies have shown, however, that only 36.6 percent of groundwater supplies demonstrate free chlorine residual (Rojas, Howard, and Bastram 1994); most water supplies do not provide protection from pathogens in the distribution system. Contamination of the Lima aquifer comes mainly from abandoned dug wells, especially those that are in industrial sites and are not sealed; currently used dug wells that are not protected or do not have chlorinators; and inefficient and unlined waste-stabilization ponds and effluent irrigation in Callao, Lima's port. As is common in developing countries, the lack of reliable data to describe the groundwater quality in Lima makes groundwater quality assessment difficult. This, undoubtedly, underestimates the situation.

About a third of those without connections rely on standpipes or group taps, another third on water vendors, and the rest on sources such as wells. The community we describe here uses purchased water delivered in tanker trucks and stored in barrels. Vendor water is expensive, about US$2.50–$2.75 per cu m in 1989. Persons who rely on vendors consume less water, estimated at about 30 liters per day (lpd) per person (World Bank 1994). Contrast this with a European average of 150–200 lpd. In addition, one-third of barrels sampled during the period of study in Canto Grande were positive for *E. coli* (Kendall and Gittelsohn 1994).

Water shortage and contamination are associated with high levels of diarrheal disease. Research was being conducted simultaneously with fieldwork by the Institute of Nutrition Research, Lima, and is reported in Kendall and Gittelsohn (1994). In 1987 infants in this community had nearly ten episodes of diarrhea before their first birthday (some of the highest reported rates in the world). These infants had high rates of diarrhea from birth, unlike infants in some other developing countries, who have been found to be relatively protected during their first six months of life. Of the 1,299 episodes of diarrhea identified in a cohort of 153 children less than one year of age, 953 (73 percent) were studied for enteropathogens. Routine cultures from children who were not ill were also collected. *Campylobacter jejuni* and enterotoxigenic *E. coli* were the most commonly isolated pathogens in both cases and controls. Enteropathogenic *E. coli*, rotavirus, and shigella were significantly associated with diarrhea in comparison with controls. Dehydration was identified in twenty-eight episodes (2.2 percent).

Diarrhea was associated with contamination, in water and in food and utensils. Samples taken from raw foods indicated that cereals, dairy products, and meats were the most frequently contaminated. Teas, often given to infants during the first month of life, had a low frequency of contamination after preparation by heating (3 percent of 87 specimens). If served in a cup, they also had low levels of contamination (2 percent of 49 specimens). If served in bottles, however, 31 percent (74 specimens) were contaminated, and 20 percent had counts of 10,000 coliform per ml or more ($p < 0.01$). Water present in homes for direct consumption or food preparation was analyzed: 33 percent (252 specimens) of the samples of unboiled water had fecal contamination. A high proportion of baby bottles and nipples was contaminated. Other potential sources of contamination were food preparation utensils and food preparers' hands. Close contact with pets and other domestic animals is another apparent source of diarrheal disease. Organization of the community and households necessitates that chickens and other animals share the house with their human owners during the day and every evening. Guinea pigs spend their entire lives in the house. The dirt floors provide little opportunity for cleaning up after them. Forty-six percent of the rectal samples taken from animals living in houses were positive for *C. jejuni* or *P. shigelloides* (Kendall and Gittelsohn 1994).

Remarkably, given the high rates of diarrheal disease, infant deaths due to dehydration are minimal, which may represent another adaptation to this environment. Lunch and supper consist of two courses: the *sopa* and *segundo*. The first course for each child and adult is a huge bowl of salty broth, an excellent rehydrating solution. Children are required to finish their broth before moving on to a plate of rice and other solids. Although not ideal for infant and child growth, this may account for a relatively low rate of dehydration-associated mortality. For Peru as a whole, the annual proportion of deaths in children less than five years of age attributed to intestinal infectious disease (ICD 9 codes 001–009) is 5/1,000 (PAHO 2002). These and other adaptations are discussed below.

## FORCES: INTERNATIONAL DEBT

The literature on underinvestment and underdevelopment in Peru and South America in general is substantial but needs to be mentioned (Fitzgerald 1979; Figueroa 1984; M. Reid 1985; Gootenberg 1989). The history of Peru's participation in the international economy is a sad one. Peru was among the first Latin American countries to open themselves to global capitalism in the nineteenth century, and the long and troubled relationship with W. R. Grace that followed is well documented (Clayton 2002; James 1993). During the 1980s debt crisis, Peru was among the worst-affected countries. External debt doubled during the decade as the country borrowed to finance its current account deficit. Negative economic growth during this period made it difficult for the government to pay back even the interest on existing loans. Total debt stood at $30.5 billion in 1997, more than 50 percent of the GNP. Half the debt is owed to bilateral creditors, mainly Japan, France, United States, Italy, and Germany. The ratio of debt service to exports is far above what even the IMF considers sustainable. The government paid $2.5 billion in debt service in 1996. This is more than was scheduled, more than 30 percent of government revenue, and is more than what was spent on national healthcare (Jubilee 2000). Meanwhile, the population we describe here lives without basic human needs.

## PUEBLOS JOVENES

The majority of Lima, approximately half of its geographical area, has been developed completely outside formal urban planning, in what Peruvians euphemistically refer to as "young towns," or pueblos jovenes. During the past fifty years, these marginal urban neighborhoods cropped up as migrants invaded public and private lots.

The pueblos jovenes of Lima have been well described by Lloyd (1980), Mangin (1957, 1959), Matos Mar (1961, 1966), Gianella (1970), and others. They lack piped water and sanitation, among other necessities. Unemployment is high, and inhabitants are desperately poor. Housing ranges from shelters constructed of flattened drums, to huts made of woven *estera* mats and packing lumber, to houses of fired brick with cement floors. Because these communities are relatively new and widely dispersed, few health services are accessible, and the burden of disease is high, as mentioned earlier. Personal and household security remains a problem. All of these conditions contribute to difficulties with water security and use.

## CONNECTIONS: THE ORGANIZATION OF CANTO GRANDE

The study reported here was conducted during the 1980s, and Peru has undergone substantial change since then. Canto Grande in the 1980s presented a synchronic picture of biology and culture: lessons can be learned from the lives of its inhabitants then. This is not meant to portray Canto Grande as it is today.

Canto Grande is organized into settlements, and settlements are organized into blocks, which constitute the smallest organizational unit of these land invasions. Blocks cooperate under circumstances that require joint presentation, under the leadership of directors or mayors of sites. In daily affairs, however, blocks most often compete for official status and services such as electricity and water. Houses are constructed around the perimeter of the block and line up facing houses on other blocks—their competitors. Blocks try to fill all the space on the perimeter to lay claim to the interior space and reduce traffic through the block. If latrines exist, they are hidden in the center of the block. Not visible from the street, latrines are also "hidden" from any obligation to maintain them.

Because traffic moves along the rectangles around the blocks, the corners of each block are where the water barrels are stored. Each family keeps a 55-gallon barrel or two, but the barrels in Canto Grande are most often left in the crossroads because the water trucks refuse to deliver to each house. Barrels are in various states of repair and with or without covers. A lively business in barrel cleaning and sales exists. Clumped in the crossroads, water barrels cannot be protected from the predations of neighbors or from people who live on other blocks. Needless to say, the opportunities to steal water are plentiful, especially if a family has "too much." One can only depend on neighbor support to prevent theft.

In reality, each family is on its own. Residents of Canto Grande maintain well-documented networks with rural family that serve as a base for migration to the city, as well as with family and friends in similar sites elsewhere in the city. Most residents have few ties to wealthier settings or to their direct neighbors. Lobo (1981) details the social resources available to families in the 1970s and the quest for a bourgeois lifestyle, that is, home ownership, purchased brick by brick over a long time by individual households. Neighbors are competitors and potential threats, not support.

*Global connections* implies links across borders, but local connections are problematic here. As pointed out above, there is a "poverty" of connectedness, of social capital, even given the corporativist rhetoric of community organizers (see Wiarda 2001). As domestic field and domain, not only neighborly connections are suspect, but intrahousehold connections as well. Unstable domestic arrangements and lack of services create a world where some children are locked in a house while their parent(s) commute to work in a distant locale. The domestic environment contains many competitors and few allies.

## HOUSING

Houses are constructed of three kinds of materials. The cheapest and most temporary materials are woven mats of estera. Bamboo poles or substitutes are driven into the ground at the corners of the house and are connected to form a frame for the roof. Mats suspended from this frame enclose the house. Houses are square or rectangular, 3–4 m on a side and measured to accommodate the sizes of the mats. The roof most often consists of black plastic sheeting. This house of straw is very vulnerable to theft. A burglar needs only to cut through the wall with a knife to remove the house's contents. Owners of straw houses therefore adopt a proven strategy: they have nothing to steal. Contents of the house might consist of two or three plastic bowls, a table and two chairs, a bed, a few utensils, and usually nothing else. If the owners have a radio, for example, they often take it with them when they leave the house.

Whether the owner upgrades house materials depends on many factors. One factor is the likelihood that the block or land invasion will receive legal status. This is a long and complicated process, well elaborated after more than half a century of these land invasions. Another factor has to do with one's neighbors. Are these the sort of people you want to live with for the rest of your time in the community? Although groups of people often participate in the same invasions, they have very little control over membership in the entire group. New immigrants to the city occupy houses alongside older migrants from the slums in the city center or from another pueblo joven and alongside recently released criminals from the notorious prisons of Lima. Settlers might participate in a number of invasions, simultaneously trying to occupy three or four houses with the rouse of moving from house to house over the course of a month. In Canto Grande, up to a third of the houses were unoccupied during fieldwork. Betting on the possibility of a given site, the family might sell or simply abandon its house in a community that is not working out.

Having selected a site, the residents might decide to upgrade the wall and roof materials, first substituting wood and windows with shutters that can be locked and purchasing a wooden door and metal roof. Cement floors are common at this stage and add property value. The final stage is the construction of a house using brick or cement. Residents begin this stage by purchasing a few bricks every week and stacking them around the outside of their house. Because the region is seismically active, they also have to purchase and install metal construction rods. These houses, with their wire antennas of building rods, are seen throughout Lima and usually represent a two-decade-long process of occupation and ownership. After the house of brick is complete and a metal door installed, possessions become visible. TV antennas spring up and stereos, washing machines, and other appliances appear.

The story seems to be that of the Three Little Pigs, with the Big Bad Wolf being one's neighbor, envy, and theft. The difference is that in the story there are three pigs. Such levels of cooperation are relatively unheard of in Canto Grande. Governments and nongovernmental organizations have organized community kitchens—and these land invasions are community activities—but when it comes to improving house sites and houses or stopping theft, each household is on its own. The cycle of migration and community development means that few or no kin are nearby and one's neighbors—in the competing block across the street and often on the same block—are potential enemies. This is one reason that families often speculate on house sites. This process of careful and financially painful accumulation and construction represents a penny consumerism (see Tax 1963), and each family strives to build both its nest egg and house, trying to avoid expensive communal obligations and the predations of neighbors.

This informal economy—which extends to trading and manufacturing—is lauded in the famous works of Hernan De Soto and considered a neoliberal triumph of the petite bourgeois against the state (De Soto, Ghersi, and Ghibellini 1986). Whereas this form of accumulation might be prized as an economic strategy in such a flawed statist regime aspiring to the free market, it works less well when individuals are trying to satisfy their needs for water.

Water, as well as all other commodities, is purchased and owned individually, reflecting the logic of the economy and the values of individualism. Users need to calculate quite carefully their daily water use and what to do if the water truck does not show up. Water is not borrowed and is rarely resold. Instead, the only guarantee of not running out of water is to use as little as possible. Local practices have adapted remarkably to achieve this. First, water is extensively reused for washing and bathing and is discarded only after three or four washes and rinses of dishes and utensils. Water is also reused for clothes washing and bathing. I witnessed a mother finish dressing her nine-year-old son before sending him off to school. His white shirt had not been washed in a month, but the terrifically dry environment guaranteed dryness. His sweater and slacks had not been washed for a much longer time, but she did not feel that they required cleaning. Before he left for school, she said, "Come here so I can wash your face." Reaching for the rag hanging from her apron string, she ran this small piece of towel over his face. As far as I could tell, the dirty and perfectly dry rag did little but organize the fine layer of dust covering the child's face into regular patterns, but, satisfied, the mother sent her son off to school.

The reality of living in a desert environment with lots of dust blowing around has created an accommodation even in the classification of dirt. Observe in the descriptions below how water use is minimized.

## LOCAL IMAGINATION: CONCEPTS OF CLEANLINESS, DIRTINESS, AND DISEASE

The word "to clean" (*limpiar*) has spiritual, as well as physical, connotations in Canto Grande. It refers not only to the physical cleaning of a baby's bottom or the "cleaning" of the gut via administration of a purgative, but also to the spiritual cleansing produced by passing an egg over the baby's body to protect against the evil eye. Furthermore, dirtiness embraces dust from the street or dirt floors, feces, and contamination. A substantial minority of mothers discussed the importance of hand washing, especially before preparing food, but few were seen to practice it. Mothers did differentiate levels of dirtiness, however, separating ordinary dirtiness (*sucio*) from *sucio mugre* (contaminated with organic waste or feces). Sucio mugre requires hand washing; sucio does not. Even when washing their hands, mothers did not differentiate between dipping hands in water and washing hands. Explicit acts of hand washing would occur only if mothers came into contact with some nonfood contaminant.

Men may wash early in the morning before work, and children who attend school are scrubbed. For others, bathing or general washing is much less common. Under these circumstances, skin infections are common, but locals associate most skin infections with bad blood (*mala sangre*) or evil humors (*mal humor*) rather than dirt or lack of washing. Several mothers expressed ideas congruent with cosmopolitan germ theory. For example, they associated food, which was dirty (*sucio*), with several illnesses, including diarrhea. Many mothers, however, expressed the idea that "dirty things don't do any harm" (*lo sucio no hace daño*) and that "poison that doesn't kill you makes you fat" (*veneno que no mata, engorda*). Proper hand and utensil washing would go a long way to reduce exposure to pathogens.

Household cleaning is routinized and follows a regular daily format, instead of responding to particular peaks of dirtiness or contamination. Dirty dishes and pots, for example, are left from the preceding evening and washed early in the morning, along with the floor of the house. This is associated with common theories of disease etiology and promotes less water use: "cold" is commonly associated with disease causation in the study area. Handling cold water at night, it is felt, could produce fever and diarrhea. These ideas fit neatly with the scarcity of water and help justify water use practices.

## CONCEPTS OF FECES AND DEFECATION

Several classes of feces are recognized, based on the producer. For example, the feces of breastfeeding infants, weaned children, adults, small animals, and large animals were all distinguished and treated differently. Although, in general, people do not think that human feces transmit diseases, they believe that large animal feces, including dog and pig feces, are dangerous. Small animal feces are not considered dangerous or bothersome, and chicken feces are collected as fertilizer. The desert-like environment provides unique, human solid-waste disposal opportunities. Hillsides, unoccupied because of the occasional rainstorm and mudslide, are places of defecation. Far from home, hills are also far from sources of water for handwashing and consequently add to the oral-fecal burden. Feces are not buried and soon dry. It is easy to see how these factors enhance contact with feces and reduce perceived necessity for hand washing.

This adaptation to life with little water in a desert environment is a remarkable achievement that demonstrates the plasticity of human behavior in response to structural violence (Farmer 2001). At the same time, it should be clear that this adaptation comes through the lens of individualism and penny consumerism rather than through developing a communal and collaborative response. After all, everyone "owns" an individual house for which he is responsible. Everyone "has" or potentially has utilities and services to pay for. As a result, communal responsibilities such as latrines get short shrift. This life entails ten times less water use than in the most deplorable international refugee camps, with levels of disease corresponding to some of the worst environments on the planet. Ultimately, this adaptation's tenuousness and unsustainability create, in contradistinction to the goals of a bourgeoisie, a sense of uncertainty that permits little in the way of planning or stability.

A reasonable response to this would be collective action and organization of water resources, but such is not the case. Instead, recently, efforts were made to privatize the water system (see Alcázar, Xu, and Zuluaga 2002; Orwin 1999). Ultimately rejected, and irrespective of the benefits of privatization, this approach is a piecemeal solution that reflects international ideological concerns. Ideological justification for privatization in Peru is found in the work of De Soto and his colleagues cited above. Take this construction, which, although concerned with housing, not water, applies *mutandis mutandi*:

> The investment people have made in their own informally built homes amounts to $8 or $8.5 billion, an investment that has been made with no government aid of any kind. Second, it is socially important because it represents the emergence of a new proprietary class. Traditionally, in Peru—as in the rest of Latin America—the less privileged classes of society had not been property owners. The access to property had been limited to the wealthy or aristocratic classes. Through this process of informal construction, however, the least privileged sectors of Latin America have been able to revindicate for themselves the right to private property and make it a reality in their cities. Finally, informal construction has had a remarkable political significance because, in the final analysis, only the property owners can fight for their rights. Only when one has a right to own something, does one have a sense of responsibility, struggle, and political challenge. Countries without private property are countries where civil society is weak and the citizenry does not confront political power because, in the final analysis, there is very little room left for individual development. (Ghersi 1997)

This argument is being made because the residents of towns like Canto Grande do not legally own their homes. They cannot leverage financial resources, nor, while beseeching the government for legal title, can they organize much in the way of a legal response. This argument is directed to Peru's government system—sometimes left-leaning, sometimes right, communal in rhetoric, corrupt, but facing the hard pragmatism and disillusionment of Peru's free-market pirates. This is just as much a stretch of the global imagination: individual-by-individual, a middle-class lifestyle can be created independent of the political environment. Ultimately, the cumulative effect of globalization may be to create the kind of world described here—a diffused, individualized, extra-legal response to shared needs, which produces ecological disaster after disaster. Water is the exemplar.

To summarize, global forces define the conditions of trade and work that help generate low levels of income and wealth (as well as drive people to live on a desert near international trade routes rather than in more hospitable environments). Global connections define a world in which the poor possess even fewer positive ties and endure unstable domestic arrangements and forced local connections of ambiguous status, such as neighbors. The lack of positive ties—family, neighborly, patron-client, and exogenous—defines the poverty of social capital. Global imagination is apparent in the ideology of water purchase and use, the patterned response to disease, and the individuated dreams of life's goals and the adoption of a penny consumerism.[1]

## CONCLUSIONS

Grounded globalization, linking local social fields with global trends, begins to provide the rejoinder to those who see a sharp separation between traditional ethnography and contemporary research in anthropology. Demonstrating the strong parallels across local and global social fields provides both a methodological response and a model of how anthropology can contribute to modeling globalization and its effects. The ideology of water conservation, including such things as the classification of dirt, reflects the thoroughness of the cultural and material adaptation to this environment.

The three axes of grounded globalization link the material and economic to the societal and cultural. Paralleling the contributions of an earlier anthropology, the axes permit the demonstration of the functionality and integration of modes of living—in this case, with factors that are both local and extralocal. The difference that grounded globalization offers is a refocusing on the personal and local while reporting on the penetration of extralocal forces. But grounded globalization is a lens that distorts both ways: not only does the local community manifest the impact of globalization in new ways adapted to local circumstances, but also the local cannot be understood outside those distant forces that define the moral, economic, and political parameters of choices in Lima. Canto Grande reveals new notions of bourgeois lifestyle, a religion of controlled consumption, and new notions of water use, hygiene, and health. But the lessons that Hernan de Soto and the Cato Institute draw about the triumph of the individual also distort the miserly local context of capital and ownership, certainly as it applies to water, where a focus on individual, extralegal solutions dooms communal and legal ones. Efforts to resolve this problem must address the poverty of social capital and imagination in all the communities looking through the lens.

### Notes

1. This imagination is "global," as Farmer (2001) is correct in pointing out: increasingly, expectations of optimal health, or housing, or lifestyle, may be remarkably similar around the world. Also, as Farmer argues, local material circumstances define the field in which these expectations play, often resulting in widely divergent differences between this global imagination and reality. These material circumstances, however, do create diverse and significant cultural conceptual resources that do determine behavior and outcomes.

# 6

## Whose Water Is It Anyway?

*Boundary Negotiations on the Edwards Aquifer in Texas*

**Irene Klaver and John Donahue**

"Well, the weather got the water and a snake bite took a child," Lyle Lovett (1998) sings in "Texas Trilogy." Movies and songs might picture a rough-and-tumble Texas "hotter than hell," with rustling cowboys, howling coyotes, and rattling snakes, but driving Highway 281 north from San Antonio towards Austin, the lush Hill Country opens into an Italian-like landscape. Terraced as Tuscany, it radiates the charm and calm of old culture, overgrown traditions that have transformed it into a landscape of gently intertwined nature and culture. The Texas terraces, however, are not the slow effect of cultivation over the years, but the even slower effect of geological formation. Differential erosion patterns of hard and soft strata of limestone and shale create Mediterranean radiance. Seductive as Italian Tuscany and blessed with a relatively mild climate, the Hill Country is a most desired retirement area for Texans and other Americans alike. It includes the fastest-growing counties of Texas—Bexar County and Hays County. A deluge of road signs promises everyone 5 acres of ranchette property. The Lyle Lovett of the twenty-first century will have to adjust his "Texas Trilogy" lyrics. The themes are still the same—water is still taken and children still die—but the causal actors have changed: population growth and traffic have replaced weather and snakes. "Well, the humans got the water and an SUV took a child." Somewhere along the way, the poetics are lost. Has something been gained in the process? In this chapter, we argue that something indeed has been gained: an awareness that water scarcity is not solely weather-related but is as much a cultural and political phenomenon.

In the past decades, politics in general have become increasingly complex. Processes of globalization, decentralization, and privatization have led to new policy forms of partnerships between government institutions and civic and commercial organizations. A wide variety of public and private participants find themselves involved in intricate decision-making processes, juggling local, state, national, supranational, and subnational, or regional, levels of organization. Add to this organizational complexity the increasing problem of scarce resources such as water, and it is clear that coordination, cooperation, and communication become vital ingredients for policy making. More than ever, ways of negotiating differences are necessary.

In this chapter, we deploy a specific approach to negotiating, namely, negotiation through the notion of boundary objects (Star and Griesemer 1989). We see a boundary object as a mediating agent. Through it, one can come to a practice of cooperative management. Boundary objects are meant to navigate conflicts by finding connections and emphasizing relations. In that sense, they do justice to the heterogeneity of the various entities affected by complex decision-making processes. We introduce the notion of boundary objects in the management conflicts and negotiation practices around the Edwards Aquifer, the underground freshwater body in south-central Texas that provides water for San Antonio and nine counties.

Furthermore, we explore a more specific area of water politics, namely, the negotiation of water conflicts for the health and well-being of the entire ecosystem. What is recommended is an integrative management in which the heterogeneous stakeholders come to cooperative decisions. We show how both economic and environmental concerns contribute to an overall sense of health. The health of the watershed is, in fact, a precondition for sustaining human health. Thus, this chapter itself could be seen as a boundary object between the first section of this book, with its focus on health and water, and the second section, which reverses the emphasis to water and health.[1]

## WATER AND POLITICS: BOUNDARY OBJECTS

It has been part of the American West lore that "whiskey is for drinking and water is for fighting." Indeed, the West has a long tradition of bitter water wars.[2] Texas, while blessed with more water than the arid Southwest, is facing its own water management crisis. Texas water law, like that of most states, still does not reflect the hydrological connection between surface water and groundwater. State water policy is based on regional plans in which political and hydrological boundaries are out of sync. Groundwater pumping, long enjoyed by individual private-property owners, is increasingly coming under corporate control in an emerging water market.

Faced with water scarcity, Texans must find "the last oasis," that is, "the untapped potential of conservation," but to tap into this potential requires greater efficiency, joint management, and a water ethic of equitable "sharing—both with nature and with each other" (Postel 1992:viii–x, 22). Instead, scarcity usually leads to greater competition. Cities compete with rural areas, regions fight over junior and senior water rights, and the welfare of people is pitted against that of the environment. Often regarded as an "externality" or an object for "command and control," the environment is more than a backdrop to these conflicts. We argue that central to the successful management of water resources is the concept of ecosystem health, "an integrative field exploring the interrelationships between human activity, social organization, natural systems, and human health" (Rapport et al. 1998).

Based upon earlier research, we start with the assumption that sustainable management depends on successful, ongoing negotiation of often mutually exclusive interests (see Klaver et al. 2002; Donahue and Sanders 2001). The art of this negotiation is the ability to reach practical, communally crafted decisions. Only when everyone's concerns are taken seriously can concessions be made. For everyone to understand the various concerns, these must be "translated" into one another's conceptual and practical vocabulary or framework. Boundary objects facilitate this translation: they have a specific meaning for each group, but their structure is common enough to form a leverage or connection among the various groups. They can be seen as vehicles of translation that enable coherence across social worlds; in their capacity to cross boundaries, boundary objects create a meeting ground. They invite cooperation without reducing inner diversity to a consensus that eliminates heterogeneity. In this evolution of cooperation, vested interests might shift, attracting potentially new players in the field. Cooperative management is, by definition, an ongoing process of negotiation.

In our research of the management conflicts around the Edwards Aquifer, we determine three kinds of boundary objects, all of which contribute to negotiating the different interests in the aquifer. First, and most generally, is the aquifer itself. It is a boundary object in the sense that it is an identifiable body of water, but at the same time teeming with contradictory interests and disparate meanings for different groups. On the level of political organization, we show how one governing body in particular, the Edwards Aquifer Authority, more than other political structures, functions as a model-boundary object. Again, it is solid and identifiable and, at the same time, a "container" for various interests. Last but not least, we conclude more specifically that the notion of public property, more than the notions of the commons or of private property, will be effective in negotiations around the Edwards Aquifer. Like the preceding two entities, it has the potential of a boundary object—albeit a concept and not an object proper—because it affords negotiation space for a variety of interests. We start with a cultural, geographical, and hydrological sketch of the Edwards Aquifer. Its bounty and its limits make this aquifer a fascinating boundary object.

## THE EDWARDS AQUIFER

In the early Western movies, Texas is often portrayed as dry, devoid of vegetation except tumbleweed, and populated more by coyotes than by people. This stereotype might fit the western Texas deserts, but the state enjoys a wide range of environmental zones, from the lush rice country and piney woods of the east to the Chihuahua desert around El Paso in the west. Between these two major zones is the city of San Antonio, the third largest metropolitan area in Texas after Houston and Dallas-Fort Worth and now the eighth largest city in the United

States, with 1.21 million people. Given its history, San Antonio is culturally more like Monterrey, Mexico, 280 miles to the south, than like Austin, the state's capital, some 80 miles to the north. The influence of northern Mexico can be found in San Antonio's food, music, and architecture. More than half of the city's residents can trace their origins back to Mexico—partly for the simple reason that, for a considerable period of its history, San Antonio was part of Mexico. San Antonio itself can be seen as a boundary object, mediating various perspectives of its own past.

In one important regard, however, San Antonio is unlike her neighbor to the south and more like other cities in the United States. Everywhere, spacious lawns are carpeted with water-thirsty St. Augustine grass (*Stenotaphrum secundatum*). Imported from tropical Africa, this grass accounts—together with landscape watering—for some 30–40 percent of San Antonio's annual water usage (Susan Butler, personal communication 2004) and symbolizes the ambivalences faced by South Texans in adapting to a semiarid environment. Yet, on the other side of the border, Mexicans long ago came to grips with living in a semiarid climate. Typically, their homes front directly onto the street, obviating any need for a lawn. An inner courtyard yields a common green space for the enjoyment of all in the home and with minimal watering demands.

A major hydrological difference adds to the cultural contrasts between northern Mexico and southern Texas in watering landscapes. Whereas northern Mexico depends on the surface water of rainfall and riverine sources, San Antonio and the whole semiarid region that characterizes the area between the limestone hills of central Texas and the Gulf Coast are blessed with groundwater from a rechargeable, underground aquifer—the Edwards Aquifer (figure 6.1).[3] The city relies on the aquifer for more than 99 percent of its municipal supply, giving San Antonio the dubious distinction of being the largest city in the country to rely so heavily on groundwater (Glennon 2002:89).

Human adaptation to the geology of the Edwards Aquifer region has created a socioeconomic landscape that concentrates the agricultural and ranching economic sector in the west, the more industrial and metropolitan sector in the center, and a major recreational and service sector in the east, around the springs in Comal and Hays

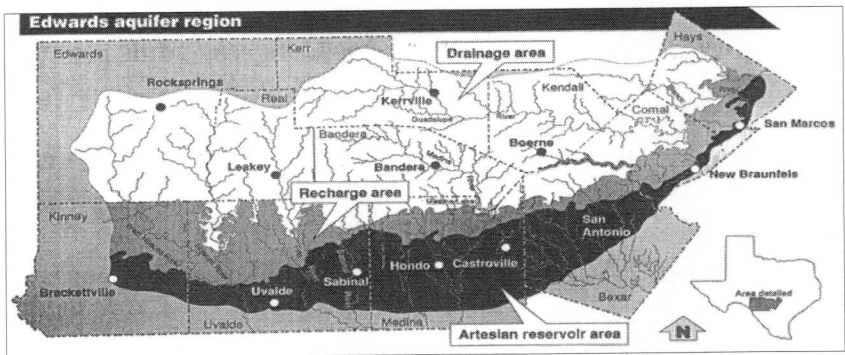

**FIGURE 6.1**
*The Edwards Aquifer region. (Map courtesy of the* San Antonio Express-News*)*

Counties. To the north of the aquifer lies an area of recharge; runoff from rainfall flows into the aquifer through porous limestone and sinkholes and percolates downward to the reservoir. Because the aquifer varies in elevation, it flows from west to east, emerging at various springs along the way (figure 6.2). Conservative estimates place the aquifer's capacity between 25 and 55 million acre-feet of water, which is more than all the surface water in the state (Maclay 1988).[4] The region's annual pumping is about 450,000 acre-feet, or 1.0 to 2.4 percent of the aquifer's capacity.[5]

Aquifer waters percolate to the surface at springs in the central (Bexar County) and eastern expanses of the aquifer (Hays and Comal Counties), which, in turn, have been sites of urban population growth. With advances in pumping technology during the early twentieth century, large tracts of irrigated farmland were opened up on the western expanses of the aquifer in Medina, Uvalde, and Kinney Counties. Currently, farmers to the west invest heavily in irrigation to grow cash crops such as corn, cotton, sorghum, and Bermuda grass, as well as fall cabbage and spinach. All are water-intensive cash crops that depend more and more on irrigation as one moves further west over the aquifer. On average, Medina and Uvalde Counties account for 38 percent of overall pumping, primarily for crop irrigation and livestock raising. Comal and Hays Counties account for 8 percent. The water then flows south in the Comal and Guadalupe Rivers to petrochemical plants downstream, where industrial effluent is discharged into the

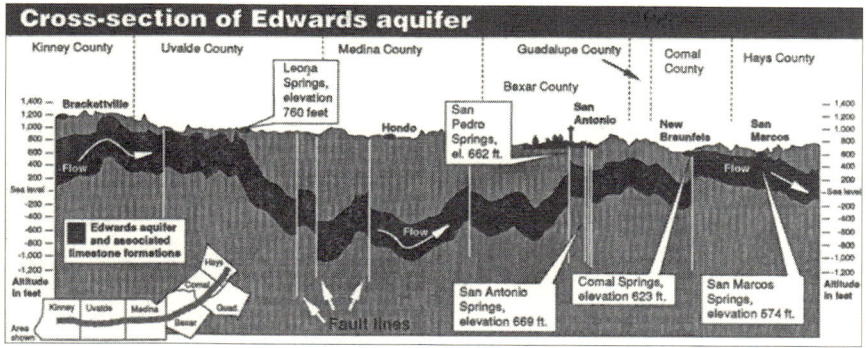

**FIGURE 6.2**
*Cross-section of the Edwards Aquifer. (Courtesy of the* San Antonio Express-News)

rivers. The major pumper of aquifer water (54 percent) is Bexar County (the City of San Antonio and the farming communities).

Tourism provides important income for the eastern counties that boast of parks and natural springs. There, endangered species could suffer if spring flows diminish because of overdrafting the aquifer. Tourism in San Antonio is now a more significant source of income than the four military bases. The River Walk alone delivers 3.5 billion a year in tourist dollars—removing the Alamo from its century-long status of tourist attraction number one in San Antonio (Glennon 2002:87). Continued building of high-density, suburban residential areas over the aquifer's recharge zone will impact water quality and quantity. The few industrial plants in existence demand substantial amounts of water in the manufacturing process. Toyota will soon make Tundra pickup trucks in a plant on the south side of the city, which will increase local demand for water. On average, it takes 400,000 liters (105,000 gallons) to make one car (Barlow and Clarke 2002:8). Kelly Air Force Base, until it was closed in 1996 as part of a Congressional cost-cutting effort, was the major depot for refurbishing cargo planes and jet engines. Large plumes of pollutants have been discovered under neighborhoods to the south of the base. Three large military bases, one Army and two Air Force, continue to be major players in the local economy—and in water issues.

In recent years, the Edwards Aquifer has become a battleground for myriad competing interests, geographical, governmental, and corporate. Regional surface-water authorities, environmental groups, municipal water purveyors, irrigators, industrial water consumers, state and county legislative bodies, and federal environmental agencies have been involved in a tug-of-war over the management of the aquifer (Donahue 1998).

The aquifer may be a hydrological given, but, as a common resource, it is also a political and cultural construction, a multivocal symbol that unites and divides people across political, economic, social, and geographical spectrums. Precisely in this context, the aquifer surfaces as a boundary object. It has a solid presence but also morphs easily into disparate meanings for different interested parties. Questions need to be addressed, such as how do the different stakeholders in the debate over management define the value of water and how is it possible to mediate among competing interests with different cultural meanings given to water? Furthermore, which power relations have been served most by which cultural definitions?

A major step in negotiating conflicts will lie in the creation of other boundary objects that facilitate communication among the several stakeholders, ensure regulation of the shared resource, and achieve ecosystem health. As noted, the Edwards Aquifer Authority and the concept of public property seem viable candidates for this.

## THE EDWARDS AQUIFER AUTHORITY

During the record drought of 1947 to 1956, the springs at San Marcos and Comal went dry, with dramatic consequences for the aquatic life, such as the San Marcos salamanders, fountain darters, Texas wild rice, and Comal Springs salamanders—all on the federal Endangered and Threatened Species List. Fears of a similar drought, combined with increased pumping from the aquifer, led the Sierra Club and the Guadalupe-Blanco River Authority (GBRA) to go to federal court in 1991. They argued that the US Fish and Wildlife Service should enforce the Endangered Species Act by setting pumping limits across the region to maintain spring flows and thus protect the various endangered species.

In response to threatened court action, the Texas State Legislature in 1993 considered three aquifer-management bills that were eventually brought together in a compromise, Senate Bill 1477. The compromise legislation called for replacing the Edwards Underground Water District with the Edwards Aquifer Authority (EAA, or the "Authority"). According to its mission statement, the EAA "is committed to manage and protect the Edwards Aquifer System and work with others to ensure the entire region of a sustainable, adequate, high quality and cost effective supply of water, now and in the future" (http://www.edwards aquifer.org/).

The Authority has fifteen directors, elected every four years by county districts. These districts have different cultural relations to groundwater, varying with agricultural, industrial, municipal, and recreational use. Agriculture and ranching dominate the western reaches of the aquifer in Kinney, Uvalde, and Medina Counties. Agricultural, municipal, and industrial uses of water are most prevalent in Bexar County. Major recreational and service sectors are found to the east around the springs in Comal and Hays Counties. The directors relatively fairly represent this diversity in water use across the aquifer.

After some initial legal challenges, the Authority began issuing permits in 2001 to pump from the aquifer according to historical usage. It is estimated that this permitting will be completed by 2005; some one hundred applications are under review. The Authority expects to grant senior rights to pump 450,000 acre-feet and some 150,000 junior rights by December 31, 2007, with further reductions to 400,000 acre-feet by 2008 and to whatever will be necessary to protect spring flow by 2012.[6] The result is that cities are seeing their future water use restricted because they do not have the history of usage enjoyed by older municipalities. Depending on the cities' rate of growth, 10–29 percent of the reductions are permanent. By 2007, cities may see total possible interruptions in pumping of 45–55 percent and by 2008, 51–62 percent (Carol Patterson, personal communication 2004).

The Authority is mandated to issue a comprehensive water-management plan for the region, including the development of alternative water supplies.[7] The Authority's operations are funded principally through management fees charged to the aquifer's users. The Authority installs meters on irrigation wells and is responsible for monitoring and protecting water quality, as well as quantitatively monitoring the actual usage. Water quality issues are now on the Authority's agenda, but the major focus in the early years was on water quantity regulation, by issuing groundwater withdrawal permits that allow farmers to sell water rights to municipal water purveyors. Irrigators can sell up to 50 percent of their allocations. Transferable rights, following the laws of supply and demand, will bring more flexibility into the system. Regulated by the EAA, these transfers not only will be determined by market mechanisms of the highest-value use but also will be subject to decision-making processes pertaining to a public resource. This approach does justice to the historic situation of our laws and political systems and to the localized context of water conflicts by acknowledging that water is subject to both private property rights and public resource policies (see also Glennon 2002:213–216).

Furthermore, the EAA is authorized to declare water use restrictions during critical droughts. Municipal purveyors have responsibility for enforcing the drought management rules; their conservation efforts have been quite successful.

A further important factor in the EAA's effectiveness is that it is structurally based on hydrological parameters and not determined by sheer political boundaries. The American West is riddled with failed water planning that did not take into account hydrological features and catered mainly to political forces (Reisner 1986).

Last, but not least, the EAA's operating procedures contribute to a sense of public property, which enhances the process of boundary negotiation. For these reasons, we argue that, more than any other organization, the EAA has proven to be amenable to sustainable management of the aquifer. The Authority provides an organizational structure that allows for multiple, equitable use of the aquifer, thereby realizing its function as a boundary object. Ultimately, the EAA may serve as a platform for a common discourse on integrated water management of the Edwards Aquifer and facilitate common decision-making processes, at the same time doing justice to the various users who place differing demands on the aquifer. Policies built on this common discourse would be a major step toward ensuring the health of the entire ecosystem.

## PUBLIC PROPERTY AS BOUNDARY OBJECT

Water as public property could be seen as a "third space" between cultural definitions of groundwater as a commons and as private property. Water as a commons is more frequently found in small-scale agricultural and fishing societies, where face-to-face interactions permit local management and enforcement of scarce water and water resources. At the other end of the spectrum is the conception of water as private property. A steadily growing global movement sees water as a commodity to be bought and sold in the marketplace (ITT Industries 1998). At the second World Water Forum in The Hague in 2000, water was explicitly defined as a commodity (Barlow and Clarke 2002:xiii). Corporations, such as Vivendi Universal and Suez/ONDEO, directly or through their subsidiaries, are buying up water rights and purchasing "privatized" municipal water systems in places as diverse as Sao Paulo and Onondaga County, New York (Barlow and Clarke 2002:109–116). Many international lending agencies are encouraging less developed countries to "privatize" their water systems and are even demanding such as a precondition for refinancing their national debt (Barlow and Clarke 2002:160–165). Such profit-making ventures may make for healthy corporate portfolios but do not necessarily contribute to a healthy ecosystem or to the health of the local population in providing affordable, equitable access to clean water.

We argue for an alternative to corporatizing water resources and management: regional and integrated water-management policies and practices, based on a cultural conception of water as public property rather than as a commons or a private commodity. As such, public property is not the same as property held by the state or federal government, as in the case of public parks. It refers, rather, to private property rights within a regulatory structure.

In the case of the Edwards Aquifer, conservation easements are a good example of public property. To stop further development of the Edwards Aquifer recharge area, various groups are advocating the use of conservation easements instead of full buyouts of private land. Private landowners keep the benefits of their property in terms of income from hunting, grazing, farming, or other activities that are not necessarily detrimental to the ecosystem. What they sell is their right to develop their property. Management of the Edwards Aquifer as a public property means, at the same time, providing an affordable and equitable access to this scarce resource, safeguarding some private interests while protecting its long-term viability. In combination, these ensure a sound public-resource policy of conservation easements (see also Glennon 2002).

Turning to Texas water policy, we ask what alternatives to the right of free capture, usually mediated by the courts, might the state create in support of public property? How might the state organize a permit system for groundwater withdrawal that would create an efficient market for water right transfers while protecting the public good?

When water law was first codified in 1840, the Republic of Texas recognized the existing surface-water rights granted under Spanish law. Yet, the legislature also adopted English common law and, with it, English riparian water law. This law applied to the vast land grants awarded to private landholders. In 1967 the Texas Legislature brought together existing rules for the allocation of surface water, riparian rights, and prior appropriation rights into a permitting system, which is now managed by the Texas Commission on Environmental Quality (TCEQ).[8] Yet, it is groundwater that accounts for 60 percent of Texas water needs. A major problem in Texas water law—as in most states—is the failure to acknowledge the hydrological connection between groundwater and surface water.

Groundwater in Texas, unlike surface water, was not seen as a public good, but rather as the property of the individual landowner. Traditionally, the face-to-face interactions of persons who shared a common resource created a commons. The creation of a commons in an increasingly urban, highly stratified, and ecologically diverse area such as Texas is highly impractical and, indeed, in all probability unachievable. The implementation of the concept of public property, however, is feasible. It can be created through democratic processes such as legislation, as well as local and regional mediation efforts. Elsewhere, one of us has discussed a successful mediation effort to craft a water plan for the City of San Antonio (Donahue and Sanders 2001). That effort looked beyond municipal boundaries to regional needs and explicitly included other species and ecosystem health in its concerns—hence, implicitly expanding the notion of public in more than a parochial way.[9] While it acknowledged the necessity of ecosystem health, unfortunately it did not have any enforcement mechanisms. Enforcement of the water plan resided in the municipal water purveyor, The San Antonio Water System (SAWS). Some of SAWS' policies, however, have placed its institutional health ahead of the ecosystem's.

## PUBLIC PROPERTY MEETS PROJECT CULTURE

SAWS was created as a public entity in 1992 through the consolidation of three predecessor agencies: the City Water Board (the previous, city-owned water supply utility), the City Wastewater Department (a department of the city government responsible for sewage collection and treatment), and the Alamo Water Conservation and Reuse District (an independent city agency created to develop a system for reuse of the city's treated wastewater). SAWS serves more than a million customers in the San Antonio metropolitan area and is a major player in securing additional surface water to supplant groundwater protected by legislatively mandated pumping limits on the Edwards Aquifer.

Although both the EAA and SAWS are constructing a new cultural definition of water in the public domain, they represent quite different and potentially conflicting institutional arrangements. The EAA is an elected body of representatives from the eight counties that draw from the aquifer. Clearly, urban and rural priorities differ on the board, but all representatives are concerned with the sustainable use and conservation of the natural resource. However, the EAA has spent most of its energies issuing permits for groundwater withdrawal based on historical usage. As noted, this has enabled farmers to sell pumping rights to excess water to needier municipal consumers, effectively making their water allocation an alternative crop. Recently, the EAA has become more involved in taking measures to protect the quality of the aquifer water as residential and commercial development proceeds at an alarming rate over the recharge zone. This is especially the case in Bexar County, where developers and city councils have historically preferred to build and extend city services northward into the picturesque Hill Country, even though such development poses a serious threat to recharge and of pollution of the aquifer. Nevertheless, the EAA has the authority to protect the public property of the Edwards and has adopted rules to do so (see http://www.edwardsaquifer.org/Pages/frames_regulations.html).

On the other hand, SAWS has a different institutional base and mission, which, in fact, has been at odds with a concept of public property. Although SAWS accepted the management plan, forged in 1997 (see note 9), its policies have not always respected needs in other watersheds or regions. Faced with legislatively mandated caps on annual pumping from the aquifer, SAWS has redefined water as a commodity, which it must purchase as a means of fulfilling its mission as water purveyor to its customers and to the city council that appoints its directors. Cost-benefit discourse dominates SAWS' efforts to obtain the greatest amount of surface water—but, it should be noted, not always at the cheapest price economically or environmentally.

A phenomenon called "project culture" can explain this anomaly (Nickum and Greenstadt 1998:4). When water rights or management is assigned to a particular institution, more expensive projects that enhance institutional maintenance may be preferred. In such cases, the original mission may become secondary to the growth of the bureaucracy. Expensive projects may become ends in themselves, and their effects on the consumer or the environment are therefore marginalized. In other words, project culture—the institutional interests of the water purveyor—takes priority over public property goals.

The pumping caps created by Senate Bill 1477 have further legitimized project culture among purveyors such as SAWS. Large capital-intensive pumping schemes are given priority over less expensive and potentially more productive alternatives to enhancing aquifer use, such as the construction of small recharge dams, augmentation of spring flows to protect endangered species, and other optimizing measures. Into the breach between supply and demand step those promoting more expensive and potentially lucrative contracts to build water pipelines and desalination plants.

A case in point is a contract between SAWS and ALCOA to purchase water mined by that company in Bastrop County, northeast of San Antonio. ALCOA is planning to build a second strip coal mine and sell underground water from the Simsboro Formation of the massive Carrizo-Wilcox Aquifer to San Antonio. Opponents, including the Austin City Council, say that the 15,000-acre project will drain the underground water supplies from two counties, devastate the land, and force landowners to sell out, (For an account of the Austin City Council Minutes and Resolution against the proposal, see http://www.ci.austin.tx.us/council/00council_012700.htm.) Even SAWS' own Citizen's Advisory Group expressed reservations about the contract. Yet, SAWS proceeded and, in so doing, violated the cultural understanding of water as public property on a regional level.

## PUBLIC PROPERTY AND THE EDWARDS AQUIFER AUTHORITY

In creating the EAA in 1993, the Texas legislature took a step toward creating public property groundwater rights, but it has yet to create a statewide body with power to mediate conflicts over private water-property rights and regulate groundwater as public property. Darcy Frownfelter (2001:5), general counsel for the EAA, notes that "no remedies exist to control the allocation of groundwater under the Rule of Capture during times of shortage." Common law groundwater use must be interpreted by the courts, which are not an effective mechanism for "groundwater management issues and administration of rights" (Frownfelter 2001:3).

Faced with the limitations of judicial interpretations of existing Texas groundwater law and an increasing demand for groundwater management, the Texas Legislature established the first of many groundwater conservation districts in 1949 in order to develop and implement comprehensive management plans. When it created the Edwards Aquifer Authority in 1993 as a groundwater conservation district, it gave the EAA significantly more regulatory powers and responsibilities concerning pumping than granted to other districts.

The EAA also has important responsibilities in the areas of conservation, water quality protection, and recharging. In other words, the EAA is obligated to develop a comprehensive integrative plan for groundwater management in the eight-county region. This means that groundwater no longer is simply subject to straightforward private-property regulation. It is embedded in the integrative processes of public resource policies that characterize a notion of public property.

## HEALTH, WATER, AND THE ECONOMY

We have argued that the discourse dominating groundwater management in Texas is cast in terms of private property. Similarly, health is seen primarily as an individual responsibility and less as a public concern (Donahue and McGuire 1995). This may help explain why health issues seem to be missing from the debate over management of the Edwards Aquifer. Nevertheless, the connection between health and water, if not explicit, is a subtext of the continuing debate over the management of the Edwards Aquifer. If public health is not a dominant theme in the discourse on groundwater management, it may be because San Antonio itself is part of a global economy in which environmental and public health concerns often take a back seat to short-term economic interests.

Health issues are present, however, and can be found in three areas that continue to be bones of contention. They are aquifer pollution hazards, the quality of additional surface water sources, and ecosystem health.

For three hundred years, the Edwards Aquifer has provided San Antonio and the region with safe, easily accessible drinking water from naturally flowing springs. In the post–World War II period, housing and population growth in San Antonio spread northward into the picturesque Hill Country over the recharge zone of the aquifer. Several citizen-organized attempts were made in the 1970s to control real estate development for fear that the aquifer would be polluted. These were unsuccessful, and building continued (Donahue 1998; Plotkin 1987). By the 1990s the threat of pollution and its impact on public health increased, and the city council passed zoning ordinances to protect the aquifer from runoff from parking lots and chemical-laden lawns. The ordinance allowed a three-month window for grandfathering. In that time, much of the remaining prime real estate was platted, thus avoiding the restrictions.

In the late 1990s the water quality issue became submerged in the debate over water quantity when San Antonio was faced with pumping restrictions, legislatively imposed in 1993 (Donahue and Sanders 2001:195). The pollution/health issue surfaced again in 2001 when the Professional Golf Association (PGA), in collaboration with Lumberman's Investment Corporation, proposed to build golf courses, hotels, and residences on a site over the recharge zone in north-central Bexar County. Several community groups opposed the plan, which had the support of the mayor and the majority of the city council. Opponents to the PGA resort argued that the economic benefits of tourism paled before the potential for pollution of the aquifer and the consequent health risks to users.

In May 2004 the PGA withdrew from a partnership with Lumberman's Investment Corporation. The reasons for the PGA withdrawal may have been primarily economic, but continuing citizen protests seem to have played a significant role. Pollution threats, however, may even increase now because Lumberman's Investment Corporation plans to develop, instead of a golf course, an even denser residential-housing project over the recharge zone.

Ironically, initiatives to protect the aquifer's water quality have come from citizens groups and not city leaders. It would be unfair to conclude that city staff and council were unsympathetic to the dangers of pollution. Yet their concern with economic growth led them to favor developers in the negotiations. As a result, public health concerns were subordinated to private interests in the name of a perceived economic good. The quality of the municipal water supply will become more of an issue when San Antonians begin to drink surface water.

The second health concern relates to the quality of surface drinking water. Faced with pumping limitations, SAWS is proposing to enter into contracts to pump water from the lower Colorado River and the lower Guadalupe River back to San Antonio. In addition to the costs of pipeline construction over 130 to 180 miles, the energy costs of running the pumps will be significant. The health concerns are even more serious. Current plans to pump water from adjacent river basins to San Antonio raise two health-related issues. Water from the lower Colorado and Guadalupe receives the effluent from petrochemical plants, and to make that water potable will be expensive. Furthermore, it is not clear whether all the toxins can be removed.

The problem of water quality leads to a third issue: the understanding of health in a broader sense than that of human health. Ecosystem health is necessary for all species to survive, including humans. Removing significant amounts of water from the rivers before they empty into the Gulf of Mexico will jeopardize ecosystem health. Estuaries and fisheries will be adversely affected when the mix of freshwater and saltwater is upset. Because SAWS' surface water plans are not yet widely known, there has been little public reaction to the health implications of the two projects.

## CONCLUSION

In modern, stratified, bureaucratically organized societies, it is difficult to speak of a commons in the traditional anthropological sense in which people share accepted rules of resource use and enforcement. In more complex and impersonal societies the commons could morph into public property, provided that the rules are democratically crafted and clearly stated, and that accountability is ensured at least through representative elections and consensual enforcement procedures.

Any water management process breaks down when water is defined more in political than hydrological terms and communities are set against one another in competition for an increasingly scarce resource. Based solely upon a cultural understanding of water resources as commodities, the alternative to commons management is for water to be privately owned, and traded in the marketplace. We argue here for a middle path between commons and private property. People depending on the Edwards Aquifer would benefit more from planning based on the cultural construction of the aquifer as public property. Conflicts would be mediated on the basis of an elected authority, which, as a boundary object, would still recognize individual water rights, not at the expense of the public access, but in support of the public good.

The public good was at the heart of health advances in the industrial world of Europe and the United States in the nineteenth and early twentieth centuries. Those efforts seemed to have been directed at safeguarding the health of the labor force, especially in the close conditions of factory and urban life. Municipal water and sewage systems were essential to the control of infectious diseases. Decisions to extend these water and waste disposal services were part of a political economy of health that was more in the redistributive than profit-making or capitalist mode. The reverse is true today.

If a commons approach to resource management is no longer viable in our modern world, the record of privatization in health care and water management is, at best, ambiguous. We conclude that a broad partnership of professionals, elected officials, and citizens, in planning and development, will lead to success in the management of our water resources. The government's role is most effective when greater responsibility is given to elected bodies that share common hydrological boundaries. Within these boundaries, changing public and private water interests can be mediated to best sustain the commonly shared resource for the health and well-being of regional ecosystems and their diverse populations. To regard an ecosystem as public property is to take the broadest and most inclusive perspective on health. This necessary step reaffirms the symbiotic relationship of all species that inhabit and share an ecosystem, which, in the last analysis, is the prime boundary object.

This last boundary object—the watershed or whole ecosystem—will bring us closest to an answer to the question, whose water is it anyway? Lyle Lovett sings the traditional "Texas River Song," which moves from the Pecos and the Nueces in the west all the way to the Trinity and the Neches in the east, showing that "there's many a river that waters the land" (Lovett 1998). Aldo Leopold, however, gives depth to these Texas rivers in his "Song of the Gavilán," about a small Mexican river just south of the American border. He writes, "The song of a river ordinarily means the tune that waters play on rock, root, and rapid" (Leopold 1949:149). And he adds, "This song of the waters is audible to every ear, but there is other music in these hills, by no means audible to all. To hear even a few notes of it you must first live here for a long time, and you must know the speech of hills and rivers. Then on a still night,...sit quietly and...think hard of everything you have seen and tried to understand. Then you may hear it—a vast and pulsing harmony—its score inscribed on a thousand hills, its notes the lives and deaths of plants and animals, its rhythms spanning the seconds and the centuries" (Leopold 1949:149). The water that resounds in Leopold's river song is the water of the whole ecosystem—from the moisture in the air to the dark depths of a silent aquifer. To hear the song of a river means to listen to raindrops falling on the surface water, but also to hear the soil absorbing the water and to know its slow percolating ways. Only when a "Texas Aquifer Song" echoes within the "Texas River Song" will we begin to learn the answer to "whose water is it anyway?"

The Lyle Lovett of the twenty-first century might already be singing a "Texas Aquifer Song." For most of us, it is still hard to hear. But, on a still night, when our sprinklers are no longer wasting the Edwards waters on St. Augustine grass, we might distinguish some faint notes from the deep distance, rhythms reflecting underground waters spanning seconds and centuries.

**Notes**

1. This chapter is part of an ongoing collaborative research project on water management. Klaver's work focuses on the cultural and political aspects of natural

resources, specifically, of water. Based on research in her native Holland, she provides a comparative perspective on public policy in natural resource management in Europe and the United States. Donahue has carried out field research in groundwater management policies on the Edwards Aquifer in south-central Texas. His research has included content analysis of official documentation and extensive interviews of the parties involved in the twice-defeated surface water project near San Antonio, as well as the subsequent successful mediation effort to craft a water policy for the City of San Antonio.

2. For an excellent account of water wars in the West, see Reisner 1986.

3. Both figures are from Donahue 1998 and are used with permission of the *San Antonio Express-News*.

4. An acre-foot of water is the amount of water than can stand in 1 acre of land at a depth of 1 foot. One acre-foot is equal to 325,851 gallons and can supply a family of five for a year. In 1993 The University of Texas Bureau of Economic Geology calculated that the aquifer holds up to 215 million acre-feet of water, four times that estimated in 1978 (*San Antonio Express-News*, October 13, 1993; July 22, 1994). Glennon (2002:91) estimates the capacity to be more than 250 million acre-feet. It should be noted, however, that much of that water is inaccessible for human use.

5. Total aquifer discharge includes pumping, but also spring flows. On the average, spring flows, primarily in Comal and Hays Counties, account for 54 percent of total aquifer withdrawal.

6. The legislature left the Authority some discretion to raise these caps if water savings accrued through conservation or other such optimizing measures.

7. For a discussion of the plan, see www.edwardsaquifer.org.

8. See http://texaswater.tamu.edu/texaswaterlaw.htm#surface, "Texas Water: Water Resources Education," Texas A&M University.

9. Among the stated criteria for effective water policy was one that would "respect, protect and support the natural biodiversity of the region by providing a sufficient volume of water to all ecosystems of the region so they can function properly" (Mayor's Citizens Committee on Water Policy 1997:7).

# Section II
# Water Management and Health

# Introduction

## Linda Whiteford and Scott Whiteford

Section II directs the reader's attention from health and disease as related to quantity and quality of water, to issues of water management that include, as Johnston posits, the creation of water scarcity. In chapter 7, which opens Section II, Johnston presents the concept of "manufactured scarcity" and how water—and public opinion about it—is manipulated to support local, regional, national, and global transformations. The multiple meanings and human experience of water scarcity and the values that shape how people view scarcity and formulate policy to address it are the focus of this chapter. The growing power of transnational corporations promotes the globalization of water, in part, by imposing a scarcity framework that employs marketplace language and analytical tools to evaluate problems and generate solutions. Local communities are losing control over their water resources as global corporations take over the supply and delivery of water. When corporate executives and commodity markets, instead of communities and watersheds, determine the value and disposition of this critical resource, profits become more important than social welfare or environmental quality. The distance grows between those who make decisions about water and the users who face the consequences of shortsighted or poorly made policy, and users are often unable to reach across that expanding gap to moderate or reverse harmful policies. Crises in water quality result all too often, severely affecting the health and well-being of hundreds of millions of people. Arsenic, perchlorate, chromium, and other byproducts of military or industrial waste have poisoned the water supplies of people around the world. In South Africa, the privatization of water ownership has led to cholera epidemics and further undermined the health of people living with HIV. Sadly, the all too apparent devastation caused by the globalization and commodification of water has not led to a reconsideration of this model of water management.

While water resource management, health, and globalization are the dominant themes of this volume, the social structuring of water management and access is the underlying leitmotif. Health disparities reflect the same, or similar, political and social processes that create scarcities, be they of water or access to health care. Johnston describes the cultural process of manufacturing water scarcity, and we have already seen the health consequences of unequal water allocation in Section I. We have also seen in Section I how the social construction of gender and power disproportionately privileges some over others. To use Farmer's term, "structural violence" results when groups are marginalized to the point that essential resources are beyond their reach.

In chapter 8, Greaves discusses a range of alternatives for resolving conflicts over water, drawn from indigenous people living on reservations in Canada and the United States. To what degree has globalization affected native peoples' water disputes, and in what ways? Water and the resources it can produce are critical to indigenous people, and they are no longer as isolated from the world beyond their reserves as in the past. The globalization of water endangers the precarious economic and political autonomy these groups have enjoyed, yet it also enables some nations to exploit the water they control to the benefit of their people.

Chapters 9, 10, and 11, by Guillet, Derman, and S. Whiteford and Cortez-Lara, respectively, turn the reader's attention to water policy reforms, demand management, and the critical role played by local communities, as well as local beliefs and practices. Their cases, from

# INTRODUCTION

Zimbabwe, Spain, and the United States/Mexico border, reflect various levels of integration with the global economy. Guillet's extensive historical analysis of his Spanish case provides an unusual depth of frame and emphasizes one type of contribution anthropological analysis can make. In chapter 9, he raises new questions surrounding the effect of water management reforms on the linkage between water for irrigation and water for health. Guillet examines potential effects of demand management on access to water in farmer-managed irrigation systems. In these irrigation systems, water often has other uses, for drinking, cleaning, personal hygiene, construction, fire fighting, and the feeding of animals. Equally important, access to water for irrigation bears directly on the health of small-scale irrigators. Water is essential to the production of food for both subsistence and trade. The response of small-scale farmers in Spain to the effects of water management reforms suggests new modes of resistance: viable interest groups created "where civil society has been restructured to facilitate stakeholder participation in the elaboration and implementation of water management policy."

Each chapter in the book pushes the conceptual envelope by asking the reader to consider, in a new light, the age-old topics of water and health—by interrelating them in the amorphous and fluid reality of globalization and then by applying domain-specific concepts to generalizable processes. Derman, in chapter 10 on water reforms in Zimbabwe, employs an analysis of the discourses being used to shape water reform policies and, in so doing, shows how discourses embed often contradictory levels of scale. He writes about Southern African nations' experimental reforms of land and water resources that combine local and international initiatives. He examines the different international and national policies and programs on the global menu of water reform and proposes that there are multiple perspectives on water policy that can and are being adjusted to Southern African contexts. Derman explores these different frameworks and uses the case of Zimbabwe as an example of how one country is attempting to accommodate the specific contexts of its national setting. He notes that when many Southern African states cry that no one is listening to them, they are referring to national-level laws and policy; ironically, they are similarly deaf to the voices of local users and customary practices. In

Zimbabwe, as elsewhere, the interconnections among water for health, the environment, irrigation, and domestic use do not shape conceptual understandings of the issues or, needless to say, bureaucratic policies. This failure means that water reforms do not resolve the problems they are promulgated to address. The ongoing crisis then hampers efforts to formulate long-term policies adequate to the scope of the problems and their resolution.

In chapter 11, S. Whiteford and Cortez-Lara take dead-on aim at how global economic agreements, in conjunction with what they term the Mexican government's "structural myopia," further the structural violence against the most marginalized population of society, the poor. Overuse and contamination of groundwater threatens this precious resource all over the world. In some cases, the contamination results from the leaching of natural substances such as arsenic or salt from the soil. In others, human activities produce industrial and animal wastes that pollute aquifers. Industrial agriculture and excessive pesticide use are manufactured risks that severely affect water security. The combination of local conditions and the globalization of agriculture can generate a contrived scarcity of water and heighten the manufactured risks. The structural myopia of the Mexican state led it to neglect of the problems of contaminated water and the burden it placed on poor people. This same shortsightedness encourages the privatization of water, including the sale of bottled waters, despite its obvious negative impact on those who cannot afford to buy this essential substance. Drawing on long-term collaborative research on the United States/Mexico border, S. Whiteford and Cortez-Lara integrate a political ecology perspective with questions of health.

The authors lay out for the reader the multiple, overlapping and separate, domains of water. It is no wonder that chasms separate the various groups of specialists, each committed to its particular domain of water. Yet, each and all of the domains are connected to health. Each and all are shaped by culturally constructed and maintained constraints, policies, practices, and histories. And each and all privilege some over others. Our attempt here is simply to make some of those connections visible and to apply analytic and descriptive contributions from the field of anthropology to help unravel these complexities.

# 7

# The Commodification of Water and the Human Dimensions of Manufactured Scarcity

Barbara Rose Johnston

In communities around the world, large corporate entities are taking over municipal and regional water-supply systems, and water resource development projects are being financed and built as private, instead of public, ventures. As the management of water supply and delivery systems moves from the community and its watershed to the corporate boardroom and its commodity markets, the prioritization of profit often trumps social welfare and environmental quality concerns. This chapter explores the varied meanings and experience of water scarcity, examines the values that shape perceptions of scarcity and related policy agendas, and describes the human dimensions of the commodification of water.[1]

The conceptual framework for this chapter was initially developed to analyze the results of archival and ethnographic field research in St. Thomas, United States Virgin Islands. Changes in rainfall, stream flow, land use, and vegetative cover over a three-hundred-year period were examined in an effort to assess the human origins of localized "drought." Subsequent fieldwork explored the historical, social, and cultural contexts and actions leading to the contamination of the island's main aquifer, demonstrating relationships between a history of slavery and racism and current inequity, poverty, and disenfranchisement in the face of a growing tourism market, as well as environmental alienation (methods and findings described in Johnston 1998). This concern with the manufacturing of critical resource scarcity and its human consequences is explored in case-specific detail in St. Thomas. Island residents experience health problems and increased cancer risks as a result of their exposure to hazardous chemicals contained in groundwater. This concern similarly structures my efforts to assess community history, conditions, and response to the consequential damages of development, militarism, and globalization-induced human rights abuse and related environmental degradation (see methods and findings emerging from global research on human rights and the environment described in Johnston 1994, 1997).

Analytical insights into the conceptual models shaping water scarcity analysis and related political economic agendas were derived from a review of current reports and policy statements developed in support of the Third World Water Forum meetings in Kyoto, Japan (March 2003); a review of reports and briefing papers developed in support of the World Commission on Dams (WCD) investigation and November 2001 Final Report; interviews in 2000–2001 with colleagues who prepared WCD briefing papers and assisted my own efforts to develop a briefing on "Reparations and the Right to Remedy" for the WCD; interviews with environmental and human rights advocacy partners (2002–2004); and interviews with consultants and project officers involved in the financing and development of large dams and water diversion projects (1996–2003). Research conducted specifically for this chapter (2002–2004) included interviews with consultants and project officers working on water management and development schemes in Bangladesh, India, Cambodia, Southern Africa, Chile, Guatemala, Canada, and the United States.

The case-specific examples described in this chapter were developed from the interviews mentioned above; a review and an analysis of case studies prepared by other colleagues, with follow-up interviews to clarify and confirm my reading of their work; a web-based review of recently published reports, news accounts, and journal articles; and follow-up research on current issues and conditions described in my previously published case studies and conceptual briefing papers

(Johnston 1994, 1997, 1998, 2001, 2003a, 2003b). In a number of cases, illustrative examples were developed from participant observation, interviews, and related document research on water crises occurring in my hometown and northern California communities (Felton, Silicon Valley, Klamath River), previous homes and adjacent communities (St. Thomas USVI and Puerto Rico), and the communities where I have conducted recent field research (the Marshall Islands and Guatemala).

## WATER SCARCITY

Water scarcity in popular terms suggests a state of immediate or impending crisis resulting from an inadequate supply of water to meet the varied demands of humans and their environment. Scarcity is relative. Freshwater supply is affected by changes in the hydrologic cycle: the amount of water entering the system; the volume of water captured and stored in surface and subsurface reservoirs; the amount of water that runs off land, enters rivers and streams, and is eventually lost to the oceans; and the amount of water held by vegetation and released into the atmosphere through evapotranspiration. Scarce supplies of freshwater are also a consequence of human activity. Some 69 percent of the world's freshwater budget is used for irrigated agriculture, which, in turn, is responsible for 70 percent of the world's water pollution (United Nations Wateryear 2003). Freshwater may be in abundance, but safe drinking water may be scarce as a result of biological and chemical contamination from agriculture, industry, and urban life.

Water demand is also a relative construct. Demand may simply reflect numbers—growing populations require greater amounts of water to meet basic human and household needs. Even in the case of increased population, however, changes in water use behavior and technology can decrease total water consumption. Perception of water scarcity due to inadequate supplies of irrigation water, for example, may dissipate when water demands are reduced with a change in the type of crops grown and the kinds of technology employed.

Water scarcity reflects not only the relative aspects of supply (the conditions and actions that affect quantity and quality) and demand (intended and projected use), but also the relative aspects of how water is valued (the cultural meanings and economic values), the relative levels of access and patterns of use, and the relative degrees of control over water resource management and distribution. Thus, scarcity might reflect the economic ability to pay for water, or the customs, social conditions, and relationships that privilege access to some while withholding access from others (Johnston 1994, 1997; Donahue and Johnston, eds., 1998).

Water scarcity may be a relative construct influenced by biophysical conditions and processes, as well as human actions and relationships, but it is also a life-threatening reality for hundreds of millions of people. Today, some 2.3 billion people suffer from diseases linked to contaminated water. Currently, water-related disease kills more than 5 million each year—ten times the number killed in wars. Assuming present trends, by 2025 some two-thirds of the world's population will face water shortages or almost no water at all. For those who have water, life will be complicated by problems with quality and reliable access (Gleick et al. 2002; United Nations Wateryear 2003; United Nations WWDR 2003). Varied causes and human consequences of water scarcity are briefly illustrated in the examples below.

## HUMAN DIMENSIONS OF WATER SCARCITY

In the Bolivian Andes, global climatic change is reflected in increased temperatures and changing rain and snowfall patterns, contributing to a 60-percent decline in glaciers and snowcaps since 1978. Decreased snowfall and glacier melt reduce reservoir levels and therefore the freshwater supply needed to sustain area agriculture and industry and to fulfill urban population needs (Forero 2002). Global warming—along with deforestation of mountain woodlands, mining, agriculture, and urban sprawl in mountain watersheds—threatens water supplies for more than half the world's people (Iyngararasan, Tianchi, and Shrestha 2002).

For the nearly thirty thousand islands in the Pacific Ocean, freshwater resources are threatened by rising temperatures in the Arctic and Antarctic, where melting polar ice caps contribute to higher sea levels. Island water resources are contaminated by saltwater infiltration of the subsurface aquifers. For low-lying atolls, rising sea levels will eventually submerge islands, even nations (Burns 2002).

While global warming and related climatic changes threaten mountain and coastal freshwater resources, economic development has, by far, the greatest impact on quality and quantity of water. Over the past fifty years, economic development and urban growth have consumed one half of the world's wetlands and have severely polluted close to half the world's lakes. In China, for example, some one hundred lakes are so polluted that 70 percent of the fluid content is untreated municipal and industrial waste (United Nations Wateryear 2003).

Economic development has also increased the short-term availability of freshwater by increasing storage capacity. Some forty-five thousand large dams have been built since World War II to capture water that would otherwise flow to the sea. The dams generate hydroelectricity, irrigate agricultural crops, and regulate river flow. Collectively, dam reservoirs cover an area of land the size of California. The overall contributions of large dam development, however, are offset by many problems, including the limited life of dams, due to sediment buildup in reservoirs, and the extreme social hardships and ecological consequences of dam development. Studies conducted for the WCD found that some 5 percent of the world's freshwater is lost by evaporation from reservoirs and that reservoirs emit an estimated 1 to 28 percent of global greenhouse gases (approximately 4 percent of $CO_2$ and one-fifth of total human-related methane emissions).

One major goal of large dam construction has been to provide a water supply to support the introduction and expansion of irrigated agriculture. Performance reviews of fifty-two irrigation dams conducted by the WCD, however, found significant failures to meet irrigation targets; salinization or water logging had occurred in some 20 percent of irrigated fields. The overall contribution of irrigation water to global food supplies is an estimated 12 to 16 percent of production, far short of the one-third figure cited by the water resources industry. Dams flood some of the most productive agricultural land in the world. Dams and water diversions constitute the primary cause of endangerment or extinction of one third of the world's freshwater fish. Dam development has contributed to the loss of livelihood and of a sustainable way of life for an estimated forty to eighty million people. Millions more living downstream suffer from dam-related changes, including loss of natural resources and increased incidence of disease. Indigenous people and women have disproportionately suffered from dam construction while being excluded from the benefits (WCD 2000; Imhof, Wong, and Bosshard 2002; McCully 2001).

Efforts to develop a public health infrastructure by improving public drinking-water supplies have also had unforeseen consequences. Water sanitation programs initiated in the 1970s and 1980s by the Bangladesh government—with development funding, project design, and technical support from the United Nations and various aid groups—encouraged the abandonment of surface water sources in an effort to reduce the public health consequences of exposure to biological contaminants. Millions of rural residents participated in public education campaigns. Surface water sources were forsaken as tens of thousands of tube wells were installed and the tap was turned on in villages across the nation. Before this intervention, diarrheal disease was responsible for the death of some quarter of a million children each year. With reduced exposure to biological contaminants, public health initially improved (Pearce 2001). But other health problems began to emerge.

In the mid-1990s the presence of arsenic, a naturally occurring mineral in Bangladesh's subsurface aquifer, was disclosed. No one had tested the subsurface aquifer for chemical or mineral contaminants. Arsenic is deadly at high doses. Over time, low doses through continued exposure produce health effects that include debilitating pain in muscles and joints, lethargy, skin sores and rashes, and, eventually, cancers of the liver, lung, bladder, or kidney. In 1998, World Bank funds provided $32.4 million for an arsenic mitigation project. As of 2003 most of the nation's estimated eleven million wells have yet to be tested, and many are unaware of the presence or danger of arsenic in their water. Safe alternative sources have yet to be introduced in a large-scale, effective way. According to World Health Organization estimates, some thirty-five to seventy million people in Bangladesh are victims of the largest mass poisoning in history, and their consumption of arsenic-contaminated water places them at high risk for skin lesions, internal cancers, and other fatal diseases (Bearak 2002; Stephenson 2002).

Industrial development over the past fifty years has consumed increasing amounts of water, generated hazardous wastes that pollute rivers and lakes, and introduced toxic chemical and mineral contaminants into groundwater supplies. By 2025 an estimated 24 percent of all freshwater in the world will be used to support industrial processes. More than 80 percent of the world's hazardous waste is produced in the United States and other industrialized countries. In developing countries, 70 percent of all industrial waste is dumped untreated into water where it pollutes the useable water supply (United Nations Wateryear 2003). High-tech industry is perhaps the most water-dependent and water-damaging sector of industry in the world.

In Silicon Valley, for example, electronics companies consumed 24 percent of Santa Clara's city water (1994–1995) and produced 65 percent of the wastewater discharged. A 1997 study found that each 6-inch silicon wafer chip requires 2,275 gallons of deionized water, 20 pounds of chemicals, and 22 cubic feet of gases (The Electronics Industry Good Neighbor Campaign 1997). Arsenic, trichloroethylene, and one thousand or more chemicals are used to manufacture silicon chips. Trichloroethylene, for example, is a known carcinogen and a suspected cardiovascular or blood toxicant, developmental toxicant, gastrointestinal or liver toxicant, kidney toxicant, neurotoxicant, reproductive toxicant, respiratory toxicant, and skin or sensory organ toxicant (Environmental Defense Fund 2003). Thanks to a history of using underground storage tanks and solvents so powerful that they leach, leak, or slip through the molecules of storage containers, these chemicals have found their way into the valley's water table. Health consequences include a documented pattern of miscarriage, birth defects, increased cancers, and a host of debilitating disorders (argued in Silicon Valley Toxics Coalition 2004; outlined in EPA 2004, http://www.epa.gov/safewater/mcl.html; documented in, for example, Chang et al. 2003 and Lee et al. 2003).

Silicon Valley groundwater contamination and related health consequences were first publicly reported in 1982, when the Fairchild Semiconductor facility in San Jose was charged with leaking underground tanks and resulting trichloroethane contamination of groundwater supplies. Residents sued Fairchild Corporation, and the resulting lawsuit stimulated epidemiological, environmental geology, and toxicology studies. The California Department of State found three times the expected number of birth defects in the neighborhood near the plant. The Regional Water Quality Control Board found 85 percent of the underground tanks in Silicon Valley to be leaking. In 1983 the

County of Santa Clara developed the first Hazardous Materials Storage Ordinance in the United States, regulating underground storage tanks and enacting public-right-to-know legislation. A statewide initiative was passed in 1984, based on the county ordinance, and similar federal legislation was adopted in 1986 (Johnston 1994:231–232).

Lawsuits, the eventual plant closure of the responsible party, and increased regulations concerning the use of solvents and other hazardous chemicals and underground facilities have resulted in profound changes in the way high-tech businesses are run. When Fairchild closed its plant, other high-tech companies took notice: improved environmental protection meant greater costs. Companies began to move the dirtier aspects of manufacturing to more hospitable political settings. The groundwater problems originally concentrated in Silicon Valley are now emerging in the many manufacturing sites of a globalized industry.

The problems of high tech–generated groundwater pollution and related environmental health risks are not restricted to the manufacturing process. As of 2004 almost all components of the desktop personal computer, including microprocessor and software, are manufactured in places such as China and shipped back to the United States for final processing and sale. Rapid improvements in the technology produce a limited life for computers and products containing computer components. Many functional products are discarded as "out-of-date" electronic waste. An estimated 50 to 80 percent of electronic waste collected in the western United States is shipped to scrap brokers in developing countries, with the largest portion going back to China. Labeling this waste "recyclable materials" legally allows the United States to transport and dump hazardous materials that otherwise would be prohibited by the restrictions of the Basel Convention.

Recycling electronic waste is a messy and dangerous business, with by-products including heavy metals, radioactive elements, and a wide variety of toxic chemicals. For example, in Guiyu, China, a town located on the banks of the Lianjiang River that hosts a large electronics waste scrap industry, samples from the public water supply showed levels of lead to be 190 times higher than World Health Organization drinking-water thresholds, and river sediment samples demonstrated high rates of lead, zinc, and chromium. Residents in Guiyu increasingly rely on water trucked in from a town 30 miles away (Schoenberger 2002 and Puckett et al. 2002).

Toxic contaminant threats to freshwater resources also occur as a result of militarism. In Kwajalein, Marshall Islands, perchlorate contaminates the water supply after forty years of United States missile defense testing. Perchlorate is a component of rocket fuel, and solid propellant debris is deposited near launch sites, even more in failed launch attempts. Marine habitat, including reef fish on which the local population relies, is also contaminated (Yokwe Online 2002). Perchlorate is a known carcinogen. It disrupts the thyroid gland and inhibits hormone function. Perchlorate impairs neurological development in fetuses and small children. It is estimated that the drinking water for millions of United States residents has been contaminated by perchlorate. Perchlorate contamination has also entered the food chain, with recent studies demonstrating uptake and bioaccumulation in lettuce and other crops grown with irrigation water tainted by military base pollutants and in milk from dairy cows (Environmental Working Group 2002, 2004).

The presence of toxic chemicals and heavy metals in groundwater supplies has been documented at military sites around the world. For example, at the Massachusetts Military Reservation on Cape Cod, the drinking water supply for five hundred thousand people has been contaminated with chemicals and heavy metals leaching from exploded and stored munitions. On the island of Vieques, Puerto Rico, where the United States Navy uses three-quarters of the island as a military base and bombing range, heavy metals and other munitions toxins were first noted in civilian drinking-water supplies in the late 1970s. By 2000, medical surveys demonstrated the presence of mercury in the hair and fingernails of 45 percent of the survey population. Epidemiological studies examining childhood cancer rates (1985–1989) found that Vieques children age 0–9 were 117 percent more likely to contract cancer than children of the same age living on the island of Puerto Rico (Military Toxics Project 2002).

## CULTURE AND POWER DIMENSIONS OF SCARCITY

This chapter explores some of the anthropogenic factors that negatively affect water quantity and quality. It is important to recognize that resource scarcity and systemic response also reflect societal values, economic behavior, and power relationships. The perception of scarcity emerges when ecosystemic factors and processes fail to produce customary supplies, when human actions and activities influence supply and/or increase demand, when changes in power and economy affect access, and when valued human uses conflict with valued ecosystemic needs. At times, the scarcity is created as a by-product of resource decision making that prioritizes one use over another. At other times, the perception of scarcity is manufactured to fuel and further various political agendas.

These points are clearly illustrated in the events and water governance decisions leading up to the September 2002 salmon kill on the Klamath River in northern California. Klamath River Basin water-management priorities established during President Clinton's administration, first, met endangered species needs, second, met treaty-based obligations to Native American tribes, and, third, met farmers' irrigation needs. These priorities were reversed in 2001 when the Bush administration responded to public protests and the lobbying efforts of farm and property rights groups by establishing governance priorities that ignored the Endangered Species and Clean Water Acts, ignored legal obligations to tribes, and diverted Klamath River water to provide temporary drought-relief water for farmers.

This prioritization was institutionalized in 2002 as part of a new Bureau of Land Management ten-year plan, with water for fish, tribes, and wildlife refuges diverted to allow full flow to farmers in the Klamath Basin. In mid-September 2002 the salmon run hit low, warm, deoxygenated water, and some 33,000 fish died—25 percent of the total run, an estimated one half of spawning fish, and the largest die-off of adult salmon ever recorded. The loss threatens the future viability of salmon on the river, the socioeconomic health of coastal fishing communities, and the health and sociocultural integrity of Klamath River area tribes (Williams 2003; California Department of Fish and Game 2002).

Conflict over Klamath River water use and the biodegenerative effects of policy change suggests some of the problems associated with development and management of complex watershed systems, especially when development involves transformations in the loci of power

## THE COMMODIFICATION OF WATER

over resource value, access, use, and control, from resident peoples to external power structures. In the face of greater competition for scarce resources, user group access to water reflects relative priorities and power in distant political realms. In this case, a federal administration that valued the contribution of economic commodities to the national economy over environmental and cultural rights and needs abruptly disenfranchised stakeholders whose former access reflected years of hard-won political struggle.

The Klamath River Basin is an example of conflict and consequences of ecopolitics in publicly controlled water-management systems where economic values are prioritized over all other concerns. Increasingly, the management of water resource systems involves private, not public, structures that prioritize economic performance over ecosystemic and sociocultural values and, in doing so, transform the social meaning of water, from an essential element and commons resource to a privately owned commodity. When water is commodified, its meaning and the prioritization of use values shift from household subsistence and regional markets to the national and global economic arena. Accompanying this centralization of authority and capital is a widening gap between those who decide water resource development, management, and distribution and those who experience the consequences of the former's decisions. Disenfranchisement—when a community or stakeholder is alienated from meaningful access, use, and control over its environment—is often the end result. This environmental alienation generates and shapes local conflicts and crises (Johnston 1998; Klare 2003).

In Felton, California, for example, 1,350 householders received news in October 2002 that California-American Water Company, which had purchased the Felton water district from Citizens Utilities in late 1999, was actually owned by the German transnational RWE Aktiengesellschaft. News of the ownership change in Felton accompanied notice of a proposed three-year rate increase totaling 71 percent. The community discovered that environmental alienation occurs not only in distant third-world communities but also, with the expansion of transnational utility companies and protective trade agreements, in hometown America. Proposed rate increases for Felton users would support regionwide costs, including the costs of building a desalinization plan to serve customers in the Carmel River Valley, some 65 miles south of Felton.

Hundreds of residents attended a town hall meeting and organized a grassroots effort to protest the rate increase in ways that might return control of the utility to community hands. In researching the ownership change, residents learned that RWE had originally owned coal power plants in the late 1800s, had built the German power grid across Europe during World War II, had expanded into a wide array of waste management enterprises (including NUKEM Nuclear Ltd., a company that has been cited for dumping nuclear waste in the North Sea), and is the fourth largest private water utility in the world. RWE's purchase of the London-based Thames Water Company, and that company's subsequent acquisition in late 2002 of the American Water Company, has made it the largest investor-owned water utility company in the United States, the fourth largest water utility company in the world.

Felton community protests resulted in the scheduling of community-based hearings hosted by the California Public Utilities Commission. Comments focused on three main concerns: that the takeover of US community water utilities by a German-owned company constituted a homeland security issue; that management would prioritize shareholders' need for profit over the water district's social and ecological needs; and that Felton water—a relatively clean source of spring water in a state park–protected watershed—would be bottled and sold as "designer water" on market shelves, with rate payer profits used to subsidize a commercial enterprise while the local watershed would be drained dry.

In these hearings, California Public Utility Commissioners (PUC) acknowledged that they had no jurisdiction over the bottling and sale of water. Lacking the protection of state regulations restricting the export of water and recognizing that foreign-owned companies are protected by international trade agreements that view water as a commodity, Felton residents requested the Santa Cruz County Board of Supervisors and the neighboring San Lorenzo Valley Water District to initiate an eminent domain case with the hope of regaining public control over the utility (Chesky 2003; Johnston 2003a). The PUC approved the rate increase in May 2004 but delayed implementation while residents attempted to pass a bond initiative to finance studies that would support condemnation proceedings.

## The Commodification of Water

Similar efforts to regain local control over water distribution and supply systems now owned by transnational corporations are occurring across the United States (American Water Company assets included water districts in some thirteen hundred US communities). Long-term success in reclaiming local public control over water resources is significantly inhibited, however, by the immense pressures on local governments to privatize their public utilities. As the delivery systems age and become susceptible to biological and chemical waste contamination, many US water supply and delivery systems are struggling with the expensive problems of increased demand due to population growth and the rising costs of providing a healthy water supply (see Tsybine 2001).

Traditionally, the federal government has played a supportive role in helping local communities develop and improve water supply and delivery systems. The Water Investment Act of 2002 passed by the US Congress, however, limits federal funding for water-system improvement projects to those jurisdictions that consider selling their public utility to for-profit corporations (Miess 2002). Furthermore, the provisions of the North American Free Trade Act (NAFTA) and the General Agreement on Trade and Tariffs (GATT) established by the World Trade Organization identify water as a commodity and provide market protections for transnational investors, significantly inhibiting local and state efforts to enforce environmental protection and social welfare laws (Barlow 1999, 2001).

Not only does the privatization of water supply and distribution systems generate conflict over the loci of management control and the prioritization of management values, but also, when the public resource of water becomes a privately managed commodity, the increased costs required to recover full costs and generate profit can limit access, with very real health consequences.

One of the stronger examples illustrating this point comes from South Africa, where World Bank assistance in drafting government policy resulted in infrastructure development plans and policy emphasizing privatization as postapartheid policy. Implementation of this policy in communities lacking the means to pay resulted in reduced access to safe water and contributed to the spread of cholera.

In 1995 World Bank advisors encouraged the South African government to adopt a "full cost recovery" principle—requiring public services such as water, electricity, and telecommunications to generate sufficient income to cover the full cost of services and encouraging the transfer of public utilities to private corporations to ensure management that more effectively focuses on cost recovery. Eventually, the full cost recovery principle was included as a condition in loan and aid agreements between the South African Government and the World Bank, the International Monetary Fund, and US, British, German, and European Union donor agencies. In 1998 local councils began commercializing their waterworks by forcing consumers to pay the full cost of drinking water. Many families paid up to 40 percent of their monthly income to keep the water taps flowing (ICIJ 2003).

Over the next few years, an estimated ten million South African households had their water cut off, and more than two million South Africans were evicted from their homes—because they could not pay their water bill (*afrol News* 2002). Unable to afford tap water, many South Africans met daily household needs by taking water from streams, ponds, and lakes polluted with manure and human waste. Use of biologically contaminated sources led to an increase of waterborne disease. Cholera appeared on South Africa's Dolphin Coast in August 2000. According to some estimates, by January 2002 two hundred and fifty thousand people were infected, and close to three hundred died (ICIJ 2003). This cholera epidemic has been directly linked to the government's cost-recovery water policies, and the high mortality rates accompanying the outbreak have been ascribed to high levels of HIV/AIDS in the affected population. In addition to the AIDS patients who died while infected with cholera, many more people infected with HIV survived the initial cholera infection only to experience a rapid deterioration and the onset of full-blown AIDS. In these cases, subsequent death is ascribed to AIDS, but exposure to cholera triggered the immune system failure (Bond 2004; Cottle and Deedat 2003).

## MANUFACTURED SCARCITY

The perception of critical resource scarcity—current crisis or impending doom—can also be manufactured and exploited to meet various agendas. For example, in 1971, when the James Bay Hydroelectric Projects were first proposed as necessary to offset an impending energy crisis, critics questioned the assumption of scarcity in a

Canadian region with few energy demands. By the 1980s, Hydro-Quebec, the provincially owned utility that developed the series of dams on rivers feeding into James Bay, refined its notion of scarcity to reflect export market opportunities associated with current energy consumption and projected population growth in the northeast United States. Environmental activists responded by developing an effective education and conservation campaign dramatically reducing consumption in the proposed energy market. Nevertheless, the project proceeded with Canadian government approval and an infusion of investment from West Germany, where the development of cheap energy suggested a means to produce hydrogen efficiently for an emerging alternative transportation industry.

In 1990, plans were announced to build a $125 million joint-venture liquid hydrogen plant in Sept-Illes, funded by West German investors, with provincial government help (Picard 1990). Operating for a number of years, the Euro-Quebec joint venture supported two pilot projects that refined fuel and cooling capabilities to allow ocean transport and created a hydrogen export market between Canada and Germany. In 2003 Canada announced the launching of a new corporation, E-H2, to commercialize and extend technologies developed under the Euro-Quebec Hydro-Hydrogen Pilot Projects (Hydrogen and Fuel Cell Letter 2002). Energy scarcity was the original rationale supporting proposals for hydroelectric dams in the James Bay region. When the demand estimates were shown to be flawed, however, the project rationale was reformulated from a scarcity model that addresses an impending energy crisis to an investment model that supports innovative development and creates export market opportunity.

The issue of water scarcity received extensive media coverage in the months and weeks before the March 2003 Third World Water Forum meetings in Kyoto, Japan. The news summarized the findings from a series of reports published by the agencies of the United Nations, International Monetary Fund, World Bank, the water resource industry, and various water crisis commissions whose members come from these agencies and institutions. These reports depict the human consequences of water scarcity in its many forms, typically framing causality and solutions as matters of water governance. For example, the March 2003 UN World Water Development Report frames water crises as problems "of water governance, essentially caused by the ways in which we mismanage water" (Executive Summary, UN WWDR 2003:1) and encourages solutions that include social and environmental priorities, while prioritizing full cost recovery (27–28; see also World Bank 2004). Such language legitimizes the top-down, centralized, imposed, and privatized megaprojects that produce adverse social and ecological conditions and fail to deliver promised benefits (see WCD 2000; McCully 2001, 2002; Shiva 2002).

Few of the 2003 water assessment reports cite the World Commission on Dams in their framing of problems, nor the findings emerging from the WCD assessment of the projects represented by the water resources industry as sustainable solutions, WCD major findings, or WCD suggestions for remedy (see UN WWDR 2003). In fact, the exhaustive, transparent, equitable approach taken by the WCD to assess the efficacy and effect of large dams produced findings that, at some levels, contradict the definition of problem and sustainable solutions articulated in the 2003 water assessment reports. The WCD analysis led to recommendations encouraging small-scale, decentralized alternative solutions that involve the equitable participation of project-affected peoples. Also recommended was a ban on additional megaproject development until the obligations and problems remaining from previously built dams are addressed. The recommendations accompanying many of the 2003 water assessment reports called for massive investment of public funds to support large public/private venture investment projects.

In public/private partnerships, the public financier's primary obligation is to ensure the financial success of its investment. Protecting business interests increasingly means restricting public access to plans, development-monitoring data, and the day-to-day operations of the resulting enterprise. Multinational corporations are not signatories to international treaties and conventions. They do have the obligation to comply with the laws of the countries where they do business, but ensuring compliance is the state's responsibility. Monitoring and enforcing state laws in a private/multilateral development process is particularly difficult, given the peripheral location of many projects, the lack of state funds to support regular and intensive scrutiny, and the state's limited or nonexistent role in negotiating forums. Without meaningful oversight, culpability for ensuing social and environmental crises is difficult to assign.

Furthermore, when the state or multilateral funders attempt to apply leverage and renegotiation agreements or actions, private corporations can simply refinance their loans. When projects are funded completely by private capital (investment banks, hedge funds, and so forth), contractual relationships between the private funder and the private corporation are confined to a specific set of obligations. The developer has the legal duty to meet those terms but is very rarely obligated to ensure that goals are actually met. Institutions such as the World Bank have established social and environmental policies and review procedures to provide some measure of public interest protection, but policies and guidelines are not the same as legally enforceable contractual obligations. Governments, as well as project-affected communities, can be and have been excluded from the information and decision-making loop in projects funded this way (as illustrated in Downing 1996; Johnston and Turner 1998; Johnston 2002:115).

In Bolivia, Aguas del Rtunari, a subsidiary of the privately held Bechtel Corporation, instituted a cost recovery program involving massive water hikes. Wide-scale social protests, with injuries and death caused by military efforts to quell the protests, led the Bolivian government to rescind its privatization agreements. Bolivia had agreed to privatize the public water system of its third largest city in the late 1990s after the World Bank threatened to withhold a development aid and debt relief package. When privatization contracts were rescinded, Aguas del Rtunari and its parent company, the Bechtel Corporation, sued Bolivia for $25 million, filing a complaint with the International Center for the Settlement of Investment Disputes, a tribunal administered by the World Bank. Amicus briefs were prepared by national and international public interest organizations and filed with the support of the Bolivian president; these requested public participation in the suit, transparent meetings, and site-based meetings to receive public testimony (Earthjustice Fund 2003). In February 2003 the tribunal panel ruled that citizens did not have the right to participate in the case, and it would not allow the public or media to participate in or witness any of the proceedings (CIEL 2003).

Strong intersects appear to exist among the multilateral agreements defining water as a commodity, the utility privatization requirements increasingly accompanying development loans and aid packages, the growth of free market/privatization incentives in national contexts, and the long-term desire articulated by financial and energy analysts and reflected in corporate investments and partnership agreements to effect a substantive transformation in the ownership of water development, management, and supply projects, especially those that generate hydroelectric energy. In late 2002 the Bush administration pushed through the US Congress a water resources act encouraging the privatization of public utilities, limiting development and improvement funds to those entities that considered privatizing public utilities. As of June 2003 the only environment-friendly initiative announced by the Bush administration was fiscal support for research and development of hydrogen fuel–powered transport. In March 2003 the World Bank announced a new water-resource investment strategy that boosts spending on big dams, interbasin transfers, and other water megaprojects, encourages privatization of utilities, supports full cost-recovery schemes, and encourages investments through public/private partnerships. Currently, the majority of the world's hydroelectric facilities are publicly owned and operated. From an energy-industry point of view, if the future is hydrogen, then substantive transformations need to take place in loci of control over potential hydrogen-production facilities if corporate entities are to make a profit.

## CONCLUSION

The case-specific examples discussed in this chapter illustrate the relative nature of water scarcity. The conditions and actions that affect water supply and water demand are relative to a myriad of factors, including biophysical conditions and hydrologic processes, cultural meanings and economic values, social relationships and histories that influence patterns of access and use, and power relationships and agendas that determine who manages and distributes water resources, and how. Although many people experience water shortages and crises, this chapter argues that scarcity—even the very perception of scarcity—can be manufactured or manipulated to support political and economic agendas.

In reviewing case-specific examples of the human dimensions of water scarcity, this chapter also suggests several consequences of employing flawed or shortsighted conceptual models. As Linda Whiteford describes in this volume, water supply and sanitation systems evolved from a public health perspective: the desire to reduce or eliminate biological contaminants was linked to the social and economic crises associated with epidemic outbreaks of waterborne disease. The conceptual models supporting sanitation and public health policy are largely concerned with these immediate threats, rather than with the long-term threats or risks associated with ecological and environmental contaminants. Resulting development agendas encourage the construction of large, centralized water storage and delivery systems that may fail to incorporate or prioritize ecological conditions and environmental contaminants and, while solving some problems, may introduce or exacerbate others. To "pay" for these facilities, communities around the world are being asked or forced to privatize their municipal and regional water-supply systems. National governments are encouraged or forced to finance their water-resource development projects as private instead of public ventures.

The transformation of a socioeconomic perception of water as a natural element to that of water as a privately owned commodity involves not only the increasing dominance of transnational corporations in building and running water supply and delivery systems, but also the global imposition of a scarcity framework that uses the language and analytical tools of the market to assess water problems and to support preferred solutions. The globalization of water supply and delivery systems involves fundamental transformations in the loci of control over water resources. Globalization increases the distance between those who make and profit from water management decisions and water user communities who must live with any adverse consequence of shortsighted or flawed resource-management policy. Increased distance weakens or renders meaningless the feedback mechanisms that operate when control over water is situated within the watershed. These conceptual flaws or shortcomings can generate water quality crises affecting the health and longevity of hundreds of millions of people, as illustrated in the case of arsenic poisoning in Bangladesh and the perchlorate, chromium, and other chemical and metal contaminants from military base contamination of subsurface aquifers. Some case studies clearly document the consequential damages associated with a flawed conceptual model. In South Africa, for example, where privatization and "full cost-recovery" programs led to cholera epidemics and rising death rates associated with the unique vulnerabilities of immune-compromised populations, these case studies have yet to demonstrate an obvious impact on the policies being promulgated.

Our ability to respond effectively to current water crises and avoid new crises is complicated by the contradictions between agendas and actions that value water as a public good and human right and those that value water as an essential and profitable commodity. In recent years, the United Nations, the World Commission on Dams, the scientific community, and civil society have shaped and attempted to apply, through international law and regulatory policy, a rights-based approach that includes decentralization and place-based water resource development, with management reflecting human environmental conditions and needs. This rights-based approach incorporates the values and concerns of placed-based peoples and resonates with a watershed approach to resource management. At the same time, the political mechanisms of trade agreements, of financial institution and government lending policies, push through—with incredible speed and authority—privatization processes and projects that operate within regional, national, and international economic frameworks having little or nothing to do with local ecosystemic dynamics and social needs. These contradictions suggest a future of messy conflict over water access, use, and quality and over the questions of culpability for legacy issues associated with flawed decisions and inept actions.

**Notes**

1. In September 2003, an abstracted version of this chapter, titled "The Political Ecology of Water: An Introduction," was published in the journal *Capitalism, Nature, Socialism*, vol. 14, no. 3, pp. 73–90.

# 8

# Water Struggles of Indigenous North America

Tom Greaves

Whether or not we Americans understand globalization, all of us are certainly familiar with its effects. The media, the organizations that employ us, the work we do, the products we consume, our recreations, all reflect globalization. We are also well aware of the political realities of a globalized world as we form opinions on AIDS in Africa, the nuclear intentions of North Korea, international trade agreements, terrorist networks, international petroleum supplies, and overseas sources of illegal drugs. We may be less aware of globalization's effects within third world countries, but it is hard not to notice that one's new sneakers were made in Malaysia or Honduras, that many familiar American occupations have decamped to sources of cheap labor overseas, and that immigration pressures push fiercely at American borders. Our planet is a small and interconnected place.

This chapter focuses on a distinctive part of North American society, reservation-dwelling American Indians.[1] Indian reservations in the United States (and "reserves" in Canada) are commonly located on hardscrabble land in remote places, a product of the power advantage that privileged the colonizers to designate reservations in places they did not then value. Geographic remoteness, however, is only one source of isolation for Indian reservations. Government paternalism, grinding poverty, underdevelopment, and social discrimination also have set them apart from the surrounding dominant society. Today, however, the embrace of globalization reaches out to reservations and reserves.[2]

At the core of this chapter is an examination of current and recent water disputes involving reservation-dwelling North American Indians. In these disputes, we will see that globalization shapes both the threat to American Indians' water resources and their response to this threat. Indeed, as we shall find, no reservation or reserve is immune to the powerful forces of globalization. We also need to be aware that, when focusing on water disputes, we are examining only one arena of reservation life that is affected by globalization. Local politics, alcoholism, and unemployment on a reservation may have nothing in particular to do with water yet may be buffeted by the forces of globalization. Nonetheless, water disputes are a productive focus of our attention, first, because water is fundamental to the present and future of Indian society and culture and, second, because water issues ramify across a broad spectrum of reservation life, health, and well-being.

## GLOBALIZATION AND INDIGENOUS PEOPLES

What is globalization? Like other large-scale social processes, globalization defies succinct definition. Arjun Appadurai (1990:324) pointed out that globalization operates within five broad "landscapes," or domains of contemporary human life: ethnoscapes, mediascapes, technoscapes, financescapes, and ideoscapes. His five-part classification need not be further examined here, but Appadurai makes clear that globalization affects whole societies in profound and multiple ways.

Globalization is not to be confused with modernization. It is not some sort of broad social evolution. It is quite specific. At its heart, globalization involves corporations, technology, and capital. More precisely, it is a process of rapid internationalization and integration of commercial enterprises, supported by global communication technologies and new management techniques, and global deployment of financial capital. Governments of the most powerful countries collaborate with globalizing corporations, smoothing the way for corporate success (for example, by forcing developing countries to adopt and enforce favorable intellectual property rights laws). The globalization process is not new. Mercantilism and colonialism were major forms of globalization in past centuries. What is new about the process is the amazing speed globalization has attained over the past forty years, as well as its truly transformative scale.

Much scholarly attention has been focused on the loss of economic control that governments experience as their economies and societies become organized around the interests of transnational corporations, a trend evident both in leading industrial countries and in third world countries. Within globalization's wide spectrum of social impacts, of particular interest in this volume are those affecting the natural environment, culture, and health. Globalization precipitates a planetwide process of preempting and commercializing scarce, economically valuable resources (such as timber, minerals, oil, and tourist sites) and prime agricultural and grazing land. These, in turn, have direct impacts on the health of the local peoples who depend on these resources.

How are indigenous peoples affected? Globalization increases acculturative pressures on indigenous groups and challenges their ethnic survival, especially by targeting them as potential customers for products and services. Also, their communities are disrupted as their lands and natural resources are appropriated for corporate exploitation. In response to the attractions of cash-based urban life, to the eroding economic base of their traditional lifeway, and to the frequent political violence (often exacerbated by globalization pressures) in their homelands, indigenous people relocate, though with continuing links to home localities and cultural bases.

As we will see, globalization dramatically affects the health of indigenous peoples. By fragmenting traditional societies, globalization replaces largely self-sufficient lifeways with impoverishing, marginalized dependency on cash economies. Globalization redistributes native populations, often into dense settlements clustered around sources of paid work or refugee assistance, with diminished nutrition, sanitation, hygiene, and food and health security. Globalization elevates the abuse of alcohol and drugs and the spread of disease and leads to dietary change, contributing to a broadening incidence of morbidity.

This chapter asks the question, to what extent are the effects of globalization on North American Indians similar to, or different from, those experienced by indigenous peoples on other continents?[3] The answer we find is that there are certain similarities in the experience of indigenous peoples everywhere because they share a common structural position as dependent ethnic groups within a nation-state dominated by a larger, contrasting social group and society. The larger dominant group controls national political, economic, and legal institutions, putting internal indigenous societies at a continuing disadvantage. Indigenous groups across the world grapple with this structural reality. Yet, because they exist in sharply contrasting, specific situations, with differing legal statuses and contact histories, their responses to globalization must be analyzed at more specific levels as well.

Indigenous groups in North America share a number of features that are, as a set, specific to North America. For instance, in the United States and Canada they are confronted with the world's most developed economies with respect to technology investment, capital concentration, communication and media use, and sheer size. The legal frameworks of the United States and Canada assign indigenous societies to subordinate status but accord them limited collective sovereignty and certain enforceable rights. In the United States, these rights are based mostly on historical treaties, cast as agreements between independent nations; in Canada, state/tribe relations employ the same principle (that is, limited collective home rule and certain enforceable rights), deriving from legal assumptions established within French and British colonialism.[4] Thus, the situations of North American Indians are at once similar and dissimilar to those of indigenous peoples elsewhere, and the conclusions we reach from studying their responses to globalization are likewise circumscribed. Keeping those limitations in mind, let us proceed to examine the water disputes of North American Indians. In the last section, we will explore their connections to globalization and health.

## DEFINING INDIGENOUS NORTH AMERICA

Who and where are North American Indians? Unfortunately, answering those questions raises various complexities. The 2000 US census allowed responders to identify themselves as Indian purely by their personal criteria. Some 4.1 million US citizens—a record number—said that they were American Indians or Alaska Natives. About 75 percent identified a specific tribe; the rest did not. A more plausible figure is obtained when we define *Indian* as people listed on the membership roll of a federally recognized tribe. Then the number is about 1.8 million (*Indian Country Today* 2004). This, however, omits the members of tribes who do not have federal recognition. It omits individuals who, although having Indian ancestors, cannot qualify for membership in any specific tribe—as well as people in various other circumstances. There are about 563 (the number fluctuates) federally recognized Indian entities in the United States, organized into tribes, nations, bands, villages, and rancherias. Some 334 are in the "lower forty-eight" states, and another 229 in Alaska (Federal Register 2002).[5] Of some 1.8 million enrolled in federally recognized tribes, those living on US reservations and trust lands during the 2000 census numbered about 538,000.[6] Less than a third of US tribal members live on reservations.

In Canada, the percentage living on reserves is higher: as of 2002 about 55 percent of the roughly 675,000 "registered" Indians (similar to being enrolled in a federally recognized US tribe) reside on reserves, organized into some 613 bands. These numbers do not include about 41,000 Inuit and perhaps 210,000 Métis.[7]

What are US reservations and Canadian reserves like? Reservations in the United States range greatly in size. The largest is the Navajo reservation, with more than 27,000 square miles in Arizona, New Mexico, and Utah. It is home to some 175,000 people (Fogarty 2003:A2). The size of the Navajo reservation is atypical, however. Although there are other large reservations, for example, in South Dakota, Montana, and several other states, many Indian reservations comprise only a few tens of square miles. Some, notably the rancherias in California, can be even smaller, sometimes supporting a resident population of just a few dozen people. In Alaska, the Inuit (Eskimo) groups typically reside in "native villages," with lands available for their use through membership in federally established native corporations.[8]

Most Canadian native reserves are small. Many are only a few square miles surrounding a village. Typically, reserve-based groups also have use rights to adjacent Crown lands for hunting, fishing, and other purposes. Over the past century, Canadian Indian lands have been much reduced, often by dubious means, and a legacy of claims to formerly occupied lands is being slowly addressed through a complex administrative process. Recent negotiated land-claim settlements and judicial decisions have resulted in sizable additions to the lands of certain reserves (Mills 2002). Reserves are self-governing entities and, like reservations in the United States, are usually located in outlying locations (see the Indian and Northern Affairs web site, appendix 3: http://ainc-inac.gc.ca).

## WATER DISPUTES AND GLOBALIZATION'S EFFECTS

Over the past several decades, certain water-related struggles of North American Indians have become notorious cases very much in the consciousness of Indian people today. Thus, although our focus in this chapter is on contemporary water disputes, these historic cases inevitably contextualize current disputes. In 1957 the US government completed The Dalles Dam on the Columbia River between Oregon and Washington, flooding the celebrated aboriginal fishing site Celilo Falls. For perhaps ten thousand years, people of many regional tribes had come to this politically neutral place on the Columbia River to dip great salmon from the thundering cataracts. The Dalles Dam is part of a massive dam-building program that transformed the main portions of the Columbia and Snake Rivers into an almost continuous series of stair-step reservoirs. The dams have, as expected, caused an enormous drop in the salmon runs. But, despite protracted protests by Indians and their supporters. The Dalles Dam could not be stopped and Celilo Falls was destroyed.

In 1965 in northwestern Pennsylvania, the Corps of Engineers dedicated another dam, Kinzua. In the name of protecting downstream Pittsburgh from potential flooding, the project forced the removal of the Allegany Seneca from the bulk of their treaty lands on the Allegheny River (McGrath and Greaves 2000; Josephy 1982:127–150). The Seneca's campaign to stop the dam was elaborate and carefully planned, but the dam went in, uprooting their burial grounds and destroying riverside villages and places of deeply important cultural history. The Seneca still mourn the losses caused by Kinzua Dam.

A third example lies in Canada. In 1975 the James Bay hydroelectric development on the southeastern shore of Hudson's Bay was initiated by Hydro-Quebec, the largest power company in Canada. Ignoring Indian land rights and protests, Hydro-Quebec constructed a vast network of dams, reservoirs, and power stations, displacing the resident Eastern Cree. In a subsequent lawsuit, the court ordered Hydro-Quebec to indemnify the Cree for despoiling their lands, but the project was allowed to proceed.[9] Later in the chapter, I discuss this case further.

Today, water is at the center of dozens of struggles that engage reservation-dwelling American Indian groups across the continent. The basic reality is well summarized by Josephy (1982:175): "The Indians need their water to survive. The Whites want not only to keep the water they have, but to secure as much Indian water as they can get for their expanding needs."

## DATA SOURCES

How does one study contemporary water-related disputes involving North American Indians? There are no systematic compilations of these disputes. The information presented in this chapter derives from the author's interest over the past decade in water disputes involving Indians and from an intensive survey mainly of the contents, across nine consecutive months, of the most important weekly newspaper devoted to American Indian affairs, *Indian Country Today*. The newspaper, while certainly an advocate for Indians, adopts national standards of journalism in its coverage of events concerning Indians throughout North America.[10] To assemble this chapter's core data set, I have used the newspaper's coverage of more than sixty water-related disputes between June 2002 and March 2003, supplemented by a substantial amount of information across a broader time frame, on these and other cases, garnered from various other sources.

As one might suppose, water disputes involving reservation Indians are more common in the areas west of the Mississippi River, mirroring the general scarcity of water in these more arid continental areas and the competition among users for what water there is. However, as the following review makes plain, water issues have arisen in all regions of the United States and Canada; indeed, water issues are as widespread as Indians themselves.

This chapter examines water disputes from a wider perspective than the reader might suppose. In this chapter, water disputes may concern surface water (rivers, lakes, streams) or groundwater pumped from wells. The issue may be the purity of water supplies, a factor strongly associated with health. Water disputes may involve fresh water or sea water. Water disputes may arise over water as a scarce consumable substance or over the resources that derive from a water habitat (for example, salmon, lobsters, shellfish). Disputes may be over water to drink or water necessary for income activities, such as raising hatchery salmon or running a casino. Water disputes may be motivated by commercial or other pragmatic concerns, but they may also be concerned with symbolic or spiritual qualities of bodies of water. And disputes may arise not over present water, but over water for the future, as tribes and non-Indian users compete to assemble the resources needed to meet their future aspirations. In these instances, the disputes usually focus on Indians' legally enforceable water rights, the source of some of the bitterest civil disputes in our time. This great diversity among water disputes stems from water's centrality in the lives of all human beings.

The following section reviews the types and forms of water disputes on North American reserves and reservations, with illustrations drawn from the data set described above. Although globalization's realities mean that no water issue is entirely local, the sequence in the next section runs roughly from predominantly local disputes to those set in the regional, the national, and the international spheres.

## ON-RESERVATION WATER ISSUES

Readers might be surprised to learn that many people living on US Indian reservations are not Indians. During several periods of US history, the federal government worked to undermine reservation communities and the tribal unity they preserved. In 1887 Congress passed the General Allotment Act, also known as the "Dawes Severalty Act," which allotted parcels of reservation land (usually 160 acres) to individual tribal members, who could, after twenty-five years, sell the land to outsiders.[11] In addition to drastically reducing the size of reservations, the 1887 act began a fifty-year campaign to transfer Indian-owned land to outsiders. On many reservations today, non-Indians own as much as half the land, turning the reservation into a checkerboard of Indian and non-Indian owners. In addition, the Dawes Act authorized federal agents to lease reservation lands not actively farmed or grazed by their Indian owners, entrenching a practice of government-managed leasing of Indian land to outsiders, at bargain rates, for grazing or timbering. This practice continues today, with non-Indian leaseholders coming to view their access to the leased Indian land as perpetual and their rights on it as similar to outright ownership.[12] Because water is almost always indispensable to the use of reservation land, it is no surprise that control of reservation water ignites strong conflict among external leaseholders, non-Indian residents on the reservations, and Indians.

Sovereignty is another source of tension between Indians and non-Indians. Although Indians have always valued tribal sovereignty (the tribe's right to govern its internal affairs), feelings regarding sovereignty have strongly intensified in recent decades. Indeed, federal practice itself has nurtured tribal sovereignty. Since the Nixon administration (1969–1974), the posture of the American government has been to off-load reservation governance responsibilities to tribes. This has led to expanded tribal police forces, tribe-run schools, and tribal offices administering federal funds for housing, utility improvement, and planning on the reservation. Tribal governments increasingly feel, as a matter of sovereign right, that they should exercise governance over all reservation lands and resources and over the people who live on the reservation. Yet US law makes it clear that the reservation's tribal government has virtually no jurisdiction over non-Indians holding deeds to reservation land (Pevar 2002:109–111, 172–173). Within this matrix of sovereignty feelings, expanding tribal governance, federal lease management, and long-standing distrust between Indians and non-Indians, water disputes are apt to become very heated.

Water disputes on reservations usually center on who controls water and who decides how it will be used. Tribal councils believe that, because they are responsible for planning, managing, and preserving reservation water resources, non-Indian residents should not put in water wells or otherwise impact reservation water supplies without their permission. Meanwhile, non-Indian residents are apt to vigorously oppose any indication of Indian authority over their activities. Tensions are currently high, for example, among the Salish and

Kootenai on Montana's Flathead Reservation, where water-well drilling by non-Indian property owners is the issue (Seldon 2003a); among Maine's Passamaquoddy and Penobscot, where waste-water discharge is contested (*Indian Country Today* 2002c); among Nevada's Western Shoshone, where the tribe is not allowing state officials to cross reservation land to adjust settings that could increase river water use by non-Indian property owners (*Indian Country Today* 2003a); and among Washington's Lummis, who are waging a long battle with the non-Indian reservation residents over water-well drilling (Russo 2002:107–109).

In addition to conflicts over water use, there are many concerns about pollution, water sufficiency, and endangerment of reservation water resources. The Walpole Island Indian Community across the Canadian border from Detroit believes that the frequent chemical spills from industries upstream have harmed its water and that its shoreline may one day be the site of a major spill from Great Lakes tanker traffic passing near the island. It protests also that its beaches are often closed because of high bacteria counts, apparently produced by off-reservation agricultural runoff (see Walpole Island, First Nation, Canada 2003). The Swinomish of Washington State are working with external authorities to better protect both the fresh water and salt water on which they depend for food resources and for their highly successful, expanding, casino-related enterprises (*Indian Country Today* 2002e). The tribes of Fort Peck (Assiniboine and Sioux) in Montana are building a major, federally financed pipeline to bring better-quality potable water to the reservation (*Indian Country Today* 2002f). New Mexico's Pojoaque are said to be pumping water far in excess of state allotment limits to supply their rapidly expanding, casino-related businesses (*Indian Country Today* 2002g, 2002h). Across the country, reservation concerns about water are common.

## OFF-RESERVATION WATER RESOURCES

In many parts of the United States, especially in the West, potable water for domestic, agricultural, and industrial use is in very short supply. Indian reservations often find themselves on the defensive against powerful groups determined to maintain or expand their water rights at the expense of Indian communities. Washington State's Lummi find the limited water supplies of their area being literally sucked up by commercial development, population growth in nearby cities, and pro-development state water authorizations. For the past decade, the Lummi have been enmeshed in negotiation and court action, at heavy expense, defending their share of water in a river with a finite amount of water and multiple non-Indian users (Greaves 1998).

The US judicial system has long held that when the government set aside land for Indians to live on, it also committed to reservation water rights to make reservations livable.[13] Now, as the competition for water sources (aquifers, lakes, rivers) grows, Indians find themselves participants in regional water-regulation schemes and involved in intense regional water negotiations. The Animas-La Plata Project, involving parts of New Mexico and Colorado, has involved the Ute Mountain Utes and the Southern Utes (*Indian Country Today* 2001, 2003c). The ongoing Gila River negotiations in Arizona are another case (*Indian Country Today* 2003d; see also Pevar 2002:249). There is a bitter fight between the users of the Klamath River waters in northern California (J. May 2002), and another affects the Salish and Kootenai in western Montana (Seldon 2003b; J. May 2002). In each of these, the Indians must now defend their interests against many other water constituencies, becoming parties to the creation and modification of large-scale, regional water-management systems. Regional water politics thrust reservation communities into contentious political arenas in which they must assert their right to participate, with opponents unused to according Indians any power in decisions involving water.

In other cases, the tribal groups are seeking to preserve the availability and purity of regional aquifers on which they depend. These aquifers extend far beyond reservation boundaries and jurisdictions. In Montana, the Northern Cheyenne are protesting the Crow's plan to open Crow reservation land to methane exploration. The Northern Cheyenne worry that their own methane wells will be negatively affected, but also that the water aquifer underlying both reservations may be reduced or contaminated as a result of new methane drilling by the Crow.[14] Meanwhile, the Assiniboine and Gros Ventre in Montana are demanding that strip mines abandoned by a bankrupt mining company be fully mitigated, at federal expense, to protect their water from mine drainage pollution (Seldon 2002). A very large water dispute involves the Hopi, the Navajo, and the Peabody Energy Company.

Peabody, with joint tribal consent, mines reservation coal deposits. The coal is conveyed through a 273-mile slurry pipeline to the massive Mohave Generating Station in Nevada. The Hopi fear that the water used to convey the coal is irreplaceably draining the aquifer. The Hopi have declared that their permission for Peabody to use aquifer water will end in 2005 (*Indian Country Today* 2002l). These cases illustrate an increased vigilance in Indian country regarding the long-term viability of their off-reservation water supplies.

Some Indian tribes are experiencing growing needs for water and must amplify water sources and delivery systems far beyond reservation boundaries. Perhaps the largest current example is the Mni Wiconi Project, which will supply better drinking water to the Oglala, the Rosebud Sioux, and the Lower Brule in South Dakota. Some parts of the project are complete, but it will require more federal appropriations and time before water begins to flow (Melmer 2000, 2003).

In addition, tribes today are often highly involved in preserving or restoring wildlife habitats in regions beyond their reservations. These habitats and species are located in areas formerly used by the tribe and, in some cases, have spiritual significance. For example, the Lummi of northwestern Washington State have purchased lands in the Cascade Mountains to protect old growth forest and spawning grounds for salmon in the river that flows past their downstream reservation (Russo 2002:111–112). Northern California's Yurok and Hoopa have vigorously protested a massive 2002 fish kill in the lower Klamath River, apparently caused when the federal government decided to divert scarce water to agricultural users, reducing the river flow and allowing the temperature of the remaining water to rise (J. May 2002; *Indian Country Today* 2002a). In Montana, the Nez Perce are opposing a US Forest Service plan to allow selective logging in the Bitterroot Mountains (aimed, in part, at improving elk habitat). The Nez Perce fear that the logging will increase silt runoff, destroying salmon spawning habitats in the area (*Indian Country Today* 2003b). In southern Puget Sound, the Nisqually have purchased nearby wetlands to protect them from industrial development.

Some struggles over off-reservation water are about its cultural value as much as its utility. The Zuni, for instance, are fighting a strip mining expansion eleven miles from Zuni Salt Lake. Salt collected from the lake plays a role in Zuni religious ritual. Although there are contradictory opinions on whether the aquifer that supplies the lake will be affected, the Zuni fear that that the strip mine will do so. They expect to continue fighting the mine in the courts (Shively 2002). The Lummi of Washington State seek to maintain the quality of river water bordering their reservation, because it sustains their salmon hatchery. Their hatchery program reflects their strong commitment to the symbolic status of salmon within their culture (Russo 2002:98–100; Greaves 1998:36–37). Thus, whether for domestic use or for cultural needs, water disputes in North America often move the struggle off the reservations because water upon which Indian tribes depend originates upstream in off-reservation locales or derives from aquifers extending far outside the reservation.

It should also be noted that Indians are not always the victims. Currently, the Pojoaque, a Pueblo group north of Santa Fe, New Mexico, are reported to be substantially exceeding their water allotment, supplying their rapidly developing commercial ventures involving a casino, hotel, and golf course. The State of New Mexico has asked a judge to order the Pojoaque to cut back and to document their compliance through metered wells. So far, the Pojoaque have refused to allow their wells to be metered (*Indian Country Today* 2002g, 2002h). The Pojoaque are responding, as have more than two hundred North American tribes, to the possibilities provided by casino-driven commerce, itself a reflection of the national and global markets that offer reservation communities lucrative business opportunities.

## COMPETITION FOR WATER-LINKED FOOD RESOURCES

Disputes outside the reservation involve not only water and water quality, but also the resources that may be harvested from water environments. Many bitter, sometimes violent, confrontations between Indians and non-Indians have occurred over fish, lobsters, and shellfish. Indeed, a showdown over marine resources is the most common contemporary flashpoint for violence between non-Indians and Indians. For years, Indians, commercial fishermen, sports fishermen, state and provincial fisheries regulators, and sundry environmental groups have clashed, particularly when Indians secure court-affirmed rights to fish outside state-prescribed fishing seasons, to use fishing gear non-Indians may not use, or to be guaranteed a percentage of the total annual catch. Angry, violent confrontations have occurred in recent years over spear fishing in Wisconsin (Beno 1991), over lobster harvesting at Burnt Church in Nova Scotia (P. Fitzgerald 2002; *Indian Country Today* 2002k), and over salmon fishing, shellfish harvesting, and whaling in Washington State (Cohen 1986; Sullivan 2000).

The twenty-five federally recognized tribes of Washington State have a singularly long history of political activism and struggle over marine resources. These battles have set influential precedents and merit a brief account here. In 1954 Robert Satiacum and James Young, Puyallups, openly challenged the state's ban on salmon fishing using fixed nets. They were arrested, and the case eventuated in a 1957 State Supreme Court tie decision (4-4). The tie vote allowed them, as well as other Indians, to continue using fixed nets. In 1958 three members of the Umatilla tribe (northern Oregon) fished in the Columbia River out of season. Their case, decided in 1963, sharply limited the state's regulatory power over Indian fishing. The court said that Washington State could restrict Indian fishing only in the interests of fish conservation, and then only if the need and the regulation's beneficial effect could be fully demonstrated. Satiacum and others then embarked on a series of "fish-ins," beginning in the early 1960s. The fish-ins, which asserted Indian treaty guarantees, gained sizable public sympathy but also generated anger, gear sabotage, and violence.

Then, Yakamas Richard and David Sohappy intentionally sought arrest for net fishing on the Columbia River, and Oregon authorities obliged. The case went to federal court, and in 1969 Judge Robert Belloni ruled that treaties reserved to Indians "a fair and equitable share" of the salmon catch. The court affirmed that Washington State's only avenue of restriction is on the basis of demonstrable need to conserve the species and any such restriction must apply equitably to all fishermen.[15] Thus, by 1969 the courts had made it clear that Indians had not ceded their treaty-guaranteed rights to fish off their reservations at what were termed their "usual and customary places," that the state had only very limited rights to regulate their fishing, and that it had a duty to regulate fishing so that other groups did not deprive the Indians of their "fair and equitable share."[16]

For western Washington's Puget Sound area, the pivotal case came in 1974 when Judge Boldt ruled that the nineteen (later twenty) treaty tribes of Puget Sound had a collective right to 50 percent of the salmon caught annually, the total catch being set by state authorities in the interest of maintaining the species (Cohen 1986:83–117). The Boldt decision evoked enormous public anger against Indians, which has only slowly moderated. In British Columbia, the 1990 Sparrow case, involving Fraser River fishing, produced the same effect. Then, in 1999 the US Supreme Court affirmed a 1994 Rafeedie decision that Puget Sound Indians had the right by treaty to 50 percent of the annual harvest not only of fish, but also of shellfish (clams, crabs, mussels, and oysters) found on Puget Sound tidelands, including those on land now privately owned. This enraged many private-property owners, who bridled at the prospect of Indians digging clams on their property.[17]

Finally, the Makah, a tribe at the extreme western tip of Washington State on the Strait of Juan de Fuca, regained (with the support of the Clinton administration) the right to hunt gray whales after a seventy-year hiatus, gray whales being no longer endangered. In 1999 the Makah succeeded in killing a whale in the face of substantial public disapproval and dramatic attempts by anti-whaling groups to thwart them (Sullivan 2000).

Thus, between 1954 and 1999 the tribes of Washington State succeeded in reasserting their treaty-guaranteed rights to marine and freshwater food resources. Because these decisions were made by federal courts, the implications reach far beyond Washington State. What all the preceding cases show is that, for Indians and their adversaries, water disputes are not only about water, but also about the economic resources that are harvested from water.

## CLAIMS BEYOND RESERVATION BORDERS UNRELATED TO WATER RESOURCES

Early in this chapter, the point is made that water disputes are only one sector of ongoing contests between reservation Indians and the society that surrounds them. It is important to understand water issues within the context of this larger set of Indian claims and how they originated. The westward expansion of Euro-Americans and Euro-Canadians dislodged Indian tribes from large territories. Over three centuries, devastating diseases, the superior military power of the settlers, missionary efforts, the rapidly growing numbers of westward-moving settlers, alcohol, and various other factors converted a continent of native peoples into interned populations on mostly small reservations. As a result, the sites of their former Indian villages, burial grounds, places of religious and historical importance, and sources of vital economic resources now typically fall outside reservation boundaries. As those lands filled up with farms, ranches, and towns or were converted to national forest lands, dam reservoirs, and national parks, access to and use of those places became uncertain.

Indian reservations and reserves are now enclaves in a landscape controlled by Euro-Americans and Euro-Canadians, and their essential resources are increasingly subject to appropriation or destruction by others. The array of off-reservation resources over which Indians now assert rights is wide indeed. It includes fishing and hunting sites, ancestral burial grounds, religious sites, archaeological remains, and sources of materials for basketry and other crafts.[18]

Among the most traumatic extra-reservation conflicts in recent years was the violent 1990 Mohawk standoff at Oka in Ontario, precipitated when the town authorities of Oka decided to expand the municipal golf course over lands the Mohawk claim as their own (Claiborne 1990). The conflict resulted in the death of a policeman, intervention by the Canadian army, a seventy-eight-day siege, and more than two hundred million dollars (Canadian) in law enforcement costs. Other conflicts in Canada have included numerous blockades of British Columbia logging roads by Indians protesting timber cutting, as well as angry politics over two large land-claim awards in British Columbia.[19] Recent disputes over off-reservation matters include the bitter fight over the bones of "Kennewick Man" (Downey 2000), the continuing effort to abolish Indian-related sports mascots, numerous abrasive fights over casinos (notably in California, Arizona, New York, and Connecticut), the Indian Trust Fund scandal involving hopelessly lost records of payments owed Indians for federally managed leasing of their lands (Brinkley 2003:A14), and protracted, no-holds-barred struggles over tribal petitions seeking federal recognition.

An especially vexing example from the northern plains is the land claim of eight Sioux tribes to the Great Sioux Reservation. In 1868, by the Treaty of Fort Laramie, the federal government recognized an expanse of land that included the Black Hills and most of South Dakota west of the Missouri River as perpetually belonging to the Sioux. The treaty also allocated the Powder River Basin of eastern Wyoming and Montana exclusively for Indian buffalo hunting. The US government pledged that it would honor the Sioux's ownership in perpetuity and prevent the entry of non-Indians to both areas.

Six years later, gold was discovered in the Black Hills, and, ignoring the treaty, miners poured in. The Sioux were then militarily subdued and confined to smaller, separated reservations, and the Great Sioux Reservation became functionally moot. The eight Sioux tribes have never conceded title to the Great Sioux Reservation, however, and refuse to accept the appropriated money (now estimated to total some half billion dollars) voted by Congress in 1980 as compensation (Melmer 1996; Welch 1994:65–70). This argument shapes water and other land disputes in the region because the Siouan groups oppose any land transfer involving public agencies, insisting that such transfers imply uncontested title (Welch 1994:265–267; Melmer 2002b).

The cases and conflicts reviewed in this section show two things: First, the fights for water, the foods and resources produced in water habitats, and treaty rights are widespread, varied, and important. Second, the water-related cases are part of a much larger palette of claims and conflicts arising from the history of contact and the increasing competition for land and resources near Indian reservations. Our task now is to return to the process of globalization, sifting these contests to see where globalization is evident.

## THE PRESENCE OF GLOBALIZATION

The core data for this analysis comprise approximately sixty cases of current Indian water disputes, supplemented by various disputes from earlier periods. The intent now is to examine, through these cases, the effects globalization may be having on reservation-dwelling Indians. To repeat this chapter's definition, globalization is a process of rapid internationalization and integration of commercial enterprises, supported by global communication technologies and new management techniques, and a global deployment of financial capital. We have also found that while globalization involves corporations and capital, it affects, directly and derivatively, whole lifeways.

Already apparent is the fact that globalization has a hand in shaping and energizing many of these water-based disputes. How strong a hand? In some, globalization may not be playing any role at all or may be simply amplifying pressures and processes that would be present anyway. But globalization can so powerfully transform a local situation in intensity and scope that it is reasonable to see globalization as the central player. We can better discern globalization's role if we examine it within four domains: political, economic, cultural, and environmental.

**Political Effects**

The instances in which globalization visibly imposes political effects on indigenous water disputes are many. The paragraphs that follow explore these effects, first at the international level and then at the national and subnational (regional) levels. We have seen that globalization intensifies political conflict for water-related resources. We can also see that globalization has often evoked a readiness to meet these challenges through multitribal coalitions and organizations, overcoming traditional reticence and impediments to working together.

At a recent meeting of Amnesty International, Nigerian Oronto Douglas, director of Environmental Rights Action, declared, "Corporate-led globalization has led to development and privileges for some and anger, poverty and even starvation for us, the indigenous peoples. And that's why we have to form international alliances to protect our communities" (Taliman 2002). Indigenous groups have invigorated and invented national and international forums to express their common protests. As recently as May 2002, the United Nations inaugurated the Permanent Forum on Indigenous Issues. The Permanent Forum establishes an institutionalized, in-house channel within the United Nations through which indigenous societies can craft joint positions and present policy demands and claims directly to the world's nation-states without the intermediation of the governments of the countries within which they are individually located. This is a major development.

The same incentives make multitribal coalitions attractive at the national level in the United States. Both the scope and importance of collective involvement are reflected in advice offered by former Assistant Secretary for Indian Affairs Kevin Gover. When his successor, Neil McCaleb, suddenly resigned, Gover wrote, "It's very dangerous for

Indian Affairs to be in a transition situation when the rest of the [Interior] Department is not. If you don't have an assistant secretary at the table, you are at a disadvantage, [including how the government handles] almost any water dispute" (J. Adams 2002:A1–3). This has long been true, but the number and scale of Indian water disputes now decided in Washington DC have much enlarged, and the scale of Indian national organizations and lobbying is now continuous and very substantial.

Groupings at the regional level have also appeared, notably the Mni Sose Intertribal Water Rights Coalition, which focuses on tribal rights to the use of the Missouri River and its tributaries and to the groundwater in these areas. Twenty-seven tribes are members, with reservations and lands in twelve states.[20] The coalition not only is a central player in regional water negotiations but also hopes to lead in the development of a national Indian water policy. The growing competition for water, brought on by national and international economic development, has fostered a readiness among tribal leaders to form alliances on regional water issues.

Various ongoing water disputes readily exhibit the influence of a national and international political arena. Two examples include the Mni Wiconi water project affecting the Oglala, Rosebud Sioux, and Lower Brule in South Dakota and the Makah, whose whale allotment has been frozen by Japan's veto in the International Whaling Commission in retaliation to pressure on Japan and certain other whaling nations to reduce their own whale harvest (*Indian Country Today* 2002d). The political arena for many reservation water concerns and water-related issues is no longer local, and indigenous leaders have developed strong, effective coalitions where needed.

**Economic Effects**

North American Indians face changes in their economic prospects on a daily basis. The rising pressure on fish and shellfish stocks, fed by international demand and distribution, has led to falling catches, listings on the roster of endangered species, rapidly expanding exploitation of previously noncommercial species, and aggressive, sometimes violent, competition in local commercial fisheries. The inauguration of aquaculture and hatcheries by northwest tribes in an effort to preserve threatened species is one type of response. Another is illustrated in the active opposition of tribes to logging, mining, agricultural pesticide runoff, and land development, in an effort to protect salmon-spawning grounds.

A spectacular case, previously cited, warrants further elaboration here. In the early 1970s the Eastern Cree bordering Quebec's James Bay (a southeastern extension to Hudson's Bay) discovered that an enormous, multidam hydroelectric development was literally ripping apart the lands they used for hunting, fishing, and trapping. The project was driven by Quebec's plan to export power to the United States, dominating the electricity market for the continental northeast and providing an economic base upon which Quebec's secession from Canada could become politically viable (Coon-Come 1991; Hazell 1991). The Cree began an epic, thirty-year battle that resulted in huge damage awards and the shelving of the project's second and third phases. Recently, the Eastern Cree signed an agreement with Hydro-Quebec to proceed with a modified second phase, offset by compensation, environmental guarantees, and tribal development input (*Indian Country Today* 2002b; Krauss 2002). Here, the Cree were initially victims of the global energy market but are now embracing a planned reinvigoration of their society through the specific opportunities that negotiating the second phase presented to them.

Mention needs to be made of a singularly visible development in Indian country that has only marginal links to water: casinos (and their new configuration as gambling-centered destination resorts). Where reservations have viable commercial locations, tribes are aggressively developing these enterprises. Where reservations are too remote, tribes are strongly pushing for access to off-reservation sites.[21] Today, there are more than four hundred tribally owned casinos, large and small, in the United States. The resistance from state governments has often been strong, but with many state budgets facing major shortfalls, governors and legislatures are now cautiously willing to expand Indian casino gambling. Casino gambling—together with hotels, spas, sports betting, celebrity entertainment, transportation, and regulation—thrusts Indian tribes into a national and international industry in which financing can come from distant countries, management expertise is highly developed, and competition is fierce.[22]

The casino industry is North America's most prominent case of indigenous groups not only being affected by globalized industry but also participating in it. Something of the same effect can be seen in the thirteen Alaskan native corporations, created in 1971 as a byproduct of the Alaskan oil pipeline. After a very difficult beginning, several of the corporations have become multibillion-dollar international corporations, propelling their indigenous directors and shareholders down a similar development path.

Where casinos have become highly profitable, the effects on the owning tribes have been significant (Anders 1999). Internal voices opposing casino involvement have been overridden; new, business-savvy leaders have emerged; reservation services have expanded; tribal membership rolls have become battlegrounds; lobbying and direct involvement in state and federal politics have increased explosively; tribal politics have become strained; external challenges to tribal sovereignty have grown; and strong jealousy has developed between tribes with commercially advantageous locations and tribes whose remote locations do not attract many gamblers. Gaming tribes have found their tribal councils consumed with casino management; patronage systems have emerged within some tribes to keep top leaders in power; and occasional examples of dishonest management have come to light. Water conflicts are involved in the casino and Alaskan corporate industries only in particular instances, but globalization's effects on the Indian gambling industry are ubiquitous.

Tourism in Indian country, often water-related (fishing, hunting, canoeing, trekking, nature observation), is another activity visibly channeled by globalization's forces. Indian groups in the United States and Canada are, to a surprising extent, involved in tourism (McDowell 2001). Numerous web sites and business associations promote Indian-owned tourist companies and guide services. In addition to tourist promotions for their casino industry, many tribes in the United States operate campgrounds, with tipi- and hogan-style vacation accommodations, and offer interpretative education, guided eco- and photo-tours, and hunting and fishing trips, both on and off the reservation. Interestingly, various tribes, as well as non-Indian entrepreneurs, have courted Indian-focused tourism in Germany and other European countries, capitalizing on a substantial European romanticism about

North America's Indians (McDowell 2001). An Alaskan Tsimshian village even has a contract with a cruise line to pick up shiploads of debarking passengers, bus them to a nearby village, put on dances and entertainment, sell them various craft and native art products, and bus them back to the ship (*Indian Country Today* 2002i). Tawdry as that may appear, it illustrates the changes that are entailed when linking to the tourist industry, which has come to be globalized in terms of promotion, scheduling, financing, and standards of service.

The economic impacts of globalization today touch almost all production and consumption of goods and services. Indian reservations engage in both. The global influence may be weak, confined to the types and brands of products sold on the reservation, or obvious and far-reaching, as when a reservation participates heavily in a casino or tourism.

**Cultural Effects**

The economic and political changes described above are linked to cultural changes. Thus, the agendas, the shared terminology, the etiquette, and the tools of international political activism constitute new additions to the knowledge inventories of indigenous peoples. Further, venturing into a globalized business entails the embrace and skillful use of the off-reservation society's institutions: inaugurating a casino-anchored destination resort or building a tourist business involves the tribe in state and federal regulation, insurance, accounting, marketing, financing, safety issues, management oversight, daily decisions about investment, business risk and allocation of profits, and sometimes overheated reservation politics. When a tribe participates heavily in these arenas, then the politics, the social structure, and the character of life on the reservation are profoundly influenced, even transformed.

At the same time, some cases exhibit determined efforts to maintain traditional cultural values and identity. When the Lummi, the Puyallup, the Yakama, and the Nez Perce strive to protect salmon, traditional cultural values are strongly in evidence. To these groups, salmon affirm deep cultural roots. Cultural values also play a role in Indian opposition to development projects and flood control measures affecting the landscapes of their former territories. Washington State's Snoqualmie oppose stream modifications to their centrally important

Snoqualmie Falls; the Yankton Sioux protest flood control projects that threaten burial grounds; the Allegany Seneca still feel the wounds of Kinzua Dam; Sandia Pueblo resists recreational development on the Sandia Mountains looming over Albuquerque; and various British Columbian groups trenchantly resist the stark defacement of clear-cut logging on lands with which they identify. Yet, when they embark on large-scale involvement in casinos, tourism, and other business enterprises, they also accept lifestyle changes that sharply revise their prior cultural experience.

**Environmental Effects**

The pressures of globalization can also induce or entice tribes to damage the environmental qualities of their reservation. One case actually stems from the acute absence of water. Currently, the Skull Valley Band of Goshutes, living south of Great Salt Lake in Utah, is seeking to allot part of its desert reservation for the temporary storage of spent nuclear fuel from the nation's power plants. The Goshutes are advantaged by having desolate, arid land and a sovereignty that, they argue, exempts the land from state and national environmental requirements. They will earn a handsome fee from the multistate utility consortium that will build and run the storage facility. Enormous opposition, not least from the entire State of Utah political leadership, is implacably contesting the Goshutes' plan (*New York Times* 2003). Where is globalization in this? The Goshutes aspire to something other than poverty. Indian casinos cannot be built in Utah, and no one has identified a more attractive enterprise that will bring economic activity to the Goshute reservation.[23] To the Goshutes, their one option for economic growth is to lease a section of their reservation to the national and global energy industry to serve this singular, odious market until the eventual completion of the Yucca Mountain facility in Nevada. To date, no other political entity in the nation has agreed to allow such a nuclear storage facility to be built within its jurisdiction. That a small Indian group has stepped forward reveals its lack of more salubrious options. Globalized industry has reached the Goshutes.

We have seen in these cases that the aggressive corporate search for more economic resources and profit opportunities repeatedly threatens the resources on which Indian reservation communities depend. These include water supplies and water rights, forest and stream habitats, underground deposits of minerals and fuels, and even land for storing nuclear waste. North American tribal groups often find themselves on the offensive to mitigate these threats to their reservations' future viability and to protect the numerous places of cultural importance on the lands they formerly occupied.

## EFFECTS ON INDIAN HEALTH

The chapters of this book examine not only globalization and water, but also their impact on health. What interlinkages of these factors are evident among North American Indians? I begin with comments on the health conditions that already exist on reservations and reserves.

By any measure, health conditions on Indian reservations and reserves, though clearly improving, remain poor. While available statistics are vulnerable to many deficiencies, the following are recent estimates. Over the past half century, diabetes has grown to "epidemic proportions" (Gohdes and Acton 2000:221). American Indians have diabetes at three times the rate of Americans as a whole (Brenneman et al. 2000:106). This trend is probably linked more closely to reservation conditions that lead to alcohol consumption, obesity, and poor diet than to a genetic factor (Gohdes and Acton 2000:222–224). Liver disease associated with alcoholism is more than eight times the American average. Tuberculosis is more than five times higher. HIV infections are lower than in the population at large, but rising rapidly (Asturias et al. 2000:358–359).

Morbidity and mortality on reservations are linked to poverty, isolation, racism, and the many deprivations derived from the history of Euro-American contact and eventual domination. The unraveling of their traditional societies, the dominant society's failure to allow Indians to form strong new societies adapted to the colonial-postcolonial situation, and the intrusion of alcohol, street drugs, and youth gangs are further factors. The result has been the perpetuation of reservation societies whose troubles bring about unfulfilled and shortened lives. In 1993 the average lifespan of American Indians relative to all Americans, while much improved, remained 4.4 years less (Brenneman et al. 2000:118). Today, suicide and homicide are about one third higher than the national rate. Injuries caused by accidents, often involving alcohol, are more than three times more likely to result in death than in the general population (P. A. May 1999:232–233). Spousal abuse and other forms of interpersonal violence are an acknowledged problem among American Indians. A similar picture obtains in Canada.[24]

The quality of reservation health services, a continuing federal trust responsibility since the 1830s, has been poor for the most part—often outrageously poor. Since the mid-1970s, however, the extent and quality of health services to American Indians have much improved. Average lifespan has lengthened (Starr 1996:27–30). In recent years, government physicians have become more tolerant of native medicine and healing traditions, reducing the sense among Indian patients that going to a clinic or hospital means enduring the message, implicit or explicit, that their beliefs are bunk. The emerging holistic attitude of Western medicine toward native healing has strengthened delivery of medical services.

How does globalization, affecting many of the water disputes reviewed in this chapter, also affect health? Curiously, there is little in either the scholarly literature or journalism to guide us. Discussions and news coverage of these water disputes make almost no mention of the consequences for health, partly because the consequences are hard to discern and partly because the joint linkages among water, health, and globalization need greater attention. Too, more widespread and more visible linkages may exist between globalization and health when water issues are not a criterion. Globalization's effects on global patterns of disease and health have received useful recent attention (see McMurray and Smith 2001). Also, Brennan (2003:8) writes, "an increasingly common pattern, especially for groups marginalized by globalization, is one of a high prevalence of both infectious diseases and NCDs [noncommunicable diseases]. One of the main causes of this uneven progress in health is the impact of global capitalism and the way it has shaped lifestyles." America's Indian reservations reflect this common pattern.

On the negative side, globalization may be expected to impair health conditions when it leads to greater unemployment and lowered incomes on the reservation. For decades, the federal government has funded, with modest success, programs encouraging businesses to locate production facilities on Indian reservations. These companies are vulnerable to the same market pressures that companies elsewhere face: to reduce labor costs or relocate to overseas low-wage zones. These decisions deepen poverty on reservations, and negative health consequences surely ensue.

Globalization pressures also strengthen the use of street drugs and inhalants (glue and paint sniffing) on reservations. Very high rates of unemployment, especially among the youth, probably facilitate this flow. The health consequences are obvious. A 1985–1989 survey of American high school students found that, in addition to alcohol consumption, Indian students "had the highest use of marijuana, hallucinogens, heroin, stimulants, sedatives, and cigarette[s]" (Howard et al. 2000:282–283). Among adults, alcohol consumption is apparently the most common form of substance abuse and is the largest factor in Indian mortality. The rates of addictive drinking appear to vary substantially from one reservation to another but are typically very high (P. A. May 1999:231–232).

Globalization's effect on health also has a positive side. Cash settlements for land claims and, especially, earnings from the casino industry have brought substantial new wealth to some reservations—in many cases, the first *Indian-managed* wealth in generations. New and improved health facilities are being funded from these new moneys. Available data are insufficient to assess whether globalization's effects on reservation health are, on balance, positive or negative, but we can conclude that both are happening.

## A GLOBALIZATION CAVEAT

Our view of globalization needs to be tempered by an awareness that globalization, while showing enormous potency and effect over the past two decades, is not inexorable or immune from constraining forces. Indeed, globalization today is reportedly in a "pause," with the value of aggregate international trade as a percentage of total economic activity—a useful measure—actually falling (Leonardt 2003). At this writing, SARS and avian flu concerns have dealt tourism in the Far East a powerful blow, and political unrest in many parts of the world has had a similar effect. Meanwhile, anti-terror measures are disrupting containerized ocean shipping. European resistance to genetically modified foods has undermined corporate investment in genetically modified cultigens. Economic nationalism is evident in many countries' policy agendas, including that of the United States. Newly imposed protectionist tariffs on agriculture and forest products are much in evidence. Popular rebellions against the destruction of traditional local markets have caught the attention of various Latin American governments, and underdeveloped nations of the world are outspoken in their opposition to further free trade agreements without a better balance of economic benefits. The World Trade Organization, charged with advancing the global economy, is now rethinking founding assumptions, for example, that all parties benefit from freer trade, that no country has rational reasons to reject Western intellectual-property laws, and that national and ethnic interests will always give way to the desire to reap the economic benefits of globalization.

Despite the great surge globalization has experienced over the past two decades, the process is neither unstoppable nor beyond reshaping to accommodate offsetting political needs and national interests. Nevertheless, one can expect globalization to continue broadening and strengthening in ways that exploit the political and numerical vulnerability of North America's reservation-based indigenous communities.

In sum, water issues are very much part of the concerns and challenges faced by the indigenous peoples of North America, and, to varying degrees, these disputes reflect the powers and processes of globalization. In the main, globalization creates or exacerbates the water disputes and health challenges faced by reservation communities. Globalization reduces the relative isolation of reservation economies, societies, and cultures. It jeopardizes key resources and places of cultural significance and accelerates the intrusion of divisive change. However, globalization's influence is not uniformly negative. North American Indians have also found themselves embracing some enticing new options, despite the profound changes those options also bring.

### Notes

1. In this chapter, I use *American Indian* in preference to *Native American*, or other common terms, for the descendents of peoples resident in North America,

TOM GREAVES

including Canada and Greenland, when Europeans first encountered the continent. The term *American Indian* is the most widely used, collective label adopted by the groups themselves in "the lower forty-eight" states. *American Indian* is little used in Canada, where *natives*, *First Nations people*, and *aboriginals* are preferred. In Alaska, *American Indian* is not used for the polar peoples (Eskimos, Aleuts, or Inuits) of that state. All of the preceding terms can evoke strong feelings and can convey unintended messages. My use of *American Indian* in this chapter is for economy of expression only. I use the term *indigenous* to refer to the same populations when discussing features and challenges they share with other post-tribal peoples throughout the world.

2. Note that less than a third of American Indians live on reservations. This does not, however, diminish the importance of reservations, which serve as perpetual homelands where native culture and identity are strongly rooted.

3. Appadurai (2001:8) cautions, however, that "the trouble with much of the paradigm of area studies as it now exists is that it has tended to mistake a particular configuration of apparent stabilities for permanent associations between space, territory, and cultural organization."

4. In the United States, such treaties reflected wholly unequal political and military positions between the parties but yet provided the conceptual framework that conditions the nature of Indian law and forms the basis for sovereignty rights today. Although Canada has made more limited use of treaties, the legal framework for aboriginal relations is also one of agreements between nations.

5. Native Hawaiians, although certainly another indigenous group with many of the same problems and aspirations as mainland groups, are administered and counted separately by the US government. The total number of federally recognized groups varies from time to time as new groups are recognized or, in some cases, federal recognition is withdrawn.

6. Compiled from the web page of the Bureau of Indian Affairs 2003, Fogarty 2003, and *Indian Country Today* 2004.

7. These figures are taken from Statistics Canada 2003 and from Indian and Northern Affairs, Canada 2002. The Métis, of mixed Indian and (usually) French ancestry, are now classified as Indians in Canada.

8. Thirteen native corporations were established as part of the Alaska Native Claims Settlement Act of 1971, taking charge of some 44,000,000 acres allotted to the corporations and, thence, to their respective member villages.

9. The indemnity funds did, however, enable Eastern Cree to fund a successful campaign to stop later stages of the project and, ultimately, to specify the

conditions under which a new stage of the project could proceed. An account of the Cree and this struggle is available in Feit 2004. See also *Indian Country Today* 2002b.

10. Until 1998 the newspaper was edited and published by Tim Giago, an Oglala Lakota and winner of numerous national awards for journalism. Thereafter, members of the Oneida Nation purchased the paper. One may question whether the paper's coverage under its Oneida owners (who also own a major casino) has become skewed or less objective. I have noted little change, other than improved marketing arrangements and more coverage of national issues. In my view, the coverage of *Indian Country Today* remains similar to its content under Giago.

11. The process led to a rapid shrinkage of many tribal lands because the land "left over" after individual allotments could be declared surplus and be sold off by the government. Between 1887 and 1934 about 90,000,000 acres of former reservation lands became owned by non-Indians (Josephy 1982:132; Welch 1994:265; Pevar 2002:6–9).

12. The federal lease program has produced a contemporary scandal of huge proportions: over the years, the federal program failed to keep adequate records of lease contracts and changes in ownership of the leased parcels and failed to exercise proper stewardship of Indian lease income. Claims of funds lost, misallocated, or stolen since the Dawes allotment process began now amount to millions, perhaps hundreds of millions or even billions, of dollars. A lawsuit, Cobell *v* Norton, has resulted in allegations of records intentionally destroyed, two secretaries of the interior being cited for contempt of court, strenuous efforts by Congress to resolve the situation, and the expenditure of millions of dollars in computerized efforts to reconstruct payment histories. (See Brinkley 2003.)

13. "[Various legal] cases established for Indians what became known as the Winters' Doctrine…which held that when the United States government created Indian reservations, it also reserved, by implication, sufficient water in any streams running through or bordering on a reservation to carry out the purposes of that reservation—that is, to make the reservation livable by reserving, also, whatever water 'may be reasonably necessary, not only for present uses, but for future requirements.' Moreover, since it was ruled that treaties were 'not a grant of rights to the Indians, but a grant of rights from them—a reservation of those [rights] not granted,' the Indians, rather than the government, had reserved the water, which like the land was their property, and they were generally deemed to possess a paramount and first-priority right, ahead of any rights a state might

grant, to all the water necessary for a reservation's purposes" (Josephy 1982:155; see also Pevar 2002:241–243).

14. "Coal-bed methane is natural gas found in coal seams. Pressure from ground water holds the gas in the coal deposits. Releasing the gas requires pumping out large volumes of ground water" (*Indian Country Today* 2002j).

15. An excellent account of these cases is found in Cohen 1986:66–82.

16. These rulings were based specifically on treaty guarantees written into the treaties of the 1850s in the Washington area that ceded land in exchange for reservations and perpetual hunting and fishing rights off the reservation in all their "usual and accustomed grounds and stations" (see Cohen 1986:181–183). The rulings do not easily generalize to Indian tribes elsewhere, if such treaty clauses were not used.

17. In effect, the court affirmed that shellfishing rights had never been extinguished and that all subsequent property deeds for beaches where shellfishing can be said to have been a "usual and customary place" for prior Indian shellfish collecting carried this implicit right of Indian access. Compare the Northwest Indian Fisheries Commission newsletter at www.nwifc.wa.gov/shellfish/ with United Property Owners, Shellfish Case, at www.unitedpropertyowners.com/rafeedie-decision.htm and Holt 2000.

18. A highly relevant case involving basketry materials is described in Lerner 1987.

19. For the Nisga'a, see *The Economist* 2000, Rynard 2000, and the Government of British Columbia web pages at www.gov.bc.ca/tno//negotiation/nisgaa/default.htm. For the Gitxsan and Witsuwit'en, see Mills 2002.

20. See Melmer 2002a and also the Coalition's web site, www.mnisose.org (accessed June 11, 2004).

21. The competition among tribes for favorable off-reservation sites is especially fierce in New York State. Governor Pataki has sought legislative support for new, off-reservation Indian casinos to improve the state's budget situation and to rejuvenate the faded spa towns of the Adirondacks (see Peterson 2004).

22. Financing to establish the Mashantucket Pequot's casino, Foxwoods, came from a Malaysian entrepreneur. Major Las Vegas corporations, such as Harrah's, also provide casino financing and management.

23. The 1988 National Indian Gaming Regulatory Act stipulates that Indian tribes can qualify to open a high-stakes casino on their reservations if the state in which the reservation is located already allows or provides high-stakes gambling

(such as a high-payout state lottery). Unlike most states, Utah allows no state-sanctioned high-stakes gambling, so Utah's tribes cannot qualify under the act.

24. See Starr 1996 for a general summary of the history of health issues and government policies toward Indians in the United States and Canada.

# 9

# Water Management Reforms, Farmer-Managed Irrigation Systems, and Food Security

*The Spanish Experience*

**David Guillet**

We are in the midst of a crisis in fresh water; put simply, enough water of good quality is not available to go around. Well known forces are driving this crisis: population growth, urbanization, industrialization, and droughts. Less recognized are changes in the culture of water consumption as standards of cleanliness and health practice entail more bathing and the increased consumption of clean water.

Throughout the twentieth century, the usual response to shortfalls in water supply was to increase its availability by investing in large-scale, capital-intensive, hydraulic infrastructure such as dams and canal systems. "Augmenting supply," as this response is called, has not entirely disappeared in the new century. In Iberia, one million old-growth oak trees are being removed for the construction of Europe's largest dam, on the river Guadiana in southern Portugal. Spain's conservative government is promoting plans for the construction of 118 dams and 14 canals. In an era of high and rising economic and environmental costs, however, such projects are seen as increasingly anachronistic. At the outset of the twenty-first century, the dominant response to the crisis is to use market forces to manage the demand for water.

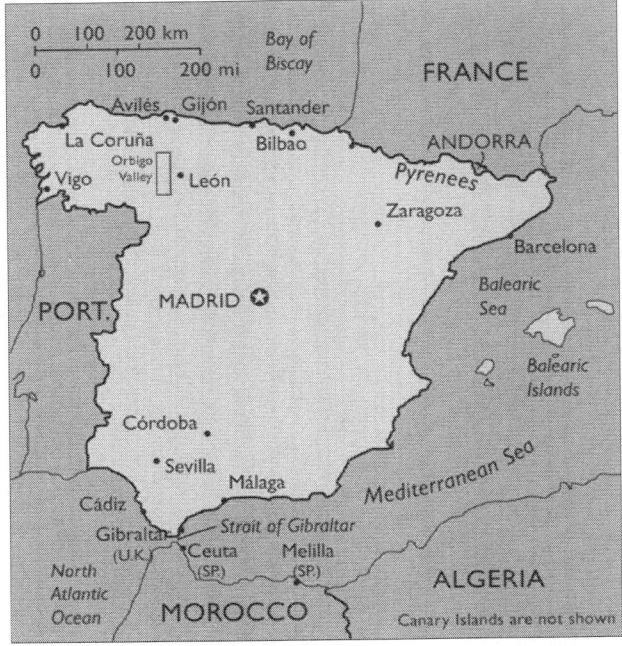

**FIGURE 9.1**
*Map of Spain.*

The most radical of demand management measures is the privatization of publicly held water and the institutionalization of water markets to allow its treatment as a commodity. Markets for federal water in the US West have been suggested as models (Anderson and Snyder 1997). A less preferable response is the recovery of the costs of operation and maintenance through volumetric pricing, measuring the amount consumed and charging users for this amount. Privatization and volumetric pricing require standardizing measures of water volume, using the new standards to recalibrate existing and new concessions, and installing physical devices to implement the new standards.

The impact of these measures on traditional farmers in the areas of water use and linkages with health raise new and unexplored questions. Three areas of potential impact of demand management have been suggested: the efficiency of water use, the direction of smallholder agriculture, and the equity of water access. I have addressed the first two elsewhere (Guillet 1997, 2000, 2002a; see also Derman, chapter 10, and L. Whiteford, chapter 2, in this volume). In what follows, I take up the potential implications of demand management for the equity of water access in farmer-managed irrigation systems (FMISs). Equitable water access is linked with health in these irrigation systems because water for irrigation often has other uses, for example, drinking, cleaning, personal hygiene, construction, fire fighting, and animal husbandry. A less obvious, but equally important, relationship of water access to the health of smallholders is its role in producing the food they consume—either directly, through subsistence production, or indirectly, through the exchange or sale of their products.

I begin with a discussion of the connection between property rights in water and land ownership and control before addressing the potential impacts of privatization and pricing on access. I then illustrate these issues with reference to the recent history of farmer-managed irrigation systems in the Orbigo Valley of northwestern Spain. Spain attempted to implement a range of demand measures in the 1879 Water Law and, since 1985, has put forth legislation and policies to provide for all the possible forms of demand management. The Orbigo Valley, after one hundred years of demand management and state intervention, can supply needed historical perspective on the response to attempts to implement water management reforms in countries with FMISs.

## PROPERTY RIGHTS IN WATER

Two basic problems are involved in irrigation. First, to extract water from the surface or the ground and transport it to the farmer without exceeding the source's productive capacity requires a technological solution. The solution can be relatively simple, such as a shallow well and a bucket lifted by a rope, or exceedingly complex, such as dam-impounded water released through a vast network of primary and secondary canals. Water's response to gravity makes it relatively inexpensive to deliver to fields and, by driving shafts, to mill grain, saw wood, and generate electricity. Lifting groundwater to the surface for irrigation and other uses, on the other hand, consumes energy. Unlike shallow wells and hand lifting, the complexity of sinking a deep artesian well can raise costs considerably. Even apparently simple technological solutions, such as digging a well and installing a lift device to exploit groundwater, can involve capital costs beyond what an individual can bear. High provision costs increase the likelihood of irrigators coalescing or the state intervening, through subsidies and in other ways, to reduce risk and capital costs.

The technological problem of obtaining water is related to a second problem, appropriation.[1] A way has to be found to exclude access to the water, lest farmers who did not contribute to the costs of the technological infrastructure divert it for their own use, a well known free-rider problem. Canal irrigation adds an additional difficulty. Upstream users can, at least potentially, take water first, leaving none for those downstream. The solution to the appropriation problem is to assign, to individuals or groups, property rights to water. Such rights could include the rights to consume, obtain income from, and transfer water to others.

Allocating exclusive rights to water directly, to farmers or to fields, requires partitioning water. Unlike other natural resources, such as animals, fields, surface ore deposits, or standing timber, water's fluid nature makes it extremely difficult to partition without costly and sophisticated absolute, volumetric measuring devices. Ownership shares of intermingled water are almost impossible to determine. The eminent jurist Blackstone put it well: "Water is a moving, wandering thing, and must of necessity continue common by the law of nature, so that I can only have a temporary, transient, usufructuary property therein" (Anderson and Hill 1975:176). Put differently, water's fluidity increases the costs of marking, monitoring, and enforcing property rights in it, particularly in comparison with stable natural resources such as land and forests. While flowing surface water most obviously fits this characterization, stationary water also can quickly become mobile. Groundwater, on the other hand, would seem similar to surface ore deposits or standing timber, for example, in adapting easily to assigned rights. Yet, aquifers and groundwater basins are much more unstable and unpredictable than commonly thought.

If private property rights are difficult to assign to water because of its fluid nature, does this mean that it must remain an open-access public good like air? No, not necessarily: smallholders throughout the world attach water rights to land and transfer them informally upon the transfer of land. Attaching water rights to land transforms permeable boundaries into impermeable by making the service area coterminous with land area. In this way, many other transaction costs stemming from the physical features of water are reduced. Attaching property rights to water as an attribute of land control and ownership is one strategy commonly found in farmer-managed irrigation systems.

## PRIVATIZING WATER

Given the association of water rights and land on the one hand and common property management on the other, privatization represents a potentially radical approach to managing demand. The process transforms water held as a public good or under communal control into a commodity capable of being transacted through sale, rental, and lease in a market. A farmer with rights to water as an attribute of his ownership or control of a field can find himself handed a piece of paper allowing him to sell or otherwise transfer the water to another, independently of the disposition of the field. Any form of direct or indirect communal control over the land through control over water distribution is lost.

In these settings, the distribution, control, and use of land govern the distribution of water rights. Land distribution is far from equitable in many agrarian societies. Demographic differentiation can, of course, contribute to inequality in farm size. Historically, however, inequalities in land distribution are often associated with inequalities in the distribution of other means of production and the coalescence of these inequalities into class divisions. Privatizing water rights in these situations does nothing to remove inherent inequalities in land distribution. Stripping water rights from land and turning water into a commodity makes it possible for a few landowners to capture all or most of the rights, creating a new class of waterlords. The lack of a requirement that the land to which water rights are attached be in use worsens the situation, rewarding absentee owners, land speculators, and lazy landowners. In the Brazilian state of Ceará, for example, large landowners own the bulk of the land; many underutilize their landed properties. Instituting tradable water rights would not only solidify their position in the economic structure but also allow them to become richer by selling their water rights. If they were unable to sell their water, then it might just accumulate in their hands with no net increase in water use efficiency (Kemper and Olson 2000:355).

The potential for introducing inequity into access to water through privatization recalls much in the agrarian history of countries of the south. In Latin America, for example, nineteenth-century reforms to privatize land laid the basis for the hacienda system and close to two hundred years of class struggle and conflict. While some *campesino* communities have managed to avoid falling within the orbit of haciendas, many retain inequities in water distribution stemming from the privatization of land. Certainly, there is no reason to believe demand management will redress existing inequities. Indeed, one can argue that it will enhance them.

Instituting tradable water property rights also raises potential third-party effects. In gravity-flow irrigation, upstream users can dramatically reduce the access to water of downstream users. Many FMISs take pains to ensure that this does not happen, rotating, for example, upstream-downstream irrigation sequences. Privatizing water rights can remove controls FMISs have exerted over upstream users and make it easier for them to abuse the system.

Moreover, surface water flowing through FMISs can have multiple, often competing, uses—for energy, cleaning, construction, fighting fires, and feeding animals—and be held under many forms of water rights. Privatizing water puts at risk water passing through the irrigation system with "hidden" uses. To avoid this, consumptive and nonconsumptive water rights can be set for nonagricultural ends. Uses can change over time, and FMISs should have the flexibility to reallocate consumptive and nonconsumptive water rights. Special rights must include continuous water delivery. Mixed uses of water in space and time put to rest the assumption behind fixed delivery volumes, that water is used only for irrigation. Fixed delivery is also opposed to the periodical cessation of agricultural activity for village festivities and pulsing supply caused by irregular precipitation in space and time. It works against those villages that specialize in certain crops and have peculiar requirements for water.

Equity principles should also be allowed to work in this regard. At one level, water trading might appear to reduce inefficient water management, but hierarchical political structures, insufficient information, and inadequate regulatory frameworks may coalesce to further marginalize the poor. For instance, the landless might attempt to improve their livelihoods through food processing or other types of cottage industries, but find themselves lacking access to adequate water, owing to monopolization of water rights by landlords.

As public water utilities are privatized and water is transacted between farmers, cities, and industries, private companies come to play a greater role in storing, managing, and transferring the water. In the United States, the sandbox of entrepreneurial extravagance, we have seen efforts by an entrepreneur to siphon rivers in northern California, fill giant bladders with the runoff, and tow the jumbo balloons with tugboats to San Diego (Bell 2002). The Texas oilman T. Boone Pickens is proposing to pump water out of the Ogallala aquifer and pipeline it to Dallas.[2] These may remain "pipe dreams," but they illustrate that a pattern of mergers of private water companies into international conglomerates is now unfolding. The three largest water companies in the United States—United Water, American Water Works, and USFilter—are now owned by the French and German conglomerates Vivendi, Suez, and RWE. Until recently, one of the big players was the water development company Azurix, a subsidiary of Enron Corp. The relentless pursuit of profit that drives these companies is now a major force in the global political economy and raises questions about water's role as a public good, its host role for endangered species, and its connection with third parties.

## PRICING WATER

Water pricing has been widely advocated by policymakers to obtain the capital to maintain existing infrastructure and install the sophisticated, costly water-measuring devices needed for standardization and volumetric pricing (Kemper and Olson 2000; Rosegrant and Binswanger 1994; Saliba and Bush 1987; Tsur and Dinar 1995; Winpenny 1994). Policymakers also argue that pricing can improve the efficiency of water use by reducing the demand for water. Pricing is rare in FMISs, but evidence suggests that, where found, it tends to be in the form of per-unit area fees. Farmers pay a fixed fee per hectare of land for the right to receive irrigation water. In a survey of 12.2 million hectares worldwide, for example, water charges were levied on a per-unit area basis in more than 60 percent of the cases (Bos and Walters 1990). Per-unit area fees do not directly influence water input and, it is argued, lead to inefficient allocation. Their chief advantages are that they are relatively easy to implement and administer and they require a minimal amount of information.

Proponents of demand management criticize per-unit area fees for their lack of influence over water input and lack of incentives to use water more efficiently. Several forms of pricing—volumetric, output, input, tiered, and two-part tariff—have been argued to meet this criterion and be efficient (Tsur and Dinar 1995). *Volumetric* refers to water charged for by the unit. In output pricing, water is priced by imposing a tax on the output produced from the application of water. With tiered pricing and two-part tariff pricing, the price rises for additional units of water (tiered pricing), or there is a fixed annual price and an additional volumetric price. Each of these pricing schemes, in its own way, influences water input and contrasts markedly with per-unit area fees.

When one moves beyond per-unit area fees to adopt pricing policies to reduce demand, a serious dilemma presents itself. On the one hand, levels must be set sufficiently high to deter demand. The International Water Management Institute has shown, in this regard, that instituting or raising the prices for water used for irrigation less than a few cents per cubic meter will have little effect on demand. Yet, prices sufficiently high to have the desired effect can be quite high proportionate to farm income. In the case of Egypt, the price required to induce a 15-percent fall in demand for water would have reduced farm incomes by 25 percent (Perry 1995, 2001). An apparently "token" charge, or increase in water pricing, to an outside observer can be an insurmountable burden to a poor farmer. For this reason, alternative strategies to pricing for increasing efficiency are being discussed. The situation described by Perry (2001:14–15) would apply to many FMISs around the world: "It is important to note that the incentives to utilize water productively are made clear to the farmer just as directly by rationing water as by trying to establish an appropriate system of water charges. In northwest India, the long-tested warabandi irrigation system (Malhotra 1982) is based entirely on ensuring an equitable distribution (over the land) of limited water resources. Water charges are not high, and not volumetric, but because all farmers are water-short, they experience directly the true value of their water ration, and strive to save every drop and maximize its productivity."

Other possibilities suggest themselves. In many instances, consumption-based fees could be charged to the FMIS rather than to individual farmers. Charging the FMIS makes use of its role as a social community by building on local knowledge and practice to allocate costs and protect vulnerable or marginal users in line with local standards of equity. Alternatively, if tariffs are charged to individuals directly, equity provisions can be built in to water pricing through an overall regulatory framework. For example, one low price can be set for a volume of water to meet basic domestic needs and minimal subsistence production, and another, full-cost rate, for water use in excess of these primary needs. Still another strategy is to ensure poor farmers access to an unpriced, prespecified quantity of water. This involves a two-step procedure. The quantity of water designated and the desired level of contribution for the deserving farmers are set on a social welfare basis. The remaining farmers are priced according to the efficiency rule. Given the social goal as expressed by the safety net, this approach tries to establish a second-best price structure that maximizes social welfare, with minimum loss (Tsur and Dinar 1995).

## STANDARDIZATION

In the demand forms of water pricing (volumetric, output, input, tiered, and two-part tariff), for prices to act as an incentive to reduce demand, measures of water volume must be standardized, existing and new concessions recalibrated, and physical devices installed to implement the new standards and measure consumption. Standardization is an issue in many traditional irrigation systems, where water rights are poorly specified and flexible and rely on approximate measures of water. Instituting more rigid, precisely defined, and absolute units of water use in these contexts raises the question of efficiency. Converting traditional rights allocated proportionally at the conveyance and distribution levels to transferable rights is possible, for example, but the transaction costs can be high.[3] It must be kept in mind that the costs of measuring quantitative and, possibly multiple, qualitative dimensions of water may be so high as to exceed the benefits (Eggertsson 1990:26). Incorporating sophisticated, absolute, volumetric measuring devices into traditional irrigation systems may outweigh the return in lowered consumption when compared with existing, low-cost methods such as allocation by proportionate shares or time. Moreover, measuring devices necessary for fixed-volume delivery have high maintenance costs. Passing on the costs of maintaining the devices to FMISs can lead to disputes.

David Guillet

## RESISTANCE TO DEMAND MANAGEMENT

Given the potential negative effects of water management reforms, small-scale irrigators are beginning to mount resistance to them. Enormous increases in the pricing of water used for domestic purposes have alerted irrigators to the implications of reforms. In Bolivia in 1999, the government responded to pressure from the World Bank to adopt structural adjustment policies by privatizing the water system of its third largest city, Cochabamba. The government granted a forty-year concession to run the debt-ridden system to a consortium led by Italian-owned International Water Limited and United States–based Bechtel Enterprise Holdings. The newly privatized water company immediately raised prices. Although the minimum wage stood at less than $65 a month, many of the poor had water bills of $20 or more. Water collection also required the purchase of permits, which threatened access to water for the poorest citizens.

The response was immediate and dramatic. A Coalition in Defense of Water and Life, known as "La Coordinadora," was formed to channel the resistance, and it quickly took a position demanding the return of the water utility to public control. In April 2000, following weeks of mass opposition, the government gave up the battle and cancelled the contract with the consortium. Control of the city's water system, including its $35 million debt, was turned over to La Coordinadora. The defeat of the privatization contract marked the first major victory against the global trend of privatizing water resources (Grusky 2001).

Following on the Bolivia turnaround, in July 2001 a $110 million structural adjustment loan for Ghana was approved, based on the country's implementing seven "prior actions," including a requirement to "increase electricity and water tariffs by 96 percent and 95 percent, respectively, to cover operating costs." Initially, the country awarded a contract to Enron/Azurix, but it was soon cancelled following public outcry over bribes allegedly paid during the bidding process. The bidding process was started over. As in Bolivia, a coalition, the National Cap of Water, is organizing public opposition to the privatization plans (Grusky 2001).

Public opposition to inequities in the pricing of water for irrigation has been much less common. Often hidden and localized in the past, it stands ready for the kind of public attention that the pricing of water for domestic use has claimed. We turn now, for an illustration of this and other issues, to the Orbigo Valley of northwestern Spain.

## DEMAND MANAGEMENT IN THE ORBIGO VALLEY OF NORTHWESTERN SPAIN

Spain would seem an unusual, if not inappropriate, choice for examining the issues related to the impact of water management reforms on smallholder irrigation. Many arid and semiarid countries of the south would envy the country's performance. Spain has managed since the 1950s to build a strong industrial base and a high standard of living. The death of the dictator General Francisco Franco on November 20, 1975, ushered in a new era of political and economic reform. For almost forty years, his regime had molded economic and political institutions to suit his ends. Following his death, many of these institutions were either scratched or reconfigured along democratic lines. The most far-reaching of the reforms was a new constitution in 1978, establishing the groundwork for a newly decentralized and democratic Spanish state. The unitary state charged with administering central government services in fifty provinces gave way to a semifederal political structure. The regional parliaments, judiciaries, and executives of seventeen newly created autonomous communities now share responsibilities with their counterparts in Madrid. The radical reconfiguring of state structure and the shift of power from the center to the periphery lack precedents in Spanish history.

Spain was rewarded for its economic and political performance by inclusion in the first wave of countries to join the European Union (EU). It has grown considerably in the years since, making difficult reforms to increase its competitiveness in world markets. Socially and culturally, Spain is fully incorporated into Western Europe. Yet, the agricultural sector, while benefiting from economic growth, still accounts for only 3 percent of the GDP of a country heavily dependent on services, particularly tourism.

Spain continues to have much in common with agrarian societies of the arid and semiarid south. Historically, irrigation has played a major role in the country's agriculture: 6,188 irrigation systems created before 1900 control 1,200,000 has, about one third of the irrigated land (Jiliberto and Merino 1997). Their time depth dates, in many instances, to the Roman and Islamic presence (Butzer, Mateu, and Butzer 1985; Glick 1970, 1979; Clot and Torres Grael 1974). These systems are largely gravity-fed and divert water from rivers to irrigate fertile alluvial terraces called *riberas* and *vegas*. The immense majority has less than 200 hectares of irrigated land, and about half have fewer than 20 members (2,000 of the 4,280 for which data exist in the official register). The large-scale, long-canal systems of Valencia, Murcia, Orihuela, and Alicante in eastern Spain have been extensively studied and are often discussed as archetypes of long-term, successful, and robust common-property regimes (Glick 1970; Maas and Anderson 1978; Ostrom 1990:69–82). While land restructuring has consolidated small, dispersed holdings, many farmers display characteristics of a classic peasantry, with a portfolio of small, irrigated fields worked by family labor. Traditional irrigation systems like these can be found throughout the European Mediterranean, in France, Italy, and Greece.

The Orbigo Valley of northwestern Spain illustrates well the range of issues associated with the enactment of demand management (Guillet 1997, 1998, 2000). In Spain, efforts to manage demand antedate the current debate, beginning more than a hundred years ago with the 1879 Water Law. The 1879 Water Law contained an explicit agenda of measures, including the standardization of water measurement, direct and indirect measurement of water consumption, and the linkage of provision costs and water access to the amount of water consumed, all of which are recognized principles of demand management today.

The enactment of these measures in the Orbigo Valley would have negatively impacted the traditional water rights of *presas*, quasicorporate irrigation associations of towns and villages formed to irrigate their lands with water diverted from the Orbigo River. Farmers resisted the implementation of these efforts, which they perceived as an attenuation of their rights. For example, the 1879 Water Law empowered state officials to force water users lacking flow-measuring devices to install these at their own expense and assume the costs of measuring their irrigated area. Municipalities resisted entreaties by the civil governor to supply information on their water consumption and, when the information failed to appear, refused to assume the expenses of obtaining the data. When the state initiated a project to install measuring devices and control demand, reengineering costs were discovered to be very high. Lacking the resources to implement direct measurement of consumption, the state adopted an indirect measure of irrigated land, in effect, laying the groundwork for per-unit area fees. The acceptance of an uncomfortably high figure of 1 liter per second per hectare reflects the state's fear of the unrest that a more "realistic" figure would have generated among Orbigo farmers.

More commonly, lacking formal channels, farmers resorted to informal, evasive actions to circumvent formal rules or procedures, negotiating "informal adjustments" or "working arrangements." For example, tariffs were imposed on one irrigation community, the Presa de la Tierra, with little outcry as that community passed the burden of collecting tariffs from end users to villages and towns. Historically, this is consistent because presas delivered water to villages and towns, which were responsible for delivering it to end users. Presas minimized expense by radically limiting the number of contracts and passing on to intermediaries the costs of contracting with end users. The solution built on the Spanish practice of municipal councils managing collectively owned pastures, forests, and threshing ground and assigning water rights to fields. This offers a model for volumetric supply: deliver water to intermediate groups—towns, villages, branch canal and irrigation organizations—and let these groups distribute the water to end users. It is interesting that this policy is identical to what many forward-thinking water policy specialists are advocating today: charge tariffs to the FMISs rather than bill individual users, in order to reduce otherwise excessive transaction costs.

Villages and towns, in turn, minimized real costs by renting harvested fields as pastures and using the proceeds to pay water fees. They were able to do this through local customs requiring landowners to open up their fields to communal pasturing after harvest. Side arrangements between municipalities and *forasteros* (outsiders) eased the potential free-rider problem caused by the village or town as the taxing unit.[4]

In 1952 the Central Irrigation Syndicate of the Barrios de Luna dam (Sindicato Central de Riegos del Embalse de Barrios de Luna) was created to manage the water of a dam that came on line in 1956. The dam reduced significant seasonal inundations and periodic and catastrophic flooding. The Central Syndicate charged a board, the Junta de Explotación, with scheduling and coordinating the release of water from the dam. Meetings to coordinate its distribution to irrigation occur weekly during the irrigation season.

While the Central Syndicate implemented proportional voting rights in its governing board, irrigation communities often ignored them in selecting their representatives. Succession to office within irrigation communities frequently diverged completely from regulatory guidelines and was adjusted informally to fit historical experience. Ancient formulas governing the obligations of villages and towns to the presa became subject to alteration. In some instances, the civil governor exercised discretionary power to force changes; in others, a tacit, informal agreement reoriented relations. The experience of negotiation and accommodation between the Presa de la Tierra and the state was replicated with minor variations in other Orbigo presas upon their organization into irrigation communities. The use of per-unit area measures of water consumption was a key axis on which these negotiations continued.

Franco's death and a new constitution in 1978 brought localized and hidden resistance into public view. In 1985 a new Water Law was implemented to correct deficiencies of the earlier law and to adjust water policy to the creation of regional autonomous communities in the 1978 constitution. It was formulated and enacted in the political space opened up to new actors and new issues long held in abeyance until the death of Franco. The 1985 Water Law emphasized water use planning. Population growth, changes in life style, urbanization, industrialization, and severe droughts had dramatically increased water demand. To meet the challenge, the 1985 Water Law charged a newly created National Water Council with overseeing the drafting of a National Water Plan and balancing the interests of regional autonomous communities and the central government. When a draft plan was released in 1993, it triggered a national debate over whether to pursue a traditional course of increasing water supply, by constructing dams and transferring water from water-surplus basins to water-deficit basins, or a new one instituting measures to manage demand and save water. The controversial measures under debate included the application of standardized volumetric measures, tariffs levied on water consumed in excess of an optimum threshold, sanctions for water wastage, and water pricing prioritized by use.

Local resistance to demand management then became subsumed in a national debate over water planning; Orbigo farmers were caught up in interest-group politics at the regional and national levels. In this debate, they found themselves included in an association of concessionary irrigators, the National Federation of Irrigation Communities (Federación Nacional de Comunidades de Regantes [FNCR]). The FNCR originated in the 1950s in reaction to Franco's large-scale program of dam construction. The government empowered the watershed authorities with executing the plans. Irrigators chafed at the power of the watershed authorities and their own inability to participate in program planning and implementation.

At the start of the 1950s, officials of irrigation syndicates in southeastern Spain initiated an exchange of correspondence complaining of the excessive interventionism. A chance meeting of representatives from the larger irrigation communities of Aragón and Valencia followed in 1952. The leadership of the Acequia Real del Júcar, a large and important irrigation community in Valencia, took the lead in organizing the federation. At the outset, the movement sought to improve the dismal relationships between irrigation communities and watershed authorities. The framers of the legislation establishing watershed authorities had sought to provide a structure to facilitate the participation of irrigation communities, but it was not working as intended. The confederations distrusted the irrigation communities and saw them as a distraction. The rare interactions were usually restricted to the provision by a watershed official of a needed signature to paperwork submitted by an irrigation community (Díez Gonzalez 1992: 51–128).

The founders of the new agrarian organization had to walk carefully. Franco approached labor movements by co-opting them into an official "vertical" labor movement, the Centro Nacional de Sindicatos, closely linked to the government. When the agricultural wing, the Hermandades Sindicales Agrarias, caught wind of the incipient irrigators federation, plans were laid to co-opt it. In the 1953 Congress of the Hermandades, officials cited provisions in legislation implementing watershed authorities, which called for the incorporation of irrigation communities into syndicates. The expressed intent to incorporate the irrigators movement into the Hermandades alerted the fledgling FNCR, which immediately sought, and won, official recognition in a June 1955 decree. It held its first general meeting the following

October and took immediate defensive action to prevent being incorporated into the Francoist labor movement. This battle was lost: a 1959 decree annulled earlier rulings authorizing the formation of the FNCR. The FNCR appealed to Spain's Supreme Court. There the appeal lapsed, putting the federation in limbo, lacking legal recognition, ignored by the power structure. Despite these problems, three national congresses (in Valencia in 1964, Seville in 1967, and León in 1972) kept the federation alive. Finally, in October 1972, the Supreme Court ruled in favor of the federation, reestablishing its legitimacy.

One of the first activities of the post-Franco regime was to issue a decree in April 1977 legalizing trade unions and introducing the rights to strike and to engage in collective bargaining. The 1978 constitution moved further, establishing the rights of unions to defend their interests and granting all citizens, except members of the armed forces and the judiciary, the right to join, or not to join, a union. The Organic Law on Trade Union Freedom of 1984 defined the negotiating role to which larger unions were entitled and prohibited any form of discrimination on the part of employers. These changes brought the FNCR, and a host of labor organizations formed in the wake of Franco's demise, into the mainstream.

One ancillary goal of the framers of the 1985 Water Law was to create a regulatory framework for irrigation communities. The process could easily have turned into a top-down exercise, drawing on the "state of the arts" debated in international congresses and academic treatises, of little relevance to the unique historical experience of Spanish irrigation communities. Fortunately, this proved not to be the case. Since their inception, the congresses organized by the FNCR had given voice to problems with the internal organization and functioning of irrigation communities, and at the 1972 congress in León, work began on a set of regulatory statutes for their internal organization. This proved to be portentous: with guidance from the FNCR, the statutes were polished and adopted into the 1985 Water Law. The FNCR support of the Water Law was considered essential, and, indeed, the organization successfully stopped the inclusion of a section on water pricing by threatening to withdraw its support for the law unless the plank was removed (Díez Gonzalez 1992; Nadal Reimat 1993:168). During the 1970s and 1980s the FNCR consulted regularly with the

Ministry of Public Works. It was given a vote on the Environmental Advisory Council when the ministry was reconfigured in 1994 to include environmental oversight. When the Ministry of the Environment was created, the FNCR was given a vote on the advisory council of that body.[5] The FNCR has collaborated in the national irrigation plan (Plan Nacional de Regadíos), the Reform of the Water Law, and the European Union's formulation of water policy (Federación Nacional de Comunidades de Regantes de España 2002). It contracts for training and technical assistance with the Ministry of Agriculture, Fishing, and Food and mentors regional confederations such as the influential Federación de Comunidades de Regantes de la Cuenca del Guadalquivir.

## THE LEÓN IRRIGATORS COUNCIL

In March 1997 a draft of a plan to reform the 1985 Water Law (Borrador del Anteproyecto de Ley de Reforma de la Ley 29/1985) led to a meeting in Hospital de Orbigo of representatives of twenty irrigation communities in the Province of León, held at the initiative of the Barrios de Luna syndicate. At that initial meeting, those attending decided to take action to found a León Irrigators Council (Concejo de Regantes de León). Two weeks later, a larger meeting was attended by representatives from all the irrigation communities in the province with more than 100 has of irrigated area. At that meeting, a vote was taken to oppose the proposed reforms and take steps to formally organize a body of Leonese irrigators. Three weeks later, the newly formed organization negotiated a contract with the University of León for an evaluation of the proposed reforms and their impact on Leonese irrigators. The cost was shared 50/50 between the irrigation communities (assessed at 5 pesetas/hectare of irrigated area) and the provincial council of León (Diputación Provincial de León). In October, a meeting was held to prepare a response (*alegaciones*) to submit to the National Water Commission concerning the Water Law reforms. The Barrios de Luna Syndicate prepared the response, fifty-one pages in all, and submitted it on the behalf of the León Irrigators Council to the regional watershed authority, the Confederación Hidrológica del Duero (Concejo de Regantes de León 1998).

The alegaciones of the León Irrigators Council make several

points. First, in a familiar criticism, irrigators decry their lack of participation in administrative deliberations. The provisions for ceding water rights are taken to task for their potential to freeze economic activity. The use of volumetric measuring devices is criticized for its inability to take into account the loss of water in transport or the reuse of excess water. The reuse of excess water, in particular, is described as confused and simplistic. The additional costs make farmers unable to compete with those in the European Union who benefit from abundant and predictable rainfall. The procedures contained in the proposed reforms for financing new hydraulic infrastructure are criticized. In sum, they rejected the proposed reforms. The position of the León Irrigators Council had little impact on the outcome of the reform, which the National Water Commission approved in April 1998. Of all the irrigators' representatives, the only vote against the reform was that of Angel del Riego, a Leonese and representative for the Duero basin.

In September 2000, the Junta de Castilla y León signed a contract with the León Irrigators Council for a six-year program to modernize the hydraulic infrastructure of 22,900 has of irrigated land in the two provinces of Castille and León.

Other actors are now instrumental in the new politics of demand management. Environmental groups became active in León in the 1970s. In 1982 enough groups existed to constitute a fragile coalition, the Coordinadora Ecologista de Castilla y León. In 1988 it was reorganized and strengthened as the Federación Ecologista de Castilla y León. The political influence of the Leonese environmental movement is out of proportion to the actual membership and financing of these groups. Only two associations, Aedenat and Tyto Alba, count more than two hundred members; two follow at around one hundred, and several minor groups have fewer than fifty members. Although most lack strong financial backing and organization, the movement has repeatedly demonstrated its power. It brought to a halt one of the last large-scale dam projects on the Omaña River by publicizing its potential impact on native habitats. It led to the creation of the first environmental advisory body in an autonomous community, the Consejería del Medio Ambiente y Ordenación del Territorio in Castile and León, with independent funding and watchdog powers, and pressured the autonomous community to enact a host of progressive environmental legislation. Astute use of print and electronic media accounts for much of the success of the Leonese environmental movement (Relea Fernández, Ríos Pacho, and Panigua Mazorra 1994).

An environmental movement respected for its successes in stopping large dam projects and weakening a coalition of Public Works Ministry officials and public works contractors finds itself courted by political parties as a new avenue to middle-class support. In recognizing the role of the environmental movement, the state is responding to pressure from the European Union to adopt demand management and retreat from supply augmentation, as well as acknowledging the political position of environmentalists.

In 1996 a government, under the conservative Partido Popular, replaced the socialist regime and took a much more favorable approach toward the use of market mechanisms in water management. The pace of the "deliverables" of water reform picked up noticeably. In 1997 the draft of a plan to reform the Water Law, Borrador del Anteproyecto de Ley de Reforma de la Ley 29/1985, was issued, followed the next year by a long-awaited White Paper on Water recommending a series of measures to increase water use efficiency and manage surface and groundwater jointly (Ministerio de Medio Ambiente 1998). In 1997 watershed authorities finally delivered management plans for each of the major river basins. The government released its long-awaited national irrigation plan (Plan de Regadíos), and the autonomous community of Castile and León issued its irrigation plan in 1997 (Junta de Castilla y León 1997).

The long-awaited national water plan, the Plan Hidrológico Nacional (NHP), and its approval by the Parliament in July 2001, entering into force in August of that year, signalled the most important development of the period by far. Spain now had on paper an overall framework for water policy and a tool for coordinating water management in each of the watersheds. The plan immediately sparked controversy, this time over the role of government agencies in water policy and the appropriate targets for water planning. The NHP contains vestiges of Franco era policy with plans for the construction of 118 dams and 14 canals, one 434 miles long. Most controversial is a proposal for the transfer of 1,050 cubic hectometers per year from the Ebro river basin—a "water-surplus" agricultural watershed housing the extremely poor mountains of Aragón and the rice-farming Ebro Delta—to four "water-deficit" basins in predominantly tourist-oriented areas along the coast. Up to one third of the total cost would come from EU funds, in particular, the European Regional Development Fund and the Cohesion Fund. This proposal has been bitterly opposed by environmentalists. The most influential environmental groups, WWF/ADENA, Ecologistas en Acción, Greenpeace, and SEO/Birdlife, came out strongly against it, objecting to the construction of costly and environmentally degrading dams and water transfers. They cited the failure to consider alternatives, including the use of market forces to make water use more efficient and save water.[6]

## WATER PRIVATIZATION: THE LEY DE MODIFICACIÓN DE AGUAS

The conservative government in 1990 issued a set of modifications of the 1985 Water Law to facilitate privatization as a measure of demand management (Law 46/1999 of December 13, 1999). The primary vehicle provided by the law is the opportunity for the contractual cessation of water rights under a set of requirements. The holder of a concession or a use right "sells" all, or part, of it temporarily. The contracts must be written and must respect the priority of uses established in the Water Law. Prior authorization from the respective watershed authority is necessary. The contract must be communicated in writing to the watershed authority, which has a time period in which to reply. If there is no answer, then it is considered authorized. The authorization can be denied if the transfer violates water use planning, public interests, or environmental parameters. Watershed authorities can establish procedures, such as setting a maximum price, to guard against speculation. The cessation of one's rights is temporary and does not result in permanent loss. Private nonconsumptive rights cannot be ceded. Parties to the transfer set the compensation through mutual agreement, although the watershed authority in question can establish a maximum amount. The law creates the possibility for establishing "water banks," centers for the exchange of water rights. Watershed authorities setting up water banks can publicize the opportunities to acquire rights and to acquire them and transfer them to a third party.

The provisions in the Ley de Modificación for the buying and selling of water generated considerable controversy and much interest among irrigators.[7] Its impact has yet to be felt, but, unquestionably, it has fomented considerable political turmoil. Environmentalists welcomed this as a move in the direction of saving water, as long as the transfer of excess capacity gives the owner benefits that compensate for his loss. In regions that are marginal for agriculture, but with strong demand from other sectors (hotels, tourism), farmers have expressed interest because they could obtain more benefits by selling their rights. In agricultural regions, farmers are much more critical and see water privatization as of a piece with water pricing.

The European Union, on December 22, 2000, issued a Water Framework Directive (WFD) furthering moves toward demand management and legitimizing the Spanish conservative government's embrace of water privatization. Measures contained in the NHP for water pricing are in line with the mandate of article seven of the WFD. Water pricing has been the subject of considerable protest by farmers in Spain and throughout the Mediterranean. The FNCR sees its best hope for defending its interests as moving beyond the national level to engage other similarly positioned irrigators increasingly threatened by EU directives. Coalescing with other Mediterranean irrigation associations to fight at the level of the European Union makes good political sense. At the 10th National Congress of the FNCR, held in April 2002, a new Euro-Mediterranean Irrigators Community made up of members from France, Greece, Italy, Morocco, Portugal, Spain, and Tunisia was launched. The objective of the new community is to strengthen the position of Mediterranean irrigators in the European Union and protect farmers against water pricing and challenges to their water rights from other sectors.

In the post 1985 era of demand management, the state finds itself with strange bedfellows. The environmental movement gained respect for its successes in stopping large dam projects and breaking a coalition of the Public Works Ministry and public works contractors following the first draft of the National Water Plan. Political parties have woken up and now court the environmental movement as an avenue for acquiring middle-class support. EU environmental directives have been a major source of power: the Spanish environmentalists act as the monitor of Spanish compliance, gathering data, publicizing shortfalls, sharing information, and so on. The environmental movement obtains financial and administrative support from an international network.

## CONCLUSION

Farmers throughout the world can be expected to resist demand management, given the threats it represents to their health and livelihood. Losing access to water puts at risk their production of food for consumption or exchange, the most obvious potential impact. But they may also think of the possible impact on "hidden" uses of water, besides irrigation. Removing the right of villages to use irrigation water can dramatically reduce that available for drinking, cleaning, and personal hygiene, with serious health consequences. The inability to draw on irrigation water for construction purposes may create difficulties in replacing rundown and inadequate housing and in building housing for new families. Insufficiently watered animals fall prey to disease and give less milk, fiber, meat, and manure, and less energy to drive farm implements. The loss of irrigation water to fight fires is a serious risk to the built environment.

In the privatization forms of demand management, the threat stems from the attachment of water rights to land. Breaking the connection between water rights and land ownership and control makes it possible to create a new class of waterlords out of landowners who capture all or most of the water rights that become available through privatization. Water managed communally often entails measures designed to ensure a "safety net" to keep smallholders afloat. Such measures are known to include indirect controls over land use through the allocation of water for irrigation by crop and restrictions on water during droughts (Guillet 1992). Turning water into a commodity and freeing it from land and communal control put at risk social welfare mechanisms working at the local level. In the pricing form of demand management, no matter how carefully one designs pricing policies, the fact remains that an increase sufficient to improve water use efficiency will still be too much for the average farmer to deal with.

Indeed, the mere mention of privatization and pricing today is sufficient to alert traditional irrigators virtually anywhere in the world. The Spanish experience suggests some paths this resistance can take. High costs and hidden or overt resistance can make volumetric pricing exceedingly difficult to implement, and planners may well decide to "fall back" on per-unit area fees. This strategy can, admittedly, provide funds for operation and maintenance. Whether it will have an effect on increasing the efficiency of water use, however, is debatable, not so much because it lacks the incentives to wring out inefficient management but rather because water use may already be quite efficient. Traditional irrigation systems, which are long-standing and display resiliency and sustainability, may be quite efficient, once one controls for the sophistication and the state of their hydraulic infrastructure. Understanding water use efficiency may require moving beyond the levels of the irrigation system and the field to the river basin as the more appropriate level of analysis. Recognition that drainage water can remain in the system and become available for use by downstream irrigators has forced a revaluation of classical approaches to efficiency. Irrigation may be relatively inefficient at the irrigation system and field levels but quite efficient at the basin level (Guillet 2002b).

Where civil society has been restructured to facilitate stakeholder participation in the elaboration and implementation of water management policy, the Spanish experience shows how irrigators can create viable interest groups. In this regard, Spain is fortunate in having a strong union of farmer-managed irrigation systems. FMISs elsewhere in the world would envy the FNCR's ability to write the section of a major national water law that regulates irrigation communities. As of yet, this experience—irrigators organizing into effective interest groups, as opposed to successful farmers organizations—is uncommon. But in the years ahead, as water demand management proceeds apace, irrigators can be expected to mobilize increasingly along lines similar to the FNCR and to the Cochabamba irrigators union formed in the context of that region's water crisis in 2000.

Indeed, irrigator mobilization illustrates the key tensions of globalization, among new forms of capitalism, organizational formations, and social formations of primary identity (Castells 1996). The Spanish experience, for example, demonstrates the conflict between the European Union's promotion of demand management principles through its regulatory authority, on the one hand, and the social formations linked to new national identities of water users, on the other.[8] Politically, the hidden and localized resistance of the past, marked by side agreements and working arrangements, is shifting to new actors sharing information and competing in public arenas where NGOs, government representatives, World Bank officials, and local stakeholders battle it out. The process is becoming increasingly transparent, participatory, and public.

**Notes**

1. I follow Ostrom, Gardner, and Walker (1994:9–15) in distinguishing between provision and appropriation problems.

2. For Texas now, water—not oil—is liquid gold (http://www.citizen.org/cmep/Water/us/bulksales/texas/index.cfm).

3. "When transactions occur in canals that are divided using fixed flow dividers (*marco partiadores*), it is necessary to measure and modify water flows through many of the individual fixed flow dividers within a canal system. For instance, if a tertiary canal delivered water to six farms (1, 2...6) in succession, and farmer 2 sold water to farmer 6, then fixed flow dividers to farms 2 through 6 would have to be modified and recalibrated by an engineer. If trades occur outside the tertiary canal, the modifications become more complicated" (Hearne and Easter 1995:39).

4. *Forasteros* contrast with legal residents (*vecinos*). Forasteros represented a potential free-rider problem because water rights are attached to land no matter where the landowner lives. Free riding can occur when a farmer claims water for land in a municipality other than his own and fails to contribute labor, cash, and kind to the maintenance of irrigation infrastructure. To resolve the free-rider problem, villages and towns charge forasteros an extra fee, added to the normal tariff calculated for a vecino. While this is not entirely legal, the state acquiesced out of a pragmatic concern for the collection of fees.

5. Government of Spain, B.O.E. no. 58, March 9, 1994; B.O.E. no. 192, August 9, 1996.

6. For the influential WWF/ADENA position, see "Seven reasons why WWF opposes the Spanish National Hydrological Plan and Suggested Actions and Alternatives," http://archive.panda.org/europe/freshwater/pdf/SNHP_seven_reasons_against.pdf.

7. See http://www.infoagro.com/riegos/ley_aguas.asp.

8. The new territorial identities forged by the transfer of water from water-rich to water-poor regions constitute yet another factor.

# 10

## The Incredible Heaviness of Water

*Water Policy and Reform in the New Millennium in Southern Africa*

**William Derman**

Southern Africa is in the midst of massive social, economic, and environmental changes. These form a mixed balance sheet of difficulties and opportunities, challenges and possibilities. On the one hand, multiple and interconnected economic, employment, environmental, and health crises are occurring. On the other hand, opportunities have arisen with the end of apartheid in South Africa and Namibia and the ending of the wars in Mozambique and Angola, and possibilities (not yet realized) of genuine development now exist in Zimbabwe, Malawi, and Zambia.[1] All parts of the region are being integrated into, and are influencing, the world economy and environmental agreements and accords, albeit in uneven ways.[2] As part of these processes, Southern African nations are experimenting with reforming the fundamental resources of land and water. These reforms blend local and international initiatives.

In this chapter, I examine some international and national policies and programs on the global menu of water reform. I suggest that the existing multiple, overlapping, and contradictory perspectives on water policy are and are not being adjusted to Southern African contexts. In

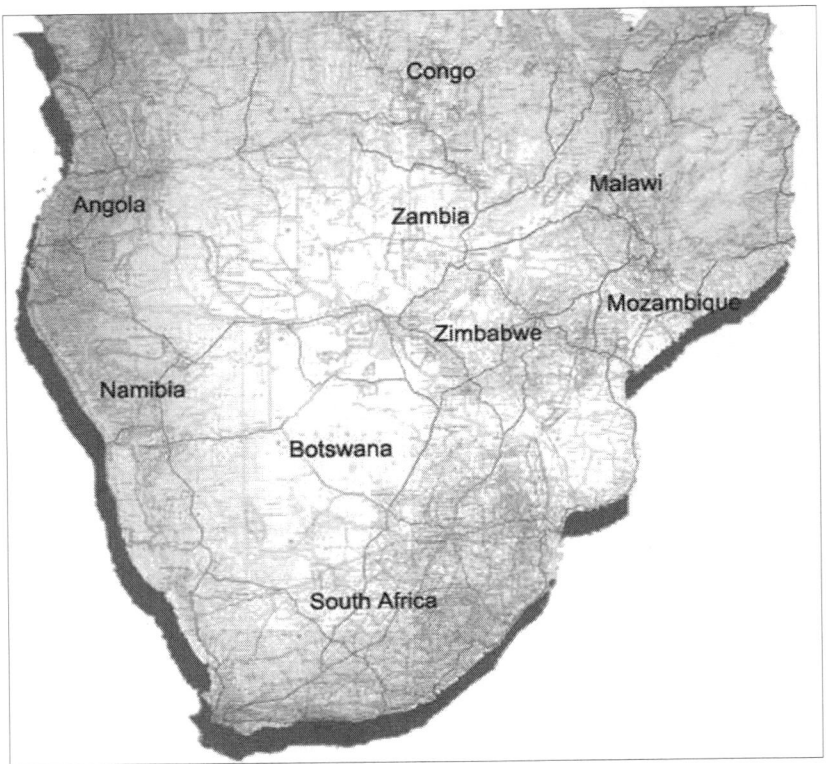

**FIGURE 10.1**
*Map of Southern Africa.*

exploring these frameworks, I present the case of Zimbabwe to demonstrate how wider changes in the political economy can derail prudent, systematic planning in the water sector. Despite the careful elaboration of new legislation and institutions, these are currently failing to attain their objectives. Zimbabwe, in particular, and Southern Africa, in general, raise the issue of how land and water reforms mesh.[3] Also, Zimbabwe illustrates that local practices and customary laws regulating water use were not of concern to Zimbabwean planners or their expatriate advisors. When Southern African states complain that their views are not being heard, they are invariably making reference to their national laws and policies, not their own local management systems.[4]

Many statements express the critical importance of water in the highly varied region of Southern Africa. For example, "water is the most strategic resource for sustaining all life forms in Southern Africa. Its effective management is an essential precondition for alleviating poverty and improving human health, food security, environmental sustainability, overall economic development and regional security" (Maro and Thamae 2002:261). In a parallel fashion, the Global Water Partnership's (2000) newly formed Southern African division envisions a water world in which there is "equitable and sustainable utilization of water for social and environmental justice, regional integration and economic benefit for present and future generations." (In a similar vein, see World Water Council 2000 and World Water Forum 2000.)

The goals for water reform and management include poverty alleviation or elimination, environmental conservation, reduction of disease, increased agricultural productivity, decreased vulnerability to droughts or floods, provision of safe drinking water adequate for all citizens, and good systems of sanitation that prevent or diminish waterborne diseases and user fees. In sum, these policies promote human and environmental well-being in Southern Africa without draining the public purse. The title of this chapter points to the complexity of the undertakings and the enormous weight that water bears on the human condition—our survival, well-being, and development.

In broad terms, what is the nature of the water crisis in Southern Africa? Is it growing scarcity, or are other significant issues involved? In Southern Africa, as elsewhere, a growing crisis is predicted in which water will become increasingly scarce unless a particular strategy for water management is adopted. But many frameworks are available for assessing the water crisis and choosing policies. Southern Africa and Zimbabwe, in particular, remind us that local and national interests remain strong enough that multilateral institutions such as the World Bank do not always get their way.

This chapter is organized into five parts. This one gives a brief introduction to Southern Africa. The second outlines the major policy options for water reform. I suggest, contrary to the notion of a single, global, capitalist water program, that the various frameworks currently being utilized for water reform are not coherent. They overlap and emphasize different dimensions of water and water reform. The third part discusses the case of Zimbabwe. Zimbabwe has particular importance in the region because it has implemented a substantial portion of its water reform. The fourth part comments on the incorporation of human health into water reform policy and practice in Southern Africa. The fifth part responds to the central question, can water reform and water policies adequately respond to so many expectations and goals?

## CURRENT INTERNATIONAL FRAMEWORKS GUIDING WATER POLICY AND WATER REFORM

The Dublin Principles form the starting point for discussions of international water policy in Southern Africa.[5] The following four principles were agreed upon in Dublin:

1. Fresh water is a finite and vulnerable resource, essential to sustaining life, development, and the environment.

2. Water development and management should be based on a participatory approach involving users, planners, and policymakers at all levels.

3. Women should play a central part in the provision, management, and safeguarding of water.[6]

4. Water has an economic value in all its competing uses and should be recognized as an economic good.

Narrative or discourse analysis constitutes one fruitful approach toward understanding the frameworks utilized for constructing water policies. As this book demonstrates, multiple frames are employed to analyze the water crisis. Political ecology has been a useful way to examine how power relations are reinforced in discourses about "the environment" maintained by powerful actors. Political ecology points toward the asymmetries of power, the unequal relations among the actors in explaining the interaction between society and environment (Adams 2001:252).

Peet and Watts (1996), in reviewing the frontiers of political ecology, observe that discursive approaches to the analysis of environment and development are central to understanding which discourses become most important or hegemonic. This area of political ecology includes research on the sociology of science and knowledge, on the history of institutions and policy on environment and development, and, what is important for the purposes of this chapter, on the globalization of environmental discourses in relation to "new languages and institutional relations of global environmental governance and management" (Peet and Watts 1996:11).

In an equivalent manner, Stott and Sullivan (2000:2) conceptualize political ecology as "a concern with tracing the genealogy of narratives concerning '[t]he environment,' with identifying power relationships supported by such narratives, and with asserting the consequences of hegemony over, and within, these narratives for economic and social development, and particularly for constraining possibilities for self-determination."

In this chapter, I suggest that several discourses exist and that they offer less hegemony and more choices than Stott and Sullivan imply. Instead of just one central or hegemonic discourse, there can (and should) be several. In addition, these discourses are not isolated; they interact with one another. The acceptance, rejection, or transformation of these discourses has real outcomes for differing sets of actors and interests. This chapter explains the discourses and their outcomes for practice, water availability, and water access. In the sphere of water management, emerging sets of global institutions are setting, or attempting to set, international water policies, strategies, and goals. One set privileges the environment; another, growing food scarcity. another, the right to water; and a fourth, the commercialization and privatization of water. Despite much theorizing about the decline of the nation-state in the era of globalization, Southern Africa points in the opposite direction. Control and management of water remain central to nation-state concerns and will not disappear any time soon (Derman 1998).

The new global institutions and networks for water, agriculture, biodiversity, health, and trade interact and compete with one another.[7] Some of these institutions oppose, for example, efforts to privatize water supply, and others support them. These new global institutions and networks attempt to enroll nations and policy makers into their programs. They provide resources, training, and networks to countries in the developing world that are employed or tasked to carry out the agendas of the global institutions and networks. They each attempt to construct institutional capacity in the nations in which they work as they exert influence on policy outcomes.

More often than not, the attempts to change international or national policies do not go unchallenged. As the World Bank (1993, 2002b), for example, promotes its approach to global water management, it is faced with analysis and critique by nongovernmental organizations (NGOs) and national governments. As the International Union for the Conservation of Nature (IUCN) puts forward its view for sustainable water use, it is critiqued by more people-oriented NGOs. Simultaneously, large private corporations are encouraging privatization in order to garner new business for themselves.

Currently, several discourses and actors with highly differentiated economic and political power are being utilized for water policy and water reform. Promoters do not describe their frameworks as discourses. Labeling them "discourses," as anthropologists do, relativizes them, from the perspective of those who accept or believe their own "discourse." Each set of organizations or institutions believes that it is promoting a "truthful" and "scientific" approach that will best solve water policy and water management institutions. Put slightly differently, the kind of deep reflexivity that anthropologists engage in is quite distinct from the approaches to water management or to political leadership that are charged with controlling a nation's water (see especially Allan 2002). In short, we return to the classic anthropological conundrum of balancing the "real world" problem of water scarcity with the interpretive one of analyzing competing discourses without necessarily judging them.

The discourses available for locating the "water crisis" crosscut the divisions between northern and southern nations, developed and underdeveloped. The institutions promoting solutions to water issues endeavor to build coalitions to generate an international consensus that their approach is the best one. In this next section, I explore four perspectives utilized in international water reform. This discussion is not meant to be comprehensive or exhaustive, but to highlight those approaches that have had greatest relevance to Southern Africa.

### Scarcity Frameworks

The major framework for understanding how to best manage water rests upon global and local water scarcities. The growing scarcity of water—both for nature and for people—can be understood within very diverse frameworks. It is not the case that the growing scarcity of water calls for a uniform response. For example, Tony Allan (2000:23), head of the Water Research Group at the University of London, states that, for the Middle East and North Africa (MENA) and Southern Africa, local water resources are insufficient to meet current and future needs. He suggests that several MENA nations have already run out of water but that this is not yet a major problem. Allan argues that "virtual water," the water embedded in food and other commodities, provides the regional answer to water scarcity. Implicitly, he suggests that such transfers can provide a solution to absolute water scarcity. As Allan (2002:29) graphically argues, "More water flows into the MENA region annually as virtual water than flows down the Nile into Egypt."

Also focusing on scarcity, Rosegrant, Cai, and Cline (2002a) argue that a crisis is escalating at the intersection of population growth; greater water needs for domestic, industrial, and agricultural use; and a stable, if not shrinking, water supply. Rosegrant and his colleagues present a sophisticated neo-Malthusian approach. They contend that water should be treated as a commodity, following the Dublin principle of water as an economic good. In turn, establishing markets for water would lead to pricing systems that reflect water's true cost and value and would result in more effective water management. Requiring people of means to pay for their water would create an incentive for them to conserve it. According to this line of argument, the financial resources necessary to provide water to those too poor to purchase it would thus be generated.[8] Given the deep poverty in Southern Africa, it is difficult to see how this solution will work in the short term.

A very divergent alternative of growing scarcity places the problem squarely on the consideration of water as a commodity and the increasing privatization of that commodity:

> As the planet dries up and water supplies are bought up by private interests, we have begun moving into a new economic configuration, where sprawling cities and agribusiness operations thrive and the wells of private citizens and local farmers run dry. Old ways of wasting water—like the rights trading that benefited a few but devastated the Owens Valley in southern California—are being revived, though they were demonstrated failures in the past. Meanwhile, in

> Third World countries, where children are already dying of thirst, the World Bank and the International Monetary Fund make privatization of water services a condition of debt rescheduling, and the poor soon find they are unable to pay for the skyrocketing costs of water and sanitation services. What lies ahead is a world where resources are not conserved, but hoarded, to raise prices and enhance corporate profits and where military conflicts could arrive over water scarcity in places like the Mexican Valley and the Middle East. It's a world where everything will be for sale. (Barlow and Clarke 2002:76)

Both these narratives locate the problem in scarcity, with strong policy statements as to how to proceed. Yet, there are water-scarce and water-abundant nations, nations that are facing immediate water scarcity and nations that will do so in the near or distant future. Freshwater distribution remains profoundly unequal. The reasons for scarcity vary within and among nations. Globalizing water scarcity often obscures more than it clarifies.

Another rendering of scarcity focuses on environmental needs and requirements. In the first three frameworks (virtual water, growing scarcity of water, and growing expensiveness and scarcity of water due to commodification), water as a human resource is privileged. In the third, nature is emphasized: "Of the more than 3,500 species currently threatened worldwide, 25 percent are fish and amphibians. The inevitable result of further human abstraction of water on this scale will be degradation or complete destruction of the terrestrial, freshwater and coastal ecosystems that are vital to life itself" (IUCN 2000:ix). Unlike many other international organizations, IUCN argues from an explicit moral, value-based position that fosters a greater intrinsic regard for nature: "Respecting the intrinsic values of ecosystems, and the benefits they provide, implies leaving water in ecosystems to maintain their functioning. This water, together with the water that is needed to meet basic human needs, is a reserve that has priority above all other water uses. Only water resources in excess of these basic needs should be thought of as 'available' for allocation to other uses" (IUCN 2000:14). With its evolving sustainable-use perspectives, IUCN has been systematically grappling with the best ways to handle scarce resources such as water in an environmentally sustainable manner. At the same time, it has been at the forefront in funding studies of water demand management in Southern Africa.

Growing water scarcity, intended by many authors to lead to greater global concerns and actions, can lead to inappropriate or alarmist actions. There can be growing global water scarcity without local problems. Indeed, Namibia stands out as water-scarce in absolute terms, but not in terms of water available per capita. In the water scarcity projections of Hirji et al., eds., (2002), Namibia has the lowest average rainfall and the highest per capita water availability in SADC, aside from the Democratic Republic of Congo.[9] This is true, according to them, in 2000 and will still be in 2025. Water scarcity can exist globally but not locally—and it can be solved by various means. I have already cited Allan, who argues that several Middle Eastern and North African nations have already run out of new waters to utilize. Yet, because they are able to import a large amount of water-intensive grains, they can have adequate water.[10]

Despite the complexities surrounding ideas of an ever-increasing water scarcity, ongoing efforts are providing global solutions to these issues. The World Bank has been a leader in supplying a global political economy of how-to-do water reform. In February 2003 it issued a new policy chapter for water resources management. The World Bank argues that it has a comparative advantage in the water sectors and that, because demands for bank services are strong, it needs to continue meeting them. Yet, because national and regional water reforms allow so much room for maneuvering, I suggest that this will continue to be the case. All water reform, in part, contains some version of water considered as an economic good.

**Water as an Economic Good**

Water as an economic good is one of the four Dublin Principles. Managing water "economically" is one of the cardinal rules of the new water-management systems. Gleick et al. (2002:37) address what it means to recognize water as an economic good: "Among other things it means that water will be allocated across competing uses in a way that maximizes its value to society. Such allocation can take place through markets, through other means (e.g., democratic or bureaucratic allocations), or through combinations of market and nonmarket processes."

Gleick et al. (2002) argue for a broad reading of what constitutes managing water as an economic good. They contend that the economic terrain should not be ceded to free marketers. Nonetheless, in the water management literature (Guillet, chapter 9 in this volume), the market and prices for water are most often cited as the "solution," or a large part thereof, to the problem of growing water scarcity. In opposition to the broad interpretation of *economic*, many scholars and practitioners argue that only the market can allocate water effectively and efficiently. The argument rests on the requirement of removing politics from water and letting allocation take place through a disinterested mechanism, within limits, of course.[11]

Even those institutions that urge an increased role for markets see markets within a wider set of policies. For example, The International Water Management Institute (IWMI), part of the Consultative Group on International Agricultural Research (CGIAR) system, currently advocates integrated water management, increased stakeholder participation, and policies that will benefit the poor, stressing the importance of markets and appropriate pricing.[12]

Conceptualizing water as an economic good does not mean that "nature" and "the environment" are ignored (Perry, Rock, and Seckler 1997). Many new management plans emphasize nature's needs. The South African integrated catchment water plan details how the Department of Water Affairs and Forestry will have to include water as a resource and describes water's part in the biotic components of a catchment or watershed. This is a historical shift in its mission. The department must now protect aquatic ecosystems in its water management policies and practices (Government of South Africa 2000). Such environmental concerns can be linked to either the growing scarcity of water or more economic uses of water.

### Water as a Human Right

Access to fundamental resources such as water moved center stage in development and human rights discourses pushed by the Johannesburg World Conference on Sustainable Development in September 2002 and in many other international settings. For many years, proponents of a rights-based development approach have argued that access to basic water should be seen as a human right (Gleick 1999; Ferguson and Derman 1999; Hellum 2001). The Convention on the Rights of the Child (CRC) gave the child a right to clean drinking water. In a reinterpretation (CRC, Article 24), the Committee on Economic, Social and Cultural Rights of the United Nations, on November 26, 2002, asserted a human right to water as part of other rights found within the International Covenant of Economic, Social and Cultural Rights.[13] The committee concluded that satisfaction of basic water needs can be interpreted as a human right implicit in the right to livelihood, as embedded in Article 11 of the Covenant on Social, Economic and Cultural Rights (see Eide 1995). From this perspective, a right to water derives from the right to life, the right to health, and the right to food (see L. Whiteford, chapter 2 in this volume; Eide 1995). Like the dictum "water should be managed as an economic good," water as a human right sets a new goal and standard but leaves open questions of how and in what time frame water will be paid for, who will pay for it, and how this right can be realized within the "real world."

The South African Bill of Rights guarantees the right of access to sufficient water. The South African Water Act reinforces the right of all South African citizens to a daily supply of clean water close to one's home. The Government of Zimbabwe continues to maintain the idea of "primary water," which means that rural peoples can continue to use water for domestic purposes without payment (Government of Zimbabwe 1998a). In short, several frameworks for water policy and reform overlap and sometimes compete with one another. This provides both opportunity and constraint for Southern African nations as they refashion theirs. Water as a human right has emerged as both a counter to and a complement of water as an economic good. How limited this right is and how it will be enforced remain to be seen. Also unknown is how many of South Africa's poor will be able to avail themselves of the courts to gain their rights. The ramifications of a right to water are staggering indeed if it is taken to be an international law that applies globally. This would produce massive priority and policy shifts. It becomes important, before dismissing this alternative, to imagine how this could happen. Before we turn to Southern Africa in greater detail, the last framework that needs to be considered is the environment.

## Water in the Environment

As all humans require water for life, so do virtually all living things. In addition, the vast ecosystems depend on a predictable (if varied) water supply. To large measure, human management of water has been for narrowly defined human purposes and has not systematically included the range of environmental needs and purposes. How to incorporate the environment into water management and policy remains a highly contested dimension of water reform. Hirji et al. (2002) provide a detailed account of the requirements for water management and planning in Southern Africa if environment were included. Among many suggestions, they name the following six for incorporating environmental sustainability (for humans also) (Hirji et al. 2002:296–310):

1. Guarantee of a minimum water requirement to maintain human health for all people.

2. Guarantee of water sufficient to restore and maintain the health of ecosystems. Specific amounts will vary, depending on climatic and other conditions. Setting and implementing the environmental flow requirements will require flexible and dynamic management.

3. Collection of data on water resources availability, use, and quality. Data will be made accessible to all parties.

4. Maintenance of water quality to meet certain minimum standards. These standards will vary, depending on the location and how the water is to be used.

5. Avoidance of human actions that impair the long-term renewability of freshwater stocks and flows.

6. Creation of institutional mechanisms to prevent and resolve conflicts over water.

The essential requirement of water for virtually all life creates an urgency for incorporating the environment into all water reform and management. As the oceans are polluted and used as sewers, with the loss of thousands of species, and as the environment in general endures multiple profound threats, this urgency intensifies. Moving from principles and ideas to implementation of new policies and laws, however, produces tensions and conflicts.

Southern Africa has become an important location for examining this movement from ideas, frameworks, and policy alternatives. It is engaged in redoing laws, creating new institutions, facilitating the acceptance of the Dublin Principles and other international documents, and proposing and implementing new systems of data gathering and information. No path to water management is easy or simple, no matter what mix of principles are selected. Using the case of Zimbabwe, what are the burdens and promises placed on changing water policies and practices?

## WATER REFORMS IN SOUTHERN AFRICA

The racial systems resulting from settler colonialism in Southern Africa continue to influence contemporary politics and national-level policy. Because Southern Africa has been characterized by profound, long-lasting fissures originating in a colonial and settler history, efforts to undue historical injustices and redress drastic inequalities have partly fueled the period of independence. Water, like other resources, was subject to appropriation by colonizers, who, in turn, became ruling minority power holders. As the new power holders, they used state resources to obtain access to and increase their annexation of the regions' relatively scarce waters. White farmers received broad and important subsidies for the establishment of irrigated farming. The Namibian (South West Africa), South African, and Zimbabwean (Southern Rhodesia, Rhodesia) colonial governments invested heavily in dams and water supply.[14]

Since independence, the redistribution of land and water has figured centrally in all efforts to diminish social inequality, as well as to reduce poverty.[15] Although land reform has received the most attention, water reform, water redistribution, and irrigation take a central place in all transformation strategies.[16] Due to the extreme dryness of Namibia and the uneven distribution of rain in South Africa and Zimbabwe, these nations do require thoughtful, careful, more long-term water reform. This subregion has attracted the attention of many water-focused organizations or ones with a strong water policy influence, such as the World Bank.[17] South Africa and Zimbabwe have new water acts and have revamped institutions to manage water.

These new water acts and policies are a mix of history, national context, and international policies (Derman 2001). All are influenced and partly shaped by the World Bank's 1993 policy statement on water management. The major donors to water reform in the three nations were also in agreement with the World Bank's policy, the Dublin Principles, and their own aims and objectives in the water sector. The major donors have included the governments of the Netherlands, Norway, the United Kingdom, Germany, and Sweden. In Southern Africa, though, they worked through an already established set of institutions, scientists, engineers, and private companies.

From a public health standpoint, Southern Africa suffers from an inadequate water supply (especially in rural areas) and poor sanitation. These are largely responsible for the high levels of waterborne diseases. Infectious waterborne diseases include schistosomiasis (bilharzias) and the diarrheal diseases of dysentery, cholera, and hepatitis. These are almost endemic in rural areas. The HIV/AIDS pandemic means that HIV-positive individuals are susceptible to waterborne diseases and others, including pneumonia and tuberculosis. Individuals and households with HIV/AIDS individuals have a reduced capacity to obtain sufficient water for drinking, washing, and other essential needs. Once again, cholera has become endemic in most Southern African countries, indicating poor sanitation and poor water supply.

Although most Southern African states have standards for the various uses of water, they cannot appropriately monitor most waters. The key proposed element for assuring water quality is polluter pay, which means that corporations, businesses, and government agencies must declare which chemicals or organic materials they are putting into waters they discharge. They are then to be charged according to the difficulty of cleaning up their discharge. This is taken up below for Zimbabwe.

For reasons of space, only Zimbabwe is considered in detail here. Zimbabwe has put in place new institutions and the accompanying acts and statutory instruments to implement water reform.

The Water Act of 1998 and the Zimbabwe National Water Authority

Act were to remedy past legal and institutional inadequacies.[18] In the following, we focus on the policy framework guiding the reforms, as well as the potential conflicts embedded in them. "Towards Integrated Water Resources Management: Water Resources Management Strategy for Zimbabwe" (Government of Zimbabwe 2000c) articulates the policy framework. Water, in these planners' view, is a critical national resource to be vested solely in the state. Unlike the earlier water acts, this stipulates that private individuals and corporations can no longer own water.[19] The policy document asserts that all Zimbabweans should have equal access to water and stakeholders should be involved in decision making in the development and management of the resource. All development of water resources should be economically viable and environmentally sustainable (Government of Zimbabwe 2000c:11). Ironically, despite the emphasis on access, equity, and state-owned water, most of the reform processes involve commercial water, not primary water. Zimbabwe attempted not only to keep control of the waters through national ownership but also to manage them economically by creating a new business-oriented, independent parastatal organization. Thus, it appears to be true to its history as a highly centralized state while seeming to incorporate new water-management global policies (Derman, Ferguson, and Gonese 2000).

Zimbabwe's waters have been divided into the categories of commercial and primary since the beginning of the twentieth century. This division of water seems to reflect the core land-tenure division between commercial (formerly European) lands and communal (formerly Tribal Trust) lands. It also reflects the dual legal system in which imported Roman Dutch law and British common law applied to the white settlers and customary law regulated relationships among black Zimbabweans. In the Water Act of 1998, but not substantially different from earlier acts, *primary water* is defined as water used for (1) domestic human needs in or about the area of residential premises, (2) animal life, (3) making of bricks for private use, and (4) dip tanks (Government of Zimbabwe 1998a, section 32, p. 1). Commercial water use is an economic concept that includes agriculture, mining, livestock, hydroelectric power, and so on. To access primary water, no one's permission is needed; to use water for commercial purposes, permits are now required (Government of Zimbabwe 1998a, section 32, p. 2). It is the obtaining of a permit that legitimizes the use of Zimbabwe's waters for commercial purposes, be they agriculture, mining, industry, or town and municipality waterworks. Turning to key provisions of the two acts (Government of Zimbabwe 1998a, 1998b), greater equality of access is to be achieved through the following five measures:

1. End the priority date system of first in, last out. This is to be replaced by a twenty-year permit system. The new allocation system remains undefined. We presume that it will be some form of proportional allocation so that in drought years all users will lose an equal proportion of their water.

2. Broaden the scope of who can apply for a permit to use water. Communal area residents can now apply for permits on their own, without having the district administrator do so on their behalf. Water to be used for agricultural purposes is still tied to land. What this means for communal area residents without individual title deeds is unclear because permits have not yet been issued. Decisions are now made on an ad hoc basis.

3. Democratize water management by increasing the participation of stakeholders, especially black communal farmers. Under the preceding act, waters were managed either by the government or by River Boards, whose membership was restricted to water rights holders, typically, white commercial farmers.[20] Representation of communal area residents' interests was left to the discretion of the government. Under the new Water Act, waters are to be managed through Catchment Councils and Subcatchment Councils, which are composed of nationally legislated stakeholder groups that include communal area residents and Rural District Councilors.[21] They are to carry out their work in coordination with the new Zimbabwe National Water Authority (ZINWA).

4. The wide definition of *primary water* remains, although Catchment Councils are empowered to limit it (Government of Zimbabwe 2000a, 2000b). In concert with global water policies, water is to be considered an economic good. In Zimbabwe, this has been captured in the phrase *user pays*. This refers only to commercial water because primary water cannot, by matter of

law, be priced. The main concern of water policy is to promote use of commercial water by encouraging business activities. Although the strategy emphasizes a uniform policy for all Zimbabwe, the development of water in communal areas still takes place under District Development Fund and Rural District Council water and sanitation programs. These remain, overwhelmingly, for primary water.

5. All commercial waters are to be levied, and all water behind government (now ZINWA) dams is to be priced.[22] In practice, everyone (including the catchment manager and staff) who receives a permit for a specific amount of water to be used is charged a levy for the costs of administering the Water Act. Any surplus is to be put into a water fund for development purposes, including the funding to run catchment councils (as opposed to the staff of ZINWA itself). The price of waters stored behind ZINWA-owned dams should be sufficient to run and maintain the dams and set aside new funds for future dam projects. This price should become more and more market-based, reflecting the real costs of water in Zimbabwe's various catchments. Ironically, water is to be paid for, but land has been given away for free in Zimbabwe's "fast-track" land reform (Hellum and Derman 2004).

## HEALTH AND THE WATER REFORM

The provision of clean drinking water was not, and is not, part of the water reform, but rather the Integrated Rural Water Supply and Sanitation program (IRWSS). Its goals are to provide adequate, safe, protected drinking-water supplies for all and to ensure that every household has at least an improved, partially enclosed latrine. The principle for providing clean water shifts to an economic-based incentive system of "polluter pay." All those with permitted water declare whether and how the water they discharge is polluted. The actual level of pollutants is determined by ZINWA. There is a fee schedule for the amount of pollutants, depending on their degree of toxicity or danger. The idea is to create incentives for businesses to prevent discharge rather than pay high fees. In the current crisis, this system has been only partially implemented.

As noted above, the supply of clean rural drinking water (IRWSS) does not fall under the new institutions of water management, but rather under the National Action Council, an interministerial committee formerly headed by the Ministry of Local Government, with participants from all the relevant ministries and departments. This interministerial program functioned well until the early 1990s but now is on the verge of collapse, despite significant donor support for many years. Multilateral and bilateral donor assistance has dried up, for the IRWSS as well, because of claims of systematic governmental human rights abuses. In addition, there have been claims that the parliamentary election in 2000 and the presidential election of 2002 were neither free nor fair.[23]

ZINWA sells water to Zimbabwe's cities, including the capital, Harare. Each city is responsible for purification and supply to urban consumers. Because of the conflict between the ruling party and the opposition party, which controls urban areas, combined with severe economic difficulties, the city of Harare has not been able to purchase the necessary chemicals for its purification plant or to provide proper maintenance. A safe water supply for urban users becomes part and parcel of the deeper economic and political crisis of Zimbabwe.

## CONCLUSIONS

Given the salience of race and history throughout Southern Africa, what hypotheses can we make about the future of water reform? Can and will water reform make a major contribution to the integration of—or at least the linkages among—environment, development, and poverty elimination? Can the experimental, simultaneous merging of the various water frameworks succeed in practice? From an anthropological perspective, how do we place struggles around water with other critical twenty-first-century issues?

Already, the notion of user pay, which has formed the cornerstone of water reform, is being challenged by the principle of water as a human right (McCaffrey 1992). This principle has been adopted in the water policies of both Namibia and South Africa, but not in any dimension of Zimbabwe's water reform to date. Because the United Nations Commission on Economic, Social and Cultural Rights has incorporated a right to water within its brief (along with the governments of

South Africa [1998] and Namibia [2004]), the terrain of debate is shifting toward how to implement such a right or even whether to do so. Can and do national, regional, and local authorities have sufficient resources to provide and manage water to actualize this right? If we, as anthropologists, adopt the view of water as a human right, does this change our ethical, political, and professional responsibilities? Experience in Zimbabwe demonstrated that the villagers (and the research team) believed that everyone has a right to drinking water. We demonstrated that the national water law had the potential to override local custom and practice, which actualized the right to drinking water.

Southern African nations, including Zimbabwe, are choosing their own water policies, blending and mixing their histories and experiences with current international frameworks. This blending of laws and policies will result in new possibilities not necessarily envisioned by the rising tide of international organizations focused on water. It is a central contradiction of ongoing globalization to emphasize stakeholder participation (including national governments, regional water authorities, and regional water and watershed management units) and provide all the answers as to how water management should be done. I find that much is to be opposed in "blueprint mandatory stakeholder participation." The question of how to balance environment and industry, basic needs and productive water, water for irrigation and water for swimming pools, does not lend itself to global answers, but to local ones. Regional pressures for privatization, especially in Namibia and South Africa, are significant. These pressures, however, will be contested by those seeking their "right to water" and by new farm owners who will not be able to afford commercial water rates.

In the Southern Africa context, the profound inequalities in access to water must be addressed. For this to occur, however, the inclusion of unions, environmental NGOs, human rights organizations, peasant unions or organizations, and farmers groups (new and old) is essential to balancing the perspectives of the new elites, who view their accession to wealth and power as establishing the new equality, not a new class of rulers. Whether and in what ways these new rulers will maintain and develop the idea of water as a human right are greatly open to question and will be increasingly politicized in the next decade. The voice of environmentalists will be challenged more and more in Southern

Africa because of worsening poverty and the profound consequences of the AIDS epidemic. More productive uses of water to be supplied for less than cost will remain a very important demand in the context of regional poverty. In my view, a human right to water will increase the political leverage of those seeking to gain greater access to water and to maintain a life of dignity. Whether or not water will be as crucial politically as it is in all other dimensions of life remains uncertain.

**Notes**

1. Precisely which nations compose Southern Africa has not been clear. Earlier divisions between Lusophone, Anglophone, and Francophone Africa have become less important. The Southern African Development Community (SADC), initially formed to oppose apartheid and to coordinate policies among nations engaged in supporting the independence struggles in Namibia and South Africa, now has been expanded. The current membership of SADC includes Angola, the Democratic Republic of Congo, Mozambique, Tanzania, Zambia, Malawi, Zimbabwe, South Africa, Lesotho, Swaziland, Namibia, and Botswana.

2. One example of environmental policy is the allowing of trade in elephant products, by modifying the Committee on International Agreements on Trade in Endangered Species (CITES) to permit Botswana, South Africa, and Zimbabwe to auction some ivory to Japan. A second example is the South African constitution's profound emphasis on human rights, including a right to clean drinking water.

3. For more information, see Derman and Gonese 2003.

4. For a more detailed consideration of this issue, see Derman and Hellum 2002.

5. See the "Report of the United Nations Conference on Environment and Development (UNCED)," UN Doc A/CONF 151/26. In 1992 five hundred participants, including government-designated experts, attended the International Conference on Water and the Environment (ICWE) in Dublin, Ireland, January 26–31. The Dublin Statement on Water and Sustainable Development was commended to the world leaders assembled at the UNCED Conference in Rio de Janeiro in June 1992.

6. In its new Water Management Strategy 2002, the World Bank reduces the Dublin Principles to three, dropping the gender component and including it in stakeholder participation. To me, this seems like male-streaming water rather than mainstreaming gender. See Cleaver 1998a and 1998b and Cleaver and Elson

1995, among several others, for some implications of what happens when women are not included.

7. The International Water Management Institute (IWMI) serves as the nerve center for promoting new ideas, new technologies, and new debates about water management and water use.

8. Critics of this approach argue that, left on its own, the market results in concentration of economic power, which, in turn, can lead to the wasteful use of water for production, for example, of high-value crops in inappropriate environments. The market's neutrality remains one of the most contentious issues in water management.

9. The Democratic Republic of the Congo has virtually no irrigation and relatively little industry. Namibia has invested heavily in water supply and in treating water both as a scarce economic good and as a commodity. Substantial concern remains, though, over whether water resources will be adequate to support the environment and economic growth.

10. In only one chapter, I cannot do justice to Allan's data and analysis. While I do not agree with much of his analysis, his concept of "virtual" water remains highly useful in its own terms and as a critical reminder that scarcity is relative and can be remedied in many ways.

11. I have not read any scholars or practitioners who claim that the market should do everything or that water is an economic good *only*. Most often, writers seek a mix of policies, with the weight of what should be done leaning toward increased markets, water pricing to reflect its real economic worth, and so on.

12. The CGIAR mission statement focuses on international research and related activities, in partnership with national research systems, to contribute to sustainable improvements in the productivity of agriculture, forestry, and fisheries in developing countries in ways that enhance nutrition and well-being, especially of low-income people. The current sponsors are the World Bank, United Nations Environment Programme (UNEP), Food and Agriculture Organization of the United Nations (FAO), and International Fund for Agricultural Development (IFAD). The IFAD, a specialized UN organization focusing on the needs of small-scale farmers, was begun in 1977 as one of the major outcomes of the 1974 World Food Conference.

13. Committee on Economic, Social and Cultural Rights, 29th session, November 2002, Geneva. "The right to water" (Articles 11 and 12 of the International Covenant on Economic, Social and Cultural Rights), E/C.12/2002/11.

14. Great Britain established the colony of Southern Rhodesia, which lasted until the declaration of unilateral independence in 1965. The former colony's government then declared itself "Rhodesia." This name lasted until independence in 1980, when it became "Zimbabwe."

15. Zimbabwe became independent in 1980 after a bitter war. Namibia achieved independence from South Africa in 1990. One can date the full independence of South Africa after the first multiracial, democratic elections in 1994.

16. For a consideration of why this is the case, see Derman 2001.

17. See the updated World Bank (2002b) water policy document titled "Bridging Troubled Waters."

18. Water Act No. 31/98, the Zimbabwe National Water Authority (ZINWA) Act No. 11/98.

19. The act states that "all water is vested in the President" and "no person shall be entitled to ownership of any water in Zimbabwe and no water shall be stored, abstracted, apportioned, controlled, diverted, used or in any way dealt with except in Accordance with this Act" (GOZ 31/98, 3 and 4).

20. The Zimbabwe government has moved to appropriate all white-owned commercial farmland. At the time of this writing, in June 2004, fewer than four hundred farmers still farmed, out of approximately four thousand five hundred in March 2000. For one woman's accurate and painful account, see Buckle 2001.

21. According to the Water Subcatchment Councils Regulations of 2000, the following stakeholder groups are to elect members of the Subcatchment Councils: Rural District Councils, communal farmers, resettlement farmers, small-scale commercial farmers, large-scale commercial farmers, indigenous commercial farmers, urban authorities, large-scale mines, small-scale mines, industry, and any other stakeholder group the Subcatchment Council may identify.

22. As part of the ongoing, fast-track land reform, all large and medium-size dams that were privately owned and all government-owned large dams are now the property and responsibility of ZINWA.

23. Amnesty International, the Human Rights Watch, the International Crisis Committee, and the Zimbabwe Human Rights NGO Forum have issued periodic reports on ongoing, government-sponsored violence and torture. For a more academic treatment of what is at stake in contemporary Zimbabwe, see Hammar, Raftopoulos, and Jensen (2003).

# 11

## Good to the Last Drop

*The Political Ecology of Water and Health on the Border*

### Scott Whiteford and Alfonso Cortez-Lara

Is your water safe to drink? How do you know? Who has guaranteed the safety of your water? Whom do you contact when you believe that there is a problem with your water, and can they correct the problem in a timely fashion? These are questions faced by people all over the world, but for the poorest, the answers are slow to come, if at all, and the human cost is staggering and growing. Water quality is difficult to assess because people cannot see harmful microorganisms or chemicals in the water they drink; furthermore, water may have a strange odor or color but be safe to drink. All things being equal, people choose water based on convenience, price, and taste. Safety, however, is the single, most important factor, yet millions must risk drinking water of marginal quality.[1]

There is a significant policy debate that transcends national borders as to whether drinking water is a public good, access to which is a human right, a natural resource, or a commodity to bought and sold by private companies. The discourse over who should control or be responsible for the quality of drinking water goes beyond the role of the state versus the private sector. Because water is basic to people's

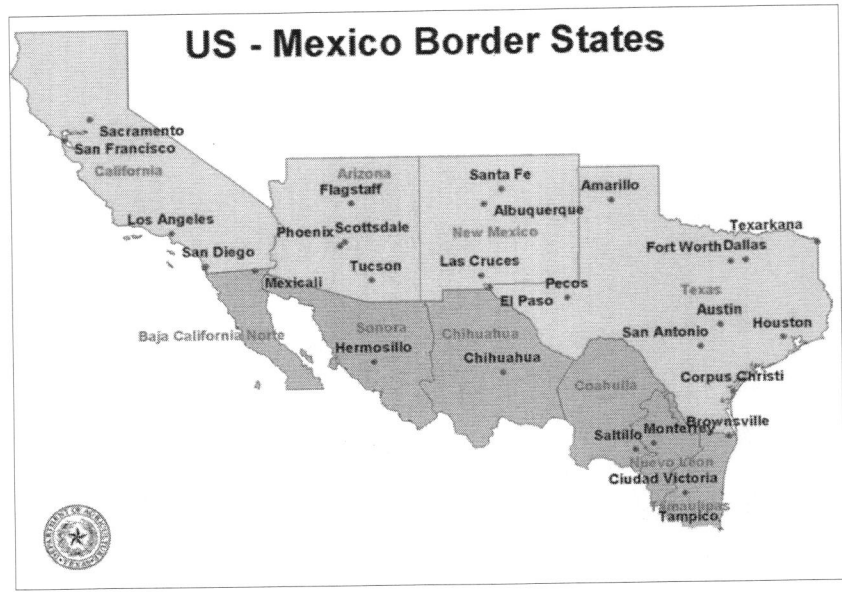

**FIGURE 11.1**
*Map of United States/Mexico border region.*

health and their control over their own bodies, the debate raises important issues about health, decision making, and trust in private and public institutions. The proponents of privatization of water include the World Bank, which claims that private companies can be "pro-poor," the Inter-American Development Bank, and private transnational companies. Those who favor the private sector herald its efficacy, while those who favor government control and responsibility believe that clean drinking water is a human right that only a government can guarantee its citizens.

In this chapter, drawing on research from the Mexicali Valley, located on the United States/Mexico border, we examine the challenges people face in evaluating the quality of their drinking water and the confidence they place in the government and private companies to provide or monitor the quality of the water they consume. In short, what assumptions do people make about their water, and how do these influence their actions? We place our questions in the context of multiple forms of globalization that influence people's lives, usually unequally, and subsequently their understanding and ability to respond. In some cases, the nation-state, state government, or community organizations filter or modify the interactive processes. In others, information flows and changes are more direct, and the nation-state and its agencies are enablers or are marginalized.

The question of who guarantees safe water leads directly to social issues of power, knowledge, and efficacy because people must consume water, whether or not they have the benefit of complete information informing their decisions. In this chapter, we use a term introduced by Anthony Giddens (1999), *manufactured risk*, risk created by human innovation and knowledge. In the case we examine, the extensive use of pesticides for high-technology agriculture resulted in contamination of water sources. Giddens contrasts manufactured risk with external risk, which comes from outside, such as regularly occurring dry seasons when there is water scarcity. Risk may be increased in a situation of water scarcity that can also be a product of social forces and unequal power, which we term *contrived scarcity*, in contrast to *natural scarcity*. Is globalization resulting in manufactured risk and water scarcity that increase people's water insecurity?[2]

"The degree of *water security or insecurity* of a population is a condition where there is a sufficient quantity of water at a quality necessary, at an affordable price, to meet both the short-term and long-term needs to protect the health, safety, welfare and productive capacity of a population (households, communities, neighborhoods or nations). The level of water security or insecurity of a population needs to be understood in both spatial and temporal terms" (Witter and S. Whiteford 1999:3). How the state, the private sector, or public organizations respond to growing water insecurity depends on a wide range of factors. In this chapter, we argue that under special local conditions, globalization of agricultural markets and production often results in contrived water scarcity and manufactured risk, increasing water insecurity and health risk.

## THEORETICAL FRAMEWORK

This chapter draws on the theoretical interface of political ecology and critical medical anthropology.[3] From the political ecology approach, we have focused our study on the ways in which environmental change is a translocal process and part of the global economy. Equally important, our study takes a historical perspective to examine large-scale social and economic structures within which unequal power relationships evolved, many extending beyond the local. These relationships influence how resources are contested, controlled, and transformed. The resources include land, water (surface water and groundwater), credit, markets, and information. We have drawn on critical medical anthropology to examine how unequal and exploitative power relationships can determine *unequal exposure* to health risks and resource benefits. This includes how health problems are defined and contested and how knowledge is developed and, ultimately, acted upon. Our research in the United States/Mexico border region of the Colorado River, where corporate agriculture has transformed the environment, explores the interface of agrarian transformation, environment, and health.

Fresh water is a vital resource in this semiarid region and the focus of international competition, which is creating contrived scarcity, reducing water for some as a result of unequal political and economic power. Drinking water comes from the Colorado River, a major aquifer that transcends the border, and bottled water companies. Part of our research examined the problems of water contamination, how people define it, what people know about it, and how they make decisions under conditions of uncertainty.

## GLOBALIZATION(S)

A range of processes creates different forms of globalization and their uneven impact on local populations. These processes include (1) the development and introduction of new communication technologies; (2) social movements organized to transcend national borders, creating new political coalitions; (3) expansion of transnational companies, incorporating global markets and material flows; (4) international agreements reducing tariff barriers and enhancing neoliberal reforms that create greater market integration; and (5) the flow of ideas, standards, and cultural forms that both link and divide countries and the people within a country. Globalization processes increase interdependence and intensify people's awareness of this interdependence. They produce solidarities in some localities and destroy these in others (Kearney 1996). Economic and technological globalization has compressed time and space. Globalization processes make state boundaries more porous and ineffective because these processes often take place beyond the control of the state. At the same time, some states become the vehicle for reconfiguring international capital to strengthen the power of state elites.

A central component of globalization is greater economic integration of the global economy. Economic globalization impacts natural resources and has been a subject of considerable debate. The World Trade Organization (WTO), for example, has worked to eliminate trade barriers and tariffs for water to enhance trade. The rationale is that, by making water a commodity, open markets will improve water conservation and decrease waste. Others have argued that deregulation and WTO rules make it increasingly difficult for communities, states, or nations to protect natural resources critical for their survival. Even protecting water for environmental purposes can be cast as a form of protectionism and made illegal by international law (Barlow 1999:35).

An important form of globalization is the spread of a dominant ideology. An example of ideological globalization has been the nearly universal adoption of national water standards and environmental regulations. The globalization of standards and regulations to facilitate trade, the gathering of comparable national statistics, and enhanced health interventions have been underway for decades, but these have gathered momentum in the past decade. Each country uniquely enforces regulations. One of the most significant engines spreading and perpetuating the ideology of privatization has been the World Bank, which has offices throughout the world. This is especially apparent in the arena of water, where the World Bank has pushed privatization by linking development formulas—a belief system about steps to development—to access to loans (World Bank 2004). The World Bank's publication program, technical program, and economic program have focused on enhancing decentralization and privatization. The World Bank has pressed for the private provisioning of infrastructure, especially for drinking water. Although this appears to contradict the World Bank's emphasis on participation, transparency, and decentralization, in fact, these latter goals are linked in some World Bank documents on privatization.

Community and nongovernmental organization activists use the new technologies to mobilize populations, to gather data, and to win political support from environmental groups and movements throughout the world. In some cases, this has helped people affected by corporate pollution to access scientific information on norms and standards so that they can enhance their negotiation leverage with companies or state representatives. In these instances, globalization may increase transparency and accountability. But this is not common. All too frequently, globalization has worked to the advantage of those with power and capital, furthering economic and political inequality.

Inherent in the frameworks of both political ecology and critical medical anthropology is what Laura Nader two decades ago called "studying up": examining unequal power and its impacts on the least powerful. In this chapter, we address five major questions: First, what factors influence the quality of drinking water in the region studied, and are they local, national, or linked to global processes? Second, what are the physical qualities of the drinking water in the region? Third, how do the consumers define good-quality drinking water, and how does that match what we found in our water tests? Fourth, in an era in which major international agencies are supporting privatization of water, do people trust the government or private companies, or both, to guarantee safe drinking water? Fifth, what can we learn from this case about the interacting forces of globalization and peoples' perception of the environment and health?

## PRIVATIZATION OF DRINKING WATER

Even though private entrepreneurs have provided water to Latin American cities since the colonial period, most have "worked within an exclusive franchise and without any subsidy or credit support from the government" (Solo 2003:1). Today, water is delivered by truck to low-income neighborhoods or delivered to homes of the wealthy in elegant bottles. Solo distinguishes between mobile water providers and fixed water providers. Usually, the poorest people, with the worst services, end up paying the most for water.

Commodification of water has taken many forms, but in all cases, "regulating the interplay between the natural and social processes of the water cycle has become increasingly articulated with the dynamics of the market, and consequently, with the spatial and institutional process associated with market forces" (Swyngedouv, Page, and Kaika 2002:6). Resource allocation decisions are becoming the domain of private actors, who may or may not operate within the system's regulator framework. This often takes place in the context of national deregulations and the "privatization of public functions including the privatization of water" (Swyngedouv, Page, and Kaika 2002:13). For our analysis, it is important to address how privatization of water is negotiated and regulated.

During the past fifteen years, water has been treated as a commodity to be bought and sold, with sources of water becoming privatized. This is due, in part, to globalization of corporate investment and the opening of markets for multinational companies. In Latin America, from the early colonial period to the present, entrepreneurs sold water and often built infrastructure, but without government subsidies, using horses and trucks to deliver water in containers to customers. Towns and cities took the responsibility of building infrastructure for water and sanitation, but population growth often outstripped public budgets, leaving the poorest to buy water from private venders at a higher price. Cash-short governments have turned to the private sector to develop, operate, and own city water systems, usually including water sources and infrastructure. Two French multinationals, Suez and Vivendi, own 70 percent of the international privatized water business (Hall and Lobina 2002:6).[4]

Bottled water companies are another type of private drinking-water enterprise. Of these, there are least two types: those that sell multigallon jugs of water in large quantities or from trucks and those that sell bottled water, as you would find in any major grocery or drug store in the United States. In Latin America and the United States, the bottled water market is rapidly expanding, aggressively marketed by major transnational companies, including Nestle, Coca Cola, and Pepsi Cola. All of them are established in the border region, where in 2004 a gallon of bottled water and a gallon of gasoline have the same price. Fifty-six companies were selling bottled water in Mexico at the time of our study. The competition among companies was, and is, fierce, and the range of ownership great, from peasant communities in the hills of Oaxaca, to traditional Mexican companies such as Garci Crespo of Puebla, to the multinationals. As a consequence of globalization, the number of companies will dwindle as the transnationals solidify their marketing.

## THE CASE STUDY: THE MEXICALI VALLEY

We began this research by examining the quality of the public water supply in the Mexicali Valley, located along the western region of the United States/Mexico border.[5] Historically, the quality of water from the United States to Mexico has been the subject of international litigation. The Mexicali Valley is a southern continuation of California's Imperial Valley. Two of the richest agricultural zones in North America, the Mexicali Valley and the Imperial Valley draw water for agriculture and drinking from the Colorado River and the Mexicali–Mesa de Andrade aquifer, which extends deep into both valleys. The agriculturalists of the Mexicali Valley live in small towns scattered throughout the valley. In contrast to many rural communities in Mexico, where modified indigenous community systems handle water, the communities in Mexicali were created with the land reform and colonization of state lands. As a result, the Mexican government has had, until recently, the dominant role in managing water for both drinking and irrigation.

The United States and Mexico have been in conflict over the quantity and quality of Colorado River water since 1922, when the Colorado River Compact was signed in Santa Fe without the participation of any Mexican delegates. This compact divided up the waters of the Colorado. In 1944 a treaty between Mexico and the United States redefined the Colorado River Compact and set water obligations of both countries along the border region. The International Boundary and Water Commission (IBWC) was established, with two independent sections, one for each country. Since its origin, the role of the IBWC has been to ensure that the treaty is carried out appropriately and to resolve technical conflicts.

One of the major conflicts managed by this bilateral institution was generated by the growing salinity of the Colorado River water that flowed into Mexico. By the 1960s, water became so saline, increasing from 800 parts per million (ppm) to more than 1,500 ppm, that it could not be used for agriculture. The devastation to Mexicali Valley agriculture mobilized agriculturalists to demand government action. The United States claimed that it was fulfilling the contract by delivering the quantity of water stipulated in the treaty and that the treaty did not specify degrees of water quality. Mexico responded that water of usable quality was inherent in the agreement. In 1974 the dispute was resolved through an addendum to the 1944 treaty, in which the United

States guaranteed that water flowing into Mexico would have no more than 115 ppm of salt.

The importance of history for our analysis is that the people of Mexicali mobilized successfully to pressure their local government and then their national government to negotiate on their behalf with the United States to protect surface water—and they were successful. Today, in 2004, groundwater is highly contested in what some journalists call "water wars." Yet, this title attributes a more active role to the Mexican stakeholders than exists. One of the questions this chapter asks is why stakeholders are responding so differently when their groundwater is threatened than they did when their surface water was contaminated? The Mexicali Valley includes a fast-growing metropolitan center, the city of Mexicali. In the 2002 census, the Mexicali *municipio* registered 813,853 inhabitants, 25 percent of them living in rural areas in more than one hundred small towns scattered throughout the valley. In the city of Mexicali, household water comes from the Colorado River and groundwater; in surrounding settlements or towns, it is almost exclusively taken from groundwater, which is recharged by water from the Colorado and irrigated fields. Loans from the World Bank have played an important role in reclaiming land and developing the irrigation system in the Mexicali Valley.

The rich agricultural region is made up of 207,000 hectares (457,000 acres) of irrigated land farmed and owned by both communal *ejidatarios* and private *pequeños propietarios*, all of whom possess an average 18–20 hectares. Eighty-five percent of the water for irrigation is from the Colorado. Additional groundwater is pumped and carried to the fields through a complex network of lined canals extending more than 4,000 lineal miles. Historically, cotton (the "white gold") was the primary crop of the region. Because of world market prices and growing domestic demand, however, wheat is now the dominant crop, followed by cotton, alfalfa, and vegetables. Major transnational companies handle the sales of cotton and vegetables, as well as provide the majority of the pesticides. The heavy use of pesticides for agriculture is a factor of risk that permeates both the Mexicali and Imperial Valleys.

Mexico has a sophisticated government program for the management of water and infrastructure, the Comisión Nacional del Agua (CNA). Irrigated agriculture plays a critical role in Mexico's agrarian strategy; in fact, Mexico ranks sixth in the world in irrigated acreage.

Much of the country is arid, so the sustainability of water resources is critical to its future. Nevertheless, much of the surface water in Mexico is contaminated by industry, urban waste, or agricultural runoff.

Mexico has aggressively incorporated itself into the global economy through the North American Free Trade Agreement (NAFTA) and twenty-three bilateral trade agreements. As a result, the country has experienced an explosion of industrial growth, urbanization, and the decline of small farm agriculture, with increased disparity of wealth within states and within regions. For example, between 1993 and 2003 Mexican manufacturing rose 43 percent while industrial wages fell 18 percent. Agricultural exports rose by three billion dollars between 1994 and 2003. During the same period, 700,000 small farmers were forced from the land to search for work in Mexican cities and in the United States. NAFTA and the General Agreement on Tariffs and Trade (GATT), globalizing ideological forces, define water as a commodity governed by all the regulatory provisions, which, in theory, means that companies can buy and sell water without local or national regulations.

As part of NAFTA, a number of binational agreements were developed to address the contamination in the border region, where 12 percent of the residents lacked safe drinking water and more than 30 percent faced health problems associated with wastewater and/or solid waste treatment. Thousands of tons of hazardous waste materials are generated in the United States and on the Mexican side of the border by the 2,889 *maquiladoras* (border assembly plants) owned by transnational companies from the United States, Asia, and the European Union.

The NAFTA Environmental Side Agreement created the North American Commission for Environmental Cooperation, designed to give voice to border citizens concerned about violation of environmental laws. The Mexican and US governments developed the Border Environmental Cooperation Commission (BECC) and the North American Development Bank (NADBANK). The BECC was designed to help state and local agencies analyze the technical, environmental, and financial dimensions of specific problems and then to certify this analysis when these agencies request funding from the NADBANK, which makes loans and guarantees. By March 31, 2002, fifty-seven projects, thirty in Mexico, had been certified as worth $1.2 billion (Nitze 2002:10).

## GLOBALIZATION ON THE BORDER

Four main types of globalization have impacted the people of rural Mexicali: (1) integration into a world agricultural market, making agriculture dependent on chemical pesticides and fertilizer; (2) access to new communication technologies; (3) multiple forms of cultural and ideological change; and (4) adaptation of worldwide grades and standards for water quality, agricultural products, and waste.

Economic globalization has integrated the region into world trade networks of agricultural commodities and products. The major crops of cotton, wheat, and, to a lesser degree, vegetables are sold in world commodity markets. Producers have access to credit from private companies and, to a lesser extent, from federal governmental agencies that sell the products on a global market. Corporate farming includes intensive use of pesticides purchased from chemical companies with a global reach. The spread of water management administration and practices defined by the World Bank as a necessary requirement for loans is a form of cultural globalization. These practices include not just privatization, but also decentralization, stakeholder participation, and great transparency. We have written elsewhere how these regulations have made some important contributions in Mexicali, but they have also led to greater inequality and recentralization within the private sector (S. Whiteford and Bernal 1996).

Accompanying the integration of commodity markets has been the globalization of the agrifood industry's grades and standards. The expansion of grades and standards worldwide and their associated social and economic imperatives are just now being studied. Increasingly, global grades and standards for agricultural produce marketed in global markets have defined not only the color and texture of agricultural products but also quality characteristics such as safety (amounts of pesticides or E. coli found on foods). Because the demands of evolving grades and standards have been further reinforced by buyers (supermarkets or wholesale chains) or by border inspections, the process has led to greater concentration and centralization of the agrifood industry (Reardon et al. 2002:1). This has happened in the Mexicali Valley at ports of entry on the Mexicali/United States border.

The globalization created by the new communication technologies, besides facilitating the spread of standards and regulations, has given individuals and communities new access to information. As economic globalization in Mexicali has led to environmental deterioration due to pollution of natural resources, people—often the poor—have mobilized to resist salinization and the dumping of waste. In some cases, these protests have led to international negotiations to protect the environment and health.

The globalization of grades and standards of water quality has had an important impact in many areas (Root, Wiley, and Peek 2000:201). The Environmental Protection Agency's standards for water quality are easily available online and have been adopted by many countries, including Mexico. Of course, Mexico has modified them to a limited degree, but Mexican regulatory agencies basically use the same standards and techniques to measure pollution or contamination as their US counterparts. Equally important, because these standards are online in both Mexico and the United States, producers and consumers can access them. Access to technology and information varies; thus, power is never equal. In a growing number of Mexican rural communities, people have computers and websites, connecting to the World Wide Web. This is the case in the Mexicali Valley, but, to date, people are not taking advantage of these resources to address water and health issues. Communication technology may make information available, but this does not mean that the information will immediately be used.

## GROUNDWATER

The water from the Mexicali–Mesa de Andrade aquifer has been a source of conflict between the United States and Mexico. Disputes over control of the Colorado River surface water were litigated and accords were developed, but cooperation on groundwater did not exist. As a result, agriculturalists on both sides of the border drilled wells, pumping water twenty-four hours a day. In 1998 the Imperial Irrigation District began negotiations to pave its canals and sell its water to the San Diego Water Authority; western cities desperately needed drinking water for the rapidly expanding population. Internal conflicts, however, have held up the agreements. Another project—the lining of the All-American Canal, which transports water from the Colorado River to the farms of the Imperial Valley—would prevent water from seeping through the ground into the Mexicali–Mesa de Andrade aquifer. Although this project would provide water for one hundred thirty-five thousand urban Californian households, it would also deprive the more than thirty thousand Mexicans in the northern area of the Mexicali Valley who are using the water seeping from the All-American Canal into the Mexicali–Mesa de Andrade aquifer. The seepage provides 10 to 12 percent of the aquifer recharge, critical for agriculture in the Mexicali Valley and households dependent on the water. Another project to save water for San Diego and Los Angeles by paving the canals of the Imperial Valley, or transferring water from the Imperial Valley, was hotly contested in 2003.

Because the Mexicali Valley is located at the lower Colorado River basin and because the river system is used to transport waste from upstream users, the surface water drawn from the Colorado, if untreated or not mixed with cleaner water, is unusable for agriculture. The most important contaminants are salts, toxic substances, mercury, bacterial strains of typhoid, and pesticides. A bitter conflict between Mexico and the United States led to an agreement in which Colorado River water had to be improved before it arrived in Mexico and was used in Mexicali. The World Bank funded a massive rehabilitation project in the Mexicali Valley (S. Whiteford and Cortez-Lara 1996).

Until recently, residents of the Mexicali Valley had seen groundwater as politically unimportant. Neither the government nor stakeholders were concerned with ownership of groundwater. It was assumed that the water was uncontaminated and important for diluting surface water to make it better for irrigation and, in some cases, for human consumption. Unlike surface water, groundwater is often not included in stakeholders' perception of the ecosystem in which they live.[6] Even school textbooks on the environment focus almost exclusively on surface water.

## PESTICIDES AND WATER

Mexicali Valley agriculture is highly dependent on the use of pesticides.[7] Each year, more than 480 tons of pesticides, including both insecticides and herbicides, are sprayed on crops throughout the valley. Some forty types of pesticides are used; most are imported from the United States and Europe, sold by twelve major transnational companies in the pesticide trade, including BASF, Bayer de Mexico, Dow Elanco, Dupont, GBM, and Monsanto. A key question in our research—do pesticides leach into groundwater?—was answered by testing the groundwater. At the time (2002) we did our tests, there was no public record that the water had ever been tested for pesticides. The general consensus was that, despite decades of heavy applications of pesticides, they posed limited health problems when mixed with water. Government officials informed us that pesticides leached out in the soil or ran into drainage canals and to the ocean, where they were broken down by oxygen and microorganisms. The groundwater was understood by most stakeholders to be free of impurities. What we found led us to ask a new set of questions.

Pesticides in groundwater can be an extremely serious problem because of the long turnover rate for groundwater. Although the rate can be as short as a few months, it is more commonly years or decades before the water in an aquifer is replaced. In fact, pesticides do get into aquifers and, if they do not break down, are difficult to remove. Oxygen is generally not present in groundwater, and the microorganisms that live in an oxygen-free environment are not effective in breaking down pesticides.

Our test of the groundwater at pumping station wells found very high levels of three agricultural chemicals: Endosulfan Sulfate, Malathion, and Clorpiriphos. The thirty wells, located in the central and southern areas of the Mexicali Valley, where many small-town residents get their drinking water, had extremely high levels of Endosulfan, a very toxic poison used in pesticides.

In the United States, Endosulfan is labeled as a restricted-use pesticide. It is highly toxic when consumed orally. People who are acutely exposed suffer from diarrhea, difficulty breathing, imbalance, and loss of consciousness. When consumed over time, it causes liver and kidney damage. Endosulfan is made by FMC Corporation and Agricultural Chemicals Group. Our studies found very high levels of Endosulfan in drainage, but more importantly, in water pumped from the Mexicali–Mesa de Andrade aquifer, which many people use for drinking and bathing. High levels of Malathion were also found in the same test. Malathion is not a highly toxic pesticide and breaks down in groundwater within three weeks; however, consumption of high levels can result in dizziness, abdominal cramps, and respiratory problems. Malathion is made by Drexel Chemical Company and is used as a pesticide for fruit and vegetable plants. A third pesticide, Clorpiriphos, is classified as moderately toxic and is used as an insecticide. Poisoning from Clorpiriphos can affect the central nervous system, the cardiovascular system, and the respiratory system; repeated or prolonged exposure can have the same effects as an acute dose. The concentration and persistence of Clorpiriphos in water depend on the type of fluoridation. Clorpiriphos is produced by Dow Elanco Company.

An internal government study of groundwater quality (CNA 1998) confirmed our concerns. The CNA has not made its study available to the public and has not been forthcoming with water users in the valley. The failure of the Mexican state is what we refer to as "structural myopia," a political decision to withhold negative information about environmental conditions that could be hazardous to the health of its citizens, while encouraging stakeholders to trust state or private sector technical knowledge to reduce health risk at a time stakeholders are exposed to abnormal risk.

The government intended to announce the findings of its study after it had a plan in place to address the problem. But, as an official pointed out, the evidence that the amount of pesticides in the water caused illness in people was murky at best. Long-term epidemiological studies are still needed.

Usually, the poor are the most vulnerable to structural myopia, but not always. In the United States, the Environmental Protection Agency (EPA) withheld information after 9/11 about the dangerous level of air pollution at the World Trade Center site, partly because it was not 100-percent sure of the meaning of its data and partly because political leaders did not want to stop the return of workers to buildings near the site, fearing the effect on the economy. This is a form of structural myopia because the government did not make public its data about the health risk of breathing the air, which contained suspended glass, metal, and chemical particles. The effects will not be known for a long time.

Why the Mexican government withheld the information from stakeholders is an important question it did not want to answer. Possibly, the Mexican government did not want to become entangled with the United

States and Imperial Valley use of pesticides while agriculturalists on the Mexican side were using the same pesticides critical to the local economy and exports. Possibly, the government was waiting to distribute the information until it had solutions in hand. Also, given the range of water-related problems the government faced, those in power might have felt that this particular issue was not a priority. Still another possibility is that the government agency was not entirely certain what the data meant and used uncertainty as an excuse to stall action, an increasingly common trend in the handling of industrial pollution.

To test whether people retained pesticides they consumed drinking water from the aquifer, we carried out a follow-up study. The results showed that people who used water from the wells had an abnormal and dangerous level of pesticides in their blood. The sample included thirty-two people (men and women between the ages of twenty and fifty) who lived in the south-central area of the valley and worked in a produce package facility, thus being in permanent contact with a local environment characterized by intensive use of pesticides.

Using a liquid-liquid technique for separating blood plasma and confirmation made with mass spectrometry, the results show the presence of two important organochlorine pesticides (among sixteen studied): Beta Isomer of Hexaclorinebencene ($\beta$-BHC) and DDT and its metabolites, both of them above the health standard norm ($< 0.001$ ppm) for adults. This was for twenty-two samples (69 percent) with values oscillating between 0.0056 and 0.160 ppm. It is important to mention that organochlorines were discontinued for agricultural use in the early 1970s. As our findings suggest, however, they remain in the environment and in the human body blood fluids, a factual and risky level of intoxication. We did not find any organophosphorus pesticides (in the sample of twenty-two) because of their natural degradation and instability in nature. The pesticides from the drinking water were accumulating in people's bodies and would inevitably cause a health problem. These findings were dismissed because the size of our sample was too small and not statistically significant; only a much larger study with a randomly selected sample would be convincing. Although we understand the need for a larger study, our research documents a clear problem, the response to which could be considered an element of the discourse of structural myopia.

## STAKEHOLDERS AND WATER USERS

Water quality has been a central issue for the people of the Mexicali Valley. They had previously mobilized to demand better-quality water, but for irrigation. Many were experts on the quality of surface water they had used for years in agriculture. Groundwater was different; it was assumed to be of great supply and high quality. How groundwater moves, connects, and is recharged and purified is little discussed and poorly understood. Until recently, the hydro-geologists and hydrologists have not paid much attention to the Mexicali–Mesa de Andrade aquifer. As a result, during the discussion about lining the All-American Canal, the Mexican users were silent, knowing that their complaints would reach deaf ears. This was seen as an American issue, as if the aquifer they used was not connected to groundwater on the other side of the border. By 2003 this changed. Wells had to be deepened to tap a rapidly lowering water table caused by the paving of the canals in the Imperial Valley. The water that had filtered through the earth canals no longer recharged the aquifer; it was being sold to San Diego.

It is important to recognize that pollution and contamination are socially defined and what is unacceptable for one person may be acceptable for another. People tolerate varying levels of contamination if these do not affect their health. Even when health is threatened, people may have difficulty explaining this in a way that captures the attention of health officials. Enforcement of contamination standards depends on many factors, including power and political pressure.

Stakeholders' lack of information about the aquifer indicated their dependence on the government to provide technical information about aquifer water quality and quantity, making it impossible for stakeholders to defend their interests. While the Mexican government had been deeply involved in litigating the Colorado River salinity crisis, more than 70 percent of the stakeholders thought that the government played a minimal role in the groundwater threat. They did not think that either their government or their water user associations would mobilize, reflecting a very low level of political efficacy (Cortez-Lara and Garcia-Acevedo 2000:28). Stakeholders perceive neither groundwater quantity nor quality as a part of their environment under their stewardship, but as a commodity managed by the government. As a result, they do not understand the nature of the aquifer or how it is threatened.

Water as a commodity is reflected in people's lack of concern about groundwater quality. For most people, groundwater was not considered a part of the desert ecology in which they live or a resource to be managed and protected. By Mexican law, groundwater belongs to the state. In Mexicali, the water belongs in practice to those who pump it, giving it quasi property status, although the government pumped groundwater for rural towns and hamlets. Pumps, in contrast to surface water, require an investment often made by family members or investors. None of the people interviewed knew that pesticides were contaminating the groundwater they were pumping and using. This partly stems from the lack of interest in and understanding of the aquifer's connection to surface water. It is also linked to their view that they could not control, as a community of stakeholders, the quality of groundwater. This was a job for the government. It is interesting to note that most people would drink groundwater only when they could not get bottled water, pointing to groundwater's smell, salty taste, and sometimes unappealing color.

In Latin America, women stakeholders are often the only people deeply concerned about the quality of aquifer water for drinking (Bennett 1995). Women are responsible for family health and acquiring drinking water. In our sample, women were twice as likely as men to distrust the safety of groundwater. As a result, they were more inclined to purchase bottled water for their families, despite not knowing for sure who checked its quality. Women had also organized protests at the offices of the CNA, demanding more information about drinking water quality, but they felt that they received little information and that the little they received was buried in technical terms. The government's failure to be more responsive has created a condition of structural myopia, an inability to deal with problems before they become crises. The protestors knew of the potential risk in drinking the aquifer water, but they could not get government officials to define the problem.

People who drank water from the wells had no idea that the water had pesticides. Some had stopped using the water because of taste and because they felt ill when they used it exclusively. Our survey of heads of households found that 40 percent of the people trusted the government to monitor the wells for water quality and 60 percent did not. Women trusted the government at a higher rate than did men, but men were less likely to buy bottled water. Men explained that they did not trust the private sector either and that, although the government should test the bottled water companies, it probably did not. We found that the government was much more systematic in testing bottled water companies than their own wells, although studies done in the United States have raised questions about the quality of bottled water (Olsen 1997; Allen and Darby 1994).

In the city of Mexicali, drinking water has become increasingly privatized. There are thirteen main sources of bottled water: Agua Santa Maria (Nestle), Estrella Azul, Suprema, Agua Anita, Purisima, Aguafiel, Bonafont, Danone, Agua Vida, Agua Azul, Agua Pura, Nestle, and Frespura. Some of the companies sell multigallon containers of water for household use; others sell water in plastic bottles for individual consumption, usually with a label that guarantees no calories and symbolizes natural purity. The companies have created an image of bottled water from nature to signal safety, portraying public water, industrially processed water, or water taken directly from groundwater they do not own as unsafe. In the case of certain towns in the Mexicali Valley, this has been true. People say that they trust the private companies to provide safe water because these are regulated by the government—the same government, however, that some do not trust to test the groundwater they use for drinking.[8]

## CONCLUSION

We began this chapter by asking whether forces of globalization were factors influencing people's access to safe water and health. In contrast to cities like Cochabama, Bolivia, where a transnational company bought the water distribution infrastructure, the case in Mexicali etches another process, a process in which water privatization came in the form of plastic bottles. People bought bottled water because of the convenience, safety, and taste. Global companies such as Coca Cola and Pepsi created a market by redefining nature and natural, but other global and local factors contributed to the degradation of groundwater that many people used for drinking.

The commitment to the industrial agricultural model of production for a global market, dependent on pesticides produced by transnational firms, ultimately transformed the environment. The high level of productivity was competitive within NAFTA and global markets. Below the surface, manufactured risk was being created by human knowledge and innovation; the aquifer was being systematically contaminated. Not everyone was equally vulnerable to the health risk being created, but few even knew that it existed. The failure caused by the Mexican government's structural myopia not only exposed people to health risks but also integrated the expanded sale of bottled water produced by global companies into its public service system, thus privatizing part of the water system.

Disentangling global processes from binational negotiations, agreements, and institutions challenges our analysis, but when studying the US/Mexican borderlands, we must try. NAFTA can be called a trinational agreement, but it has to be understood in the context of GATT and other world trade blocks. Regardless, NAFTA creates unique agreements and commitments of resources that have to be understood both on their own and as parts of larger units.

Since the very definition of the border, Mexico and the United States have been in competition for land and water. They have developed institutions to negotiate the disputes, but the challenge is almost overwhelming because the two countries have very different water laws, national institutions, and constituencies. With high rates of economic and population growth, the problems and the significance of the problems have changed. The issue is not only the finite quantity of water, but also a legal power struggle over who has the rights to the water, to define its quality, and to manipulate scarcity. The primary discourses on border water have reflected a desire for cooperation, but the reality is one of increasing contention and conflict. With the drought that has caste its shadow over the West, water will become increasingly valuable as a commodity and as a human right.

Despite the porous nature of the border, nearby communities are often left out of the official discourses between Mexico and the United States. Information about what powerful people or organizations on the other side of the border are doing is minimal. Within Mexico, the CNA's policies to decentralize costs and management of water have had positive effects, but as our case illustrates, that is not enough. Transparency, access to information, and government accountability are needed. Ironically, globalizing international institutions such as the World Bank also use these concepts. Nevertheless, citizens' right to know about the risk in their environment has never been more compelling, and it is incumbent upon governments to be accountable and share information. NGOs and academic research have a role to play as well; the research findings must be shared with stakeholders and governments, and alternative solutions offered. If the government is not going to take chemical contamination of water more seriously than it has done in Mexicali, people will turn, not surprisingly, to the private sector for safe drinking water. On the other hand, people are not sure about the quality of bottled water either. Many assumed that it would be as safe as the soft drinks provided by many of the same companies. This form of privatization seems to be acceptable for most people, as long as they have options and the price is reasonable.[9]

Water insecurity is a growing problem in many parts of the world, including the western United States, especially the lower Colorado. As the region faces surging competition for water from cities in the United States and Mexico, farmers, and nature, more sustainable use of water and other natural resources must be developed. There is still time to construct a healthier, more collaborative approach to sustainable resource management, but the early indicators suggest troubled waters ahead.

### Notes

1. People throughout the world, the most vulnerable and the poor, suffer from illnesses associated with contaminated water. More than "18% of the world's population do not have access to safe drinking water, and nearly 40% lack adequate sanitation"(UNEP 2002:47). Worldwide, more than six thousand people a year, mostly children under the age of five, die from water-related diseases (UNESCO 2003b:4). Water insecurity is growing in Mexico and Central America. The debate regarding whether clean and sufficient water should be a human right or a salable commodity is intensifying, but many other development issues are also associated with water. Agriculture and production of food and cash crops increasingly depend on irrigation. Flood control, erosion, and protection at times

of drought are critical development challenges. Twenty-three new big dams have been proposed for the region to control flooding and generate hydroelectric power, but they also require resettlement of whole communities and will transform the ecology of watersheds without providing sustainable solutions. Industrial expansion and waste and urban growth and waste management, put even greater pressure on the quality and quantity of limited water resources (S. Whiteford and Melville, eds., 2002:10).

2. In chapter 7 of this volume, Barbara Rose Johnston uses the concept of manufactured scarcity for the same condition she contrasts to natural scarcity, which occurs because of seasonal, annual, and even cyclical fluctuations of natural cycles. These constitute an interactive continuum.

3. Many disciplines share the political ecology paradigm, but each has developed its own approach. In a volume of Human Organization on this topic, Derman and Ferguson (2003:6) point to the importance of a political ecology–situated, historically aware analysis that considers the political, discursive, and ecological to be mutually constituted. At the same time, Baer (1996a) and Torres (2003), among others, have pointed to the links between political ecology and health. During this period, there has been a growing literature in other fields on environmental justice or environmental racism, linking health problems to unequal exposure to toxic environments of the poor or populations that are discriminated against. The political economy approach within medical anthropology focuses on how transitional and translocal economic or political processes impacting specific communities affect health (Ortner 1994:386). The work of Morsy (1996:24), L. Whiteford (1998), and Ferguson (chapter 3 in this volume) reflect this approach.

4. These companies, working through joint ventures, have major holdings in Latin America. To expand their markets there, they are purchasing water infrastructure such as plants and piping systems and regulatory responsibility. The World Bank has strongly advocated privatization of water (Goldman 2004). Stakeholder organizations, however, frustrated with mounting prices and lack of local control, have challenged operations in Latin America, forcing the companies to reduce new investment and, in some cases, to sell their infrastructure. In Mexico, the private French companies manage water in Aguascalientes, Cancún, and part of Mexico City. Aguas Argentinas, a major water company in Argentina, is owned by Suez, Vivendi, and Anglian Water. Together, these companies also own concessions in Brazil, Chile (Santiago), Bolivia (La Paz), and Colombia (Cartagena) and, through Agbar, the water concession in Cuba (Habana) (Hall

and Lobina 2002). In certain cases, as in Argentina (Tucuman), Puerto Rico (Vieques), and Bolivia (Cochabamba), protests have forced the companies to withdraw (Spronk 2004). In other cases, privatization has been regarded as a better option than corrupt political management (Hoops and Ashur 2004).

5. Mexican and US researchers who had worked in this region for more than twenty-five years carried out the research on which this chapter is based. They used both qualitative and quantitative techniques, including a survey of a stratified random sample of rural households, in-depth interviews with key informants, and documentary analysis. Mexican collaborators carried out tests of surface and groundwater sources, human blood tests for organochlorines and organophosphorus pesticides, a preliminary survey of attitudes toward water quality, and a set of in-depth interviews about environmental hazards and conflicts over water. Team research is challenging, but it allows researchers to address complex issues often not possible for an individual. Equally important, collaborative, binational research teams enrich the project by helping to define critical issues, interpret data, and access new sources of data. We incorporated colleagues (men and women) trained in agronomy, biology, water chemistry, and toxicology. Our Mexican colleagues are based at El Colegio de la Frontera Norte, the major Mexican research institute in the border region. Working the Mexicali Valley for twenty-five years enabled us to draw on a very large database. The historical perspective is critical for our research because the region has experienced rapid social and economic change, which is reflected in the present socio-spatial-power arrangement.

6. In some regions of Mexico, people have local or indigenous knowledge about groundwater. For example, they link groundwater to springs and hand-dig galeria filtrantes to tap veins of water, using gravity to bring it to the surface at lower elevations (Enge and S. Whiteford 1989). In chapter 6 in this volume, on the San Marcos aquifer, Klaver and Donahue report that the movement of groundwater is carefully monitored. In many other parts of the world, people do not understand the complexities of aquifer systems, which may have multiple levels, flow directions, or contamination plums. In Mexicali, where groundwater is important for agriculture, most people assume that the government is monitoring the system. Folk knowledge about the system is scant. Furthermore, people have focused on extracting groundwater for irrigation, and the groundwater has always been of a higher quality than the surface water.

7. For years, pesticides have been recognized as a serious threat to people's health in the Americas (Sparks 1988; Murry 1994; Extoxnet 2003; Gillette et al.

1998). Acute exposure by air or from drinking water stored in pesticide drums has been of greatest concern. Health risk linked to pollution and toxic waste is an increasing public issue (Steingraber 1998).

8. Academic research can contribute to structural myopia when important findings are not shared with stakeholders. As a result of this project, we are recommending a systematic educational program about water quality and the need for local monitoring of drinking water quality. Pumps used for drinking water need filters that extract pesticides relatively inexpensively. We are also recommending the preparation of educational models about the aquifer, the threats to the aquifer, and its importance to the region. Knowledge about the aquifer—a significant factor in the region's political ecology—is critical for community empowerment. Making the water hidden below the surface an important part of peoples' knowledge and politics can make a difference. We would like to thank Victor Torres (2003), whose work opened this line of inquiry.

9. Only three of these companies included on their labels information required by Mexican law: the source of the water, mineral level, inspection approval number, and year of bottling. Three of the major companies imported water from the United States: Palomar Mountain, Agua Ciel (Coca Cola), and Mount Everest. Most of the labels focused on the advertising. The quality of bottled water in Mexico has been tested and debated (Robles et al. 1999). In the United States, Nestle, Pepsi, and Coca Cola have the highest sales of bottled water marketed under many labels. In many countries, as Gleick (2004:25) points out, "standards vary from place to place, testing is irregular and inconsistent, and contaminated source water may lead to contaminated products."

# 12

## Concluding Comments

*Future Challenges*

**Scott Whiteford and Linda Whiteford**

The authors in this volume accepted the challenge to examine the water-health interface in the context of globalization. Their work documents many ways in which global processes and the discourses about these processes have been translated, facilitated, resisted, and mobilized. At the same time, the authors met the conceptual challenges of theorizing about the links among local cultures, historical legacies, ecologies, and power constellations while examining emerging governance structures, changing world markets, new technologies, and local agency. Their work underlines the reality that globalization processes are reshaping health and environmental policy, prioritization, and outcome. In the cases presented here, the people are acutely aware of change generated by globalization(s), especially when it challenges or threatens the very bases of their culture, lifestyle, or health. In some cases, people respond quickly, taking advantage of new opportunities; in others, responses require reflection and mobilization.

In examining multiple dimensions of the relationships linking globalization, health, and water, the chapters share a common theme: for us to understand evolving health and resource management policies and their effectiveness, we must see them in a historical and global context. The authors' work focuses on peoples' lives and the meanings, interpretations, and processes of structural violence, or the violence of exclusion and inequality. Critical to the analysis are the interaction of culture, resources, and power in peoples' lives and the interfacing of the social construction of diversity (gender, ethnicity, and class) with power. From the World Bank to the World Health Organization, institutions with a global reach have generated policies, programs, and projects for countries throughout the world. The chapters herein document the local within the global as people in Spain, Ecuador, China, Zimbabwe, Malawi, and the United States organize to protect locally controlled water critical to their culture, to their food security, health, and way of life.

In this concluding chapter, we highlight contributions of the volume and point to future challenges that merit deeper or new research. We begin by discussing two global organizations that play a critical role in water and health policies and influence governments, communities, and families: the United Nations Millennium Challenge and the World Bank. We use the World Bank case to highlight several forms of global-local relationship and the impact on national program goals examined in the chapters, including privatization and the modification of water and health law, decentralization of management and control, and stakeholder participation.

The World Bank and other lending organizations urge privatization of municipal water companies, river basin systems, irrigation water associations, and sanitation systems. Because of political obstacles and community opposition, though, many private companies are withdrawing from any commitment to provide water services. There is an outstanding need for investment in sanitation systems that can reduce pollution and curtail the spread of disease. Is there a private/public mix in this area that can make a difference?

Global institutions play a key role in gathering international data and articulating health and water problems in global terms, as well as facilitating the exchange of information about poverty, environmental degradation, and infant mortality. These organizations also coordinate programs to address these global problems on local terms. For example, the water strategy of twenty-four United Nations programs focuses on reducing poverty and child mortality. The United Nations organizations have established the Millennium Development Goals: (1) to halve the number of people without safe drinking water and basic sanitation by the year 2015 and (2) to stop unsustainable exploitation of water resources by developing policies that enhance equitable access and adequate supplies. The United Nations Development Program and other programs concentrate on creating effective water governance, resolving conflicts over water, and integrating a gender perspective throughout water management programs and policies. These efforts and their local consequences merit study and evaluation by social scientists, whose findings are necessary for policy revision and implementation.

The World Bank globally funds ambitious, expensive water projects. Many of its big dam projects, to generate electricity, store water, and reduce flooding, have led to relocation and displacement of thousands of people throughout the world. These projects have induced indigenous people, farmer organizations, environmental groups, and academics to protest and mobilize (Johnston and Garcia-Downing n.d.; Shiva 2001; Alexander 2002). Their criticism may have influenced World Bank funding policy, which shows the tension and complexity of global-local connections.

In its 1992 Water Policy document, the World Bank Water Development Strategy focuses on privatization of water, market mechanisms to increase efficiency, and incorporation of the private sector to modernize municipal and city water and sanitation systems. It gives scant attention to local governance, stakeholder participation, cultural rules of management, and indigenous rights or knowledge (Bayliss and Hall 2002). The 2004 World Bank Water Policy document, however, appears to demonstrate a paradigmatic change: it does not directly mention privatization. Privatization and demand-based distribution, in contrast to rights-based distribution, still have defining roles in World Bank policy (World Bank 2004), but the 2004 document also acknowledges local stakeholder participation, accountability, and transparency.

How to empower and protect local institutions through greater participation, accountability of all actors (including the nation-state), and transparency are issues raised in this volume. More importantly, the chapters document how difficult it is to defend the rights of the less powerful and most vulnerable and to protect the environment when power or access to power is distributed unevenly in society. Global capitalism, functioning in the name of efficiency, provides little support for small agricultural producers or struggling urban residents. Two chapters address the problem of manufactured or contrived scarcity, concepts that are foreign to the World Bank analyses yet are grim realities in countries throughout the world. Documenting the processes and outcomes of the paradigmatic changes in the 2004 World Bank Water Strategy is a future challenge. Without research, it will be difficult to demonstrate whether the strategy has changed or only the presentation.

Privatization and water markets are often linked in the discourse on decentralization. As the chapters reveal, the privatization of water raises many questions about long-term, equitable ownership and control, questions that demand more research. The World Bank and other regional banks have incorporated privatization and decentralization into their loan policies. Some call this "the new culture of water," complete with new principles of ownership, management, and control. Simultaneously, decentralization and privatization have been the hallmarks of health "reforms" since the 1990s; far too often, they have increased levels of malnutrition, failed to immunize, and reduced access to drinking water and health systems. Decentralization has been encouraged as a strategy to overcome the overly regulated, slow federal bureaucracy insensitive to local needs or knowledge. Decentralized programs, however, are at risk of being co-opted by local elites at the expense of the poor, or may simply exclude the poor from services altogether. Given that these processes have been in place since the final quarter of the twentieth century and that data on their consequences is available, future research on the long-term results of privatization and decentralization policies will now be possible.

Centralized water management, decision making, and regulation composed the paradigm advocated by international agencies during the 1960s–1990s. This model reflected a view that water was a public good and that the state had a welfare obligation to provide water to its citizens. Centralization was challenged because studies found highly centralized water or irrigation systems to be unresponsive to local needs, authoritarian, inefficient, and expensive for the state. Decentralization of water management became a critical component of neoliberal reform demanded by the World Bank. Justified by the assumption that water is "an economic good and input in economic activity and cost recovery and financial viability" are of paramount importance (Saleth and Dinar 1999:40), decentralization is presented as enhancing a more efficient, sustainable use of water.

While recognizing the virtues and success of decentralization, chapters in this volume question assumptions about the meaning of decentralization, what is being decentralized for whom, and the influence of local power inequalities on community and regional management systems. Often, decentralization relieves the burden of water and health management costs, reducing subsidization of water costs for poor households or for irrigation for peasants. In some cases, it means shifting the responsibility for drinking water from the state to private water companies. Nevertheless, in the chapters of this book, people want local control, where local knowledge can be used to address local problems in an equitable manner. When centralized water control systematically fails its stakeholders, in some cases, decentralization brings about reform and empowerment. When local institutions can be transparent and accountable, decentralization may be an especially powerful tool.

As reflected in a rich anthropological literature, and documented in chapters 9 and 10 on Spain and Southern Africa, respectively, decentralization is a keystone of many traditional water-management systems built on cultural practices and community agreements unfettered by central government mandates (McMillan 2003; Enge and S. Whiteford 1989). Massive dam projects created by federal governments often suffer from bureaucratic inefficiency, patronage, and closed accounting systems. When forced to be more transparent and participatory, people in these systems benefit. At a second level, however, the policy conditions for loans by the World Bank and other donor agencies are centralizing, contradicting the rhetoric of decentralization and perpetrating what could be considered another form of structural violence (Bayliss and Hall 2002).

The Millennium Challenge—the United Nations' campaign to reduce the world's child morality by 50 percent and to improve health—is directly involved in water and sanitation programs. The

United Nations Children's Fund (UNICEF), the World Health Organization (WHO), and the United Nations Development Program (UNDP) coordinate global efforts to address water, health, and sanitation problems. In conjunction with world conferences on sustainable development, such as the World Summit for Children and Water, these efforts constitute a form of globalization, spurred by the United Nations. The United Nations General Assembly proclaimed 1981–1990 the International Drinking Water Supply and Sanitation Decade. In 1995 the World Summit for Social Development focused on poverty and health, placing safe drinking water and health at the center of the problem of meeting basic human needs. In addition, UNICEF has developed a water and environmental sanitation program (WES). Despite all these programs, more people than ever have no access to potable water and sanitation. During the past decade, an estimated 1.2 billion people gained access to water supplies and 770 million to improved sanitation (UN WWDR 2003:8), but world population growth has outstripped expanding water and sanitation programs.

The nation-state receives varying degrees of attention in these chapters. Some argue that the state has lost its power to control and regulate its citizens in the era of globalization. Information flows across borders, unhindered by state control, and states have opened their borders for trade as part of GATT and other global trade agreements. Illegal immigration has transformed population demographics. At the same time, because of 9/11 and the war in Iraq, North American countries are regulating their borders in the name of security, and European countries are redefining theirs.

Government and international aid organizations develop policies and programs to protect people during floods, droughts, and water-related disasters brought on by hurricanes, which cause the largest number of natural disaster deaths. As part of these strategies, governments have built massive dams, often funded by the World Bank or major regional banks. Damming rivers has been a subject of hot policy debate in which anthropologists and other social scientists have actively participated. Massive dam projects often displace thousands of people and wildlife; however, they may also help to control flooding that has devastated populations for centuries. There is a continuing need for anthropologists to study the social and environmental impacts of

## Concluding Comments

potential dam projects. Too often, people have been sacrificed in the name of policies that claim to protect them (Johnston and Garcia-Downing n.d.).

The nation-state is still the ultimate definer of environmental and health policy, translator of international treaties and agreements, and implementer of programs and projects. The chapters in this volume describe how the nation-state may co-opt, build on, or resist global trade, information, culture, and power. The authors also point out how states differ in their policies and in their ability to negotiate with one another or with global organizations.

The importance of NGOs in water and health reform is a persistent theme in these chapters, but they now play an even more powerful role in world health and water programming. Social science theories and evaluations of the various types of NGOs should be an essential part of the future agenda. Major NGOs, many with a global reach and mandate, include Resources for the Future, the International Water Management Institute, Water Aid, Global Water Partnership, Nature Conservancy, and World Vision. The range of their contributions to communities varies tremendously, from baseline research to technical aid and loans. NGOs have taken divergent and often opposing positions on whether water should be seen as a human right or a commodity and on the implications of these positions. Because of their significance as global actors transcending levels, NGOs merit greater attention from scholars interested in worldwide health and water issues.

Another aspect of water security/insecurity examined in this volume concerns water critical for irrigation, food production, and, ultimately, the world's nutritional and health security. Worldwide irrigation for agriculture accounts for 80 percent of water consumption. With population growth increasing the demand for food, the pressure for more irrigation water intensifies (Rosegrant, Cai, and Cline 2002b:1). At the same time, aquifers are being depleted by intensive pumping, and new sources of freshwater are becoming increasingly more difficult to tap. Irrigated fields are plagued by salinization and waterlogging. As discussed, on the United States/Mexico border, these sparked massive farmer mobilization and international negotiations. Three chapters in this volume examine the competition for water among farms, cities, mines, and factories. Improving water efficiency through new irrigation technologies, building infrastructure to reduce water loss, and raising the cost of water are suggested methods for better irrigation-water conservation. Here again, international agencies and national governments are expecting the market to force people to conserve water and society to prioritize how water is distributed.

The research detailed in this volume reflects current theories and methods in anthropology. Yet, by crosscutting substantive differences in research foci (resource management and health), the authors have extended their theoretical range by considering topics previously outside their scope of inquiry. This volume is designed to address two primary substantive issues—resource management of water and water-implicated health outcomes—and how they are connected to globalization(s). One of the questions authors explore together is whether similar political, economic, and cultural forces produce the restriction of access that creates health and resource inequities. We suggest that similar local and global processes underlie patterns of access and that water management policies and water-related health outcomes are inexorably linked.

Too often, the linkage between water management and water-related diseases is invisible. In fact, researchers in the arena of water and natural resource management tend not to write about the connection between those management policies and practices and health outcomes. Rarely do discussions of water management policies and practices (water for irrigation systems, for example) influence the management of drinking water or acknowledge its direct effect on access to clean and reliable water. Public health professionals have long recognized that access to a reliable, clean supply of water is a basic requirement for essential improvements in health statistics; however, public health professionals and resource management professionals seldom consult one another when making decisions about water.

Chapters in this volume document the range of cultural, economic, and political processes that structure how water is managed, and how these processes can generate or maintain health disparities. Concepts such as the manufactured, or contrived, scarcity of water or other natural resources, illustrate how political processes are used to manipulate public opinion to privilege one group over another, resulting in structural violence toward disenfranchised groups. The artificial creation of resource scarcity has direct health implications too often ignored by social scientists. Simultaneously, anthropologists who work in the area of health, including those who focus on water-borne diseases, often fail to consider water management practices and policies as part of their larger research questions. Yet similar cultural, economic, and political forces are at work.

The reasons for this conceptual lacuna are many; differences in research orientations, levels of scale, technical methods, theoretical frameworks, research funding sources and partnerships, and even applied programming often make crosscutting discussions awkward, if not impossible. This book attempts to open up discussion regarding the similarities of processes, the role of social constructs that shape water management decisions and health access decisions, and how these two are intertwined. We recognize that this product reflects a relatively nascent level of conceptual integration, but the discussion has, at least, begun.

The chapters reflect conceptual and empirical research from several subfields in anthropology. Chapters on Malawi, the United States/Mexico border, Ecuador, and Silicon Valley, respectively, connect critical medical anthropology with political ecology, which, in turn, reflect elements of economic and political anthropology. Each chapter approaches theoretical issues differently, but the linking of political ecology with medical anthropology is most obvious, a relationship infrequently addressed (Baer 1996b). The analysis of power, discourses of power, and the body links the fields. As examined in this volume, the persistent assaults on the environment by human activity, from pesticides to industrial waste, are ultimately apparent in the physical body of all creatures, including humans. It is in the body that "the social contradictions are played out, as well as a locus of personal and social resistance, creativity and struggle" (Lock and Scheper-Hughes 1996:7). New directions in anthropology are exploring how illness, disease, and environmental explanatory narratives interact, frequently generating awareness and action (Torres n.d.).

Cultural anthropologists, like their disciplinary colleagues in archaeology, are working more in multidisciplinary teams or, at the least, are turning to other fields to examine the complex issues discussed in this volume. This is certainly the case where our understanding of environmental contamination and human health is concerned. At the same time, cultural anthropologists approach this collaboration with a critical eye, understanding that science, too, is subjective, politically bound, and a part of culture itself.

During the past decade, globalization has emerged as an important concept in anthropology and other social sciences. A rich scholarship has evolved on the topic of globalization, especially on the impact of global markets and trade, the changing role of the state, immigration and transnationalism, and whether new communication technologies influence culture, power, and identity, and vice versa. Globalization has been equally important in the fields of resource management and health. Although the authors in this volume take different tacks on globalization, all examine issues of resource management and health. The growing inequalities of power, health, and access to land, water, and wealth associated with globalization and the ways in which people have mobilized, resisted, or been overwhelmed by globalizing forces are central themes in the chapters.

The degree to which globalization exacerbated inequality and poverty in the case studies varies. Certainly, the chapters reflect struggles between state and global institutions to impose regulations and constraints on communities, as well as the diverse efforts of people to resist these pressures yet take advantage of the information resources of a global society. New products, from pesticides to bottled water, generated new patterns of consumption but also created new needs. At the same time, the discourses about the human rights of global or national citizens clashed with policies that actually subordinate people (Briggs and Mantini-Briggs 2003:324).

The chapters reflect the articulation of scholarship evolving out of two subfields in anthropology: medical anthropology, particularly critical medical anthropology, and environmental anthropology, especially political ecology. The authors engage conceptual and methodological issues from these fields, most significantly issues of scale, by linking different levels of analysis, integrating multiple research methods and data, and including power in the health/environment analyses. All the authors are deeply concerned about the people with whom they work, the applicability of their work, and the sharing of their work with colleagues in the countries where they do their research. Another important dimension of the volume is how the studies link to policy issues or direct applied actions.

The problems discussed in this volume are time-sensitive. Each day, six thousand children die from diseases associated with consuming contaminated water. The present era of globalization is a time of global markets, vast commodity chains, rapid diffusion of information, growing consumerism, and the emergence and reemergence of infectious diseases. Complex ecological systems are regularly obliterated by human activities. The cost of mismanagement and the rapid rate of pollution escalate each day. Global organizations are responding to environmental and social problems, although sometimes with too little too late. It is increasingly difficult to address "development problems" outside the context of global processes of world capitalism, expanding consumer culture(s), inequalities, and disparities. These chapters focus beyond development problems, taking aim instead at the global contexts that shape them.

Protecting the physical environment and human health must be part of a deeper change in societal values. For anthropology and other social sciences to participate in this transformation through methodologically rigorous, theoretically informed, and socially relevant research is the biggest challenge. We end this book by returning to a beginning statement: "this is a book about crimes and passions." The passions are embedded in high-stakes gambling—for future control of resources, how they are managed, and who profits and who pays. The crimes are just as real as the futures they trade: the lost futures of children without safe drinking water, the stolen futures of women caring for the elderly and ill, the sold futures of families without water and work, and the flooded futures of people displaced by dams. In this era, social science must make new theoretical understandings relevant to world problems, or it will be too late.

# References

**Adams, J.**
2002 Gover: Departure of McCaleb Is "a Bad Thing" for Indians. *Indian Country Today*, 4 December: A1, A3.

**Adams, W.**
2001 *Green Development: Environment and Sustainability in the Third World.* 2nd edition. Routledge: London.

**afrol News**
2002 10 Million Water Cuts after South Africa's Water Privatization. Electronic document, http://www.afrol.com/News?sa024_water_private.htm, accessed November 4.

**Agarwal, B.**
2000 Conceptualizing Environmental Collective Action: Why Gender Matters. *Cambridge Journal of Economics* 24:283–310.

**Ahmed, A. K.**
2002 Serious Environmental and Public Health Impacts of Water-Related Diseases and Lack of Sanitation on Adults and Children: A Brief Summary. electronic document http://www.cec.org/files/pdf/POLLUTANTS/karim_ahmed.pdf, accessed March 2003.

**Alcázar, L., L. C. Xu, and A. M. Zuluaga**
2002 Institutions, Politics, and Contracts: The Attempt to Privatize the Water and Sanitation Utility of Lima, Peru. In *Thirsting for Efficiency: Experiences in Reforming Urban Water Systems*, edited by M. Shirley. Oxford: Elsevier Press.

**Alexander, N. C.**
2002 A Critique of the World Bank Water Resources Strategy. *Global Policy Forum*. Electronic document, www.globalpolicy.org.

# References

**Allen, L., and J. L. Darby**

1994 Quality Control of Bottled and Vended Water in California: A Review of Comparison of Tap Water. *Journal of Environmental Health* 56(4):17.

**Allan, T.**

2000 *The Middle East Water Question: Hydropolitics and the Global Economy*. London: I. B. Tauris.

2002 Water Resources in Semi-Arid Regions: Real Deficits and Economically Invisible and Politically Silent Solutions. In *Hydropolitics in the Developing World: A Southern African Perspective*, edited by A. Turton and R. Henwood, pp. 23–36. Pretoria: University of Pretoria African Water Issues Research Unit, Center for International Political Studies.

**Almeda, J., M. Corachan, A. Sousa, C. Ascaso, J. M. Carvalho, D. Rollinson, and V. R. Southgate**

1994 Schistosomiasis in the Republic of Sao-Tome-and-Principe—Human Studies. *Transactions of the Royal Society of Tropical Medicine and Hygiene* 88(4):406–409.

**Anders, G. C.**

1999 Indian Gaming: Financial and Regulatory Issues. In *Contemporary Native American Political Issues*, edited by T. R. Johnson, pp. 163–173. Walnut Creek, CA: AltaMira Press.

**Anderson, T. L., and P. J. Hill**

1975 The Evolution of Property Rights: A Study of the American West. *Journal of Law and Economics* 43(1):163–179.

**Anderson, T. L., and P. S. Snyder**

1997 *In Pursuit of Water Markets: Priming the Invisible Pump*. Washington, DC: Cato Institute.

**Appadurai, A.**

1990 Disjuncture and Difference in the Global Cultural Economy. *Public Culture* 2(2):1–23. Reprinted in *The Globalization Reader*, edited by F. J. Lechner and J. Boli, pp. 322–330. London: Blackwell, 2000.

1996 *Modernity at Large*. Minneapolis: University of Minnesota Press.

2001 Grassroots Globalization and the Research Imagination. In *Globalization*, edited by A. Appadurai, pp. 1–21. Durham, NC: Duke University Press.

**Armelagos, G.**

1990 Health and Disease in Prehistoric Populations in Transition. In *Disease in Populations in Transition*, edited by G. Armelagos, pp. 127–144. New York: Bergin and Garvey.

**Ashton, P., and V. Ramasar**

2002 Water and HIV/AIDS: Some Strategic Considerations. In *Hydropolitics in the Developing World: A Southern African Perspective*, edited by A. Turtun and R. Henwood, pp. 217–235. Pretoria, South Africa: African Water Issues Research Unit, Center for International Political Studies, University of Pretoria.

# REFERENCES

**Asturias, E., G. R. Brenneman, K. M. Petersen, M. Hazme, and M. Santosham**
2000      Infectious Diseases. In *American Indian Health: Innovations in Health Care, Promotion, and Policy*, edited by E. R. Rhoades, pp. 347–369. Baltimore: Johns Hopkins University Press.

**Baer, H. A.**
1996a      Toward a Political Ecology of Health. *Medical Anthropology Quarterly* 10(4):451–454.
1996b      Bringing Political Ecology into Critical Medical Anthropology: A Challenge to Bicultural Approaches. *Medical Anthropology* 17:129–141.

**Baer, H., and M. Singer**
1995      *Critical Medical Anthropology*. Amityville, NY: Baywood Publishing Company.

**Baer, H., with M. Singer and I. Susser**
1997      *Medical Anthropology and the World System: A Critical Perspective*. Westport, CT: Bergin and Garvey.

**Bakker, I., ed.**
1994      *The Strategic Silence: Gender and Economic Policy*. London: Zed Books.

**Barbosa, C. S., C. B. da Silva, and F. S. Barbosa**
1996      Schistosomiasis: Reproduction and Expansion of the Endemic Region in Brazil. *Revista De Saude Publica* 30(6):609–616.

**Barlow, M.**
1999      *Blue Gold: The Global Water Crisis and the Commodification of the World's Water Supply*. Sausalito, CA: International Forum on Globalization. In *International Forum on Globalization Special Report*. Electronic document, www.ifg.org/bgsummary.
2001      Water as Commodity—The Wrong Prescription. *Food First Institute for Development Policy, Backgrounder* 7(3). Electronic document, http://www.foodfirst.org/pubs/backgrdrs/2001/s01v7n3.html

**Barlow, M., and T. Clarke**
2002      *Blue Gold: The Battle against Corporate Theft of the World's Water*. London: Earthscan.

**Barlow, M., with T. Clarke**
2002      *Blue Gold: The Fight to Stop the Corporate Theft of the World's Water*. New York: The New York Press.

**Bayliss, K., and D. Hall**
2002      Unsustainable Conditions and the World Bank, Privatization, Water and Energy. London Public Services International Research Unit, University of Greenwich. Electronic document, www.psiru.org.

**Bearak, B.**
2002      Bangladeshis Sipping a Slow Death from Wells: Aid Groups Racing Time to Halt "Mass Poisoning" from Arsenic. *The Miami Herald*, 14 July: 5A.

# References

**Bell, D.**
2002 Tugboats, Huge Bladders Featured in Water Plan. *San Diego Union-Tribune*, 2 February.

**Bennett, V.**
1995 *The Politics of Water*. Pittsburgh: University of Pittsburgh Press.

**Beno, M.**
1991 Treaty Troubles: The Spearfishing of Walleyes Off the Reservations by Chippewa Indians Has Inflamed Passions in the Wisconsin Wood. *Audubon* (May):102–114.

**Birrie, H., N. Berhe, S. Tedla, and N. Gemeda**
1993 Schistosoma-Haematobium Infection among Ethiopian Prisoners of War (1977–1988) Returning from Somalia. *Ethiopian Medical Journal* 31(4):259–264.

**Bond, P.**
2004 The Political Roots of South Africa's Epidemic. In *Sickness and Wealth: The Corporate Assault on Global Health*, edited by M. Fort, M. A. Mercer, and O. Gish, chapter 10. Boston: South End Press.

**Booth, M., Y. S. Li, and M. Tanner**
1996 Helminth Infections, Morbidity Indicators and Schistosomiasis Treatment History in Three Villages, Dongting Lake Region, PR China. *Tropical Medicine & International Health* 1(4):464–474.

**Bos, M. G., and W. Walters**
1990 Water Charges and Irrigation Efficiencies. *Irrigation and Drainage Systems* 4:267–278.

**Brennan, T.**
2003 *Globalization and Its Terrors, Daily Life in the West*. London: Routledge.

**Brenneman, G. R., A. O. Handler, S. F. Kaufman, and E. R. Rhoades**
2000 Health Status and Clinical Indicators. In *American Indian Health: Innovations in Health Care, Promotion, and Policy*, edited by E. R. Rhoades, pp. 103–121. Baltimore: Johns Hopkins University Press.

**Briggs, C., and C. Mantini-Briggs**
2003 *Stories in the Time of Cholera: Racial Profiling during a Medical Nightmare*. Berkeley: University of California Press.

**Brinkley, J.**
2003 American Indians Say Documents Show Government Has Cheated Them Out of Billions. *New York Times*, 7 January, A14.

*Britannica*
1998 Peru. Introduction, vol. 25, p. 506. Chicago: Encyclopedia Britannica Inc.

**Buckle, C.**
2001 *African Tears: The Zimbabwe Land Invasions*. Johannesburg: Covos Day Books.

# References

**Burawoy, M., J. A. Blum, S. George, Z. Gille, T. Gowan, L. Haney, M. Klawiter, S. H. Lopez, S. O. Riain, and M. Thayer**
2000    *Global Ethnography: Forces, Connections, and Imaginations in a Postmodern World*. Berkeley: University of California Press.

**Bureau of Indian Affairs**
2003    Electronic document, www.doiu.nbc.gov/orientation/bia2.cfm, accessed March 4.

**Burns, W. C. G.**
2002    Pacific Islands Developing Country Water Resources and Climate Change. In *The World's Water 2002–2003: The Biennial Report on Freshwater Resources*, edited by P. H. Gleick, with W. C. G. Burns, E. L. Chalecki, M. Cohen, K. K. Cushing, A. S. Mann, R. Reyes, G. H. Wolff, and A. K. Wong, pp. 113–131. Washington, DC: Island Press.

**Butzer, K. W., J. F. Mateu, and E. K. Butzer**
1985    Irrigation Agrosystems in Eastern Spain: Roman or Islamic Origins? *Annals of the American Association of American Geographers* 75:479–509.

**California Department of Fish and Game**
2002    September 2002 Klamath River Fish Kill: Preliminary Analysis of Contributing Factors. State of California, The Resources Agency, Department of Fish and Game. Electronic document, http://www.dfg.ca.gov/html/krfishkill-rpt-err.pdf.

**Castells, M.**
1996    *The Information Age: Economy, Society and Culture*. Cambridge, MA: Blackwell.

**Center for International Law (CIEL)**
2003    International Financial Institutions Program, Bechtel Lawsuit page. February 12 press release. Electronic document, http://www.ciel.org/Ifi/Bechtel_Lawsuit_12Feb03.html.

**Center for Policy Analysis on Trade and Health**
2004    The FTAA: Health Hazards for the Americas? Electronic document, Electronic document, http://www.cpath.org/CPATH-Testimony.html, accessed August 27.

**Chang, Y., C. Tai, R. S. Lin, S. Yang, C. Chen, T. Shih, and S. Liou**
2003    A Proportionate Cancer Morbidity Ration Study of Workers Exposed to Chlorinated Organic Solvents in Taiwan. *Industrial Health* 41:77–87.

**Chavula, G., and W. Mulwafu**
2001    Hazardous Water: An Assessment of Water Resource Quality in the Likangala Catchment Area for Domestic Purposes. BASIS Report. Madison, WI: Broadening Access and Strengthening Input Market Systems Collaborative Research Support Program (BASIS-CRSP) Management Office.

**Chen, X. Y.**
2002    The Challenges and Strategies in Schistosomiasis Control Programs in China. *Acta Tropica* 82(2):279–282.

# References

**Chesky, L.**
2003    Liquid Assets: Felton Fights an International Mega-Corporation to Take Control of the Town's Water. *Good Times* 13–19 (February):16–21.

**Children's Water Fund**
2004    Did You Know…Electronic document, http://www.childrenswaterfund.org, accessed May 26.

**Chilima, G., B. Nkhoma, G. Chavula, and W. Mulwafu**
2001    *Community-Based Management Approach in the Management of Water Resources by Different Organizations in the Lake Chilwa Basin, Malawi.* BASIS Publication. Madison, WI: BASIS-CRSP Management Office. Electronic document, http://www.wisc.edu/ltc/live/bassaf0112a.pdf.

**Chilton, J.**
1998    Dry or Drowning. Fresh Water. Our Planet 9.4. Electronic document, http://www.ourplanet.com/imgversn/94/chilton.html, accessed October 23, 2004.

**Claiborne, W.**
1990    Mohawks, Army Still at Standoff; Bridge to Montreal Reopens to Traffic. *The Washington Post*, 7 SeptembeR: A17, A21.

**Clarke, R.**
1993    *Water: The International Crisis.* Boston: MIT Press.

**Clayton, L.**
2002    *Grace: W. R. Grace & Co.: The Formative Years, 1850–1930.* Ottawa, IL: Jameson Books.

**Cleaver, F.**
1998a    Choice, Complexity and Change: Gendered Livelihoods and the Management of Water. *Agriculture and Human Values* 15:293–299.

1998b    Incentives and Informal Institutions: Gender and the Management of Water. *Agriculture and Human Values* 15:347–360.

2001    Institutions, Agency and the Limitations of Participatory Approaches to Development. In *Participation. The New Tyranny?*, edited by B. Cooke and U. Kothari, pp. 36–55. New York: Zed Books.

2003    *Bearers, Buyers and Bureaucrats: The Missing Social World in Gender and Water.* Sussex, UK: Institute of Development Studies.

**Cleaver, F., and D. Elson**
1995    *Women and Water Resources: Continued Marginalisation and New Policies.* Gatekeeper Series No. 49. London: International Institute for Environment and Development.

**Clifford, J.**
1989    Notes on Travel and Theory. *Inscriptions: Traveling Theories, Traveling Theorists* 5:177–188.

1992    Traveling Cultures. In *Cultural Studies*, edited by L. Grossberg, C. Nelson, and P. A. Treichler, pp. 96–112. New York: Routledge.

**Clot, S. R., and M. C. Torres Grael**
1974    *Historia de un canal 1147–1974.* Lerida: Artis Estudios Graficos.

**Cohen, F. G.**
1986    *Treaties on Trial: The Continuing Controversy over Northwest Indian Fishing Rights.* Seattle: University of Washington Press.

**Comisión Nacional del Agua (CNA)**
1998    Estudio General de Calidad del Agua en el Distrito de Riego 014, Rio Colorado (metales pesados y pesticidas). Report elaborated by O. Ríos Noriega for the CNA, contract no. MP. 14-65-3-001-97. Mexicali, Baja CA.

**Commission on Macroeconomics and Health**
2001    *Macroeconomics and Health: Investing in Health for Economic Development.* Geneva: World Health Organization.

**Concejo de Regantes de León**
1998    *Circular Informativa.* León: Concejo de Regantes de León.

**Cooke, B., and U. Kothari, eds.**
2001    *Participation. The New Tyranny?* New York: Zed Books.

**Coon-Come, M.**
1991    Where Can You Buy a River? *Northeast Indian Quarterly* (Winter):6–11.

**Cornwall, A.**
2003    Whose Voices? Whose Choices? Reflections on Gender and Participatory Development. *World Development* 31(8):1325–1342.

**Cortez-Lara, A., and M. R. Garcia-Acevedo**
2000    The Lining of the All-American Canal: The Forgotten Voices. *Natural Resource Journal* 40(2):261–280.

**Cottle, E., and H. Deedat**
2003    Cholera Outbreak: A 2000–2002 Case Study of the Source of the Outbreak in the Madlebe Tribal Authority Areas, uThungulu Region, KwaZulu-Natal. Report by Health Systems Trust. Electronic document, http://new.hst.org.za/pubs/index.php/480/.

**De Soto, H., E. Ghersi, and M. Ghibellini**
1986    *El Otro Sendero.* El Barranco, Peru: Instituto Libertad y Democracia.

**DeGabriele, J.**
2002    *Improving Community-Based Management of Boreholes: A Case Study from Malawi.* BASIS Report. Madison, WI: BASIS-CRSP Management Office.

**Derman, W.**
1998    Balancing the Waters: Development and Hydropolitics in Contemporary Zimbabwe. In *Water, Culture and Power*, edited by J. Donahue and B. R. Johnston, pp. 63–80. New York: Island Press.

## References

2001 Water Unites Us, Water Divides Us: Race and Water in Contemporary Zimbabwe. Paper prepared for the panel "The Ethics of Ethnography in the Racialized Postcolony: Choosing and Changing Sides in Zimbabwe," the American Ethnological Society and Canadian Anthropology Society Joint Meetings, Montreal.

**Derman, W., and A. Ferguson**
2003 Value of Water: Political Ecology and Water Reforms in Southern Africa. *Human Organization* 63(3):277–289.

**Derman, W., A. Ferguson, and F. Gonese**
2000 Decentralization, Devolution and Development: Reflections on the Water Reform Process in Zimbabwe. BASIS Report. Madison, WI: BASIS-CRSP Management Office.

**Derman, W., and F. Gonese**
2003 Water Reform in Zimbabwe: Its Multiple Interfaces with the Land Reform and Resettlement. In *Delivering Land and Securing Rural Livelihoods: Post-Independence Land Reform and Resettlement in Zimbabwe*, edited by M. Roth and F. Gonese, pp. 241–257. Harare: Centre for Applied Social Sciences, University of Zimbabwe; Madison: Land Tenure Center, University of Wisconsin.

**Derman, W., and A. Hellum**
2002 Neither Tragedy nor Enclosure: Are There Inherent Human Rights in Water Management in Zimbabwe's Communal Lands? *The European Journal of Development Research* 14(2):31–50.

**Devereux, S.**
2002a Safety Nets in Malawi: The Process of Choice. Paper prepared for the Institute of Development Studies Conference "Surviving the Present, Securing the Future: Social Policies for the Poor in Poor Countries," Sussex, UK.
2002b The Malawi Famine of 2002. *Institute of Development Studies Bulletin, The New Famines* 33 (October):70–78.

**DeWaal, A.**
2002 AIDS-Related National Crises in Africa: Food Security, Governance and Development Partnerships. *Institute of Development Studies Bulletin, The New Famines* 33 (October):120–126.

**Díez Gonzalez, F.**
1992 *La España del regadio y sus instituciones basicas*. Madrid: Grafica 82.

**Donahue, J. M.**
1998 Water Wars in South Texas: Managing the Edwards Aquifer. In *Water, Culture and Power: Local Struggles in a Global Context*, edited by J. M. Donahue and B. R. Johnston, pp. 187–208. Washington, DC: Island Press.

# References

**Donahue, J. M., and M. B. McGuire**
1995    The Political Economy of Responsibility in Health and Illness. *Social Science and Medicine* 40(1):47–53.

**Donahue, J. M., and J. Q. Sanders**
2001    Sitting Down at the Table: Mediation Efforts in Resolving Water Conflicts. In *On the Border: An Environmental History of San Antonio*, edited by C. Miller, pp. 182–195. Pittsburgh: University of Pittsburgh Press.

**Donahue, J., and B. R. Johnston, eds.**
1998    *Water, Culture & Power: Local Struggles in a Global Context*. Washington, DC: Island Press.

**Downey, R.**
2000    *Riddle of the Bones: Politics, Science, Race, and the Story of Kennewick Man*. New York: Copernicus.

**Downing, T.**
1996    An Overview of the International Finance Corporation Sponsored Participatory Evaluation of a Pehuenche Indigenous Development Foundation. Prepared for the International Finance Corporation, March 27 (censored report). Electronic document, http://www.ted-downing.com/Peheunche%20 summary.htm.

**Drimie, S.**
2002    The Impact of HIV/AIDS on Rural Households and Land Issues in Southern and Eastern Africa. Background paper prepared for the Food and Agricultural Organization, Sub-Regional Office for Southern and Eastern Africa, Rome.

**du Guerny, J.**
2001    Agriculture and HIV/AIDS. Paper prepared for EASE International, Copenhagen.

**Duque, M. C.**
2002    The Columbian Health Crisis: Applications from Cuba. Paper presented at the Annual Meeting of the Society for Applied Anthropology, Atlanta.

**Earthjustice Fund**
2003    Bolivia Petition. Amicus brief filed by M. Wagner (Earthjustice Fund, Oakland, CA), M. Orellana (CIEL, Washington, DC), and Jim Schulz (The Democracy Center, Bolivia). Electronic document, http://www.earthjustice.org/news/documents/boliviapetition.pdf.

***The Ecologist***
1993    *Whose Common Future? Reclaiming the Commons*. Philadelphia: New Society Publishers.

***The Economist***
2000    Canada—First Nationalism. Nisga'a Win Land Claim Case in British Columbia. *The Economist* 356(8182, August 5):38.

# References

**Eggertsson, T.**
1990    *Economic Behavior and Institutions*. Cambridge: Cambridge University Press.

**Eide, A.**
1995    The Right to an Adequate Standard of Living Including the Right to Food. In *Economic, Social and Cultural Rights: A Textbook*, edited by A. Eide, C. Krause, and A. Rosas, pp. 89–106. Dordecht: Martinus Nijhoff.

**The Electronics Industry Good Neighbor Campaign**
1997    Sacred Waters (El Agua es de Todos/Life-Blood of Mother Earth): Four Case Studies of High-Tech Water Resource Exploitation and Corporate Welfare in the Southwest. Report published by People Organized in Defense of Earth and Her Resources (Austin, TX), Silicon Valley Toxics Coalition (San Jose, CA), SouthWest Organizing Project (Albuquerque, NM), and Tonatierra Community Development Institute (Phoenix, AZ).

**Enge, K., and S. Whiteford**
1989    *The Keepers of Water and Earth: Mexican Rural Social Organization and Irrigation*. Austin: The University of Texas Press.

**Engelman, R., and P. Leroy**
1993    Population Action International. *Sustaining Water: Population and the Future of Renewable Water Supplies*. Electronic document, http://www.cnie.org/pop/pai/image2.html.

**Environmental Defense Fund**
2003    Scorecard. Trichloroethylene Chemical Profile. Electronic document, http://www.scorecard.org/chemical-profiles/summary.tcl?edf_substance_id=79 percent2d01 percent 2d6#hazards.

**Environmental Working Group**
2002    Rocket Science: Perchlorate and the Toxic Legacy of the Cold War. Report by the Environmental Working Group. Electronic document, http://www.ewg.org/reports/rocketscience.

2004    Rocket Fuel Contamination in California Milk. Report by the Environmental Working Group. Electronic document, http://www.ewg.org/reports/rocketmilk/.

**Ernould, J. C., A. K. Kaman, R. Labbo, D. Couret, and J. P. Chippaux**
2000    Recent Urban Growth and Urinary Schistosomiasis in Niamey, Niger. *Tropical Medicine & International Health* 5(6):431–437.

**Extoxnet**
2003    Extension Toxicology Network. Pesticide Information Profiles Malathion. Oregon State University. Electronic document, http://ace.orst.edu/cgi-bin/mfs/or/pips/malathio.htm.

**Farmer, P.**
1992    *AIDS and Accusations: Haiti and the Geography of Blame*. Berkeley: University of California Press.

2001    *Infections and Inequalities: The Modern Plagues.* Berkeley: University of California Press.

2003    *Pathologies of Power: Health, Human Rights, and the New War on the Poor.* Berkeley: University of California Press.

2004    An Anthropology of Structural Violence. *Current Anthropology* 45 (June):305–317.

**Farooq, M.**

1973    Historical Development. In *Epidemiology and Control of Schistosomiasis (Bilharziasis)*, edited by N. Ansari, pp. 1–16. Baltimore: University Park Press.

**Federación Nacional de Comunidades de Regantes de España**

2002    Las comunidades de regantes de España y su federación nacional. Electronic document, http://agua.geoscopio.com/empresas/fenacore2/.

**Federal Register (US Government)**

2002    Department of the Interior, Bureau of Indian Affairs, Part IV, Indian Entities Recognized and Eligible to Receive Services from the United States Bureau of Indian Affairs; Notice. National Archives and Records Administration, Friday, July 12. Washington, DC.

**Feit, H. A.**

2004    Hunting and the Quest for Power. In *Native Peoples, The Canadian Experience*, 3rd edition, edited by R. B. Morrison and C. R. Wilson, pp. 101–128. Toronto: McClelland.

**Feldmeier, H., R. C. Daccal, M. J. Martins, V. Soares, and R. Martins**

1998    Genital Manifestations of Schistosomiasis mansoni in Women: Important but Neglected. *Memorias Do Instituto Oswaldo Cruz* 93:127–133.

**Ferguson, A.**

2002    Decentralization: Whose Empowerment? Reflections on Environmental Policy Making in Malawi. Paper presented at the Annual Meeting of the American Anthropological Association, New Orleans.

**Ferguson, A., and W. Derman**

1999    Water Rights vs. Right to Water: Reflections on Zimbabwe's Water Reforms from a Human Rights Perspective. Paper presented at the Annual Meeting of the American Anthropological Association, Chicago.

**Ferguson, A., and W. O. Mulwafu**

2001    Decentralization, Participation and Access to Water Resources in Malawi. Paper presented at the BASIS Collaborative Research Support Program (CRSP) Policy Synthesis Workshop, Johannesburg, South Africa. Electronic document, http://www.basis.wisc.edu/live/water/decentralization, participation.pdf.

**Ferguson, J.**

1999    *Expectations of Modernity: Myths and Meanings of Urban Life on the Zambian Copperbelt.* Perspectives on Southern Africa, vol. 57. Berkeley: University of California Press.

# References

**Figueroa, A.**
1984     *Capitalist Development and the Peasant Economy of Peru.* Cambridge: Cambridge University Press.

**Firmo, J. O. A., M. Costa, H. L. Guerra, and R. S. Rocha**
1996     Urban Schistosomiasis: Morbidity, Sociodemographic Characteristics and Water Contact Patterns Predictive of Infection. *International Journal of Epidemiology* 25(6):1292–1300.

**Fitzgerald, E. V. K.**
1979     *The Political Economy of Peru, 1956–1978: Economic Development and the Restructuring of Capital.* Cambridge: Cambridge University Press.

**Fitzgerald, P.**
2002     Fishing for Stories at Burnt Church: The Media, the Marshall Decision and Aboriginal Representation. *Canadian Dimension* 36(4):29–32.

**Fogarty, M.**
2003     Stats say Big Apple Has Most Urban Indians. *Indian Country Today*, 26 February: D1, D2.

**Forde, C. D.**
1963     *Habitat, Economy and Society: A Geographical Introduction to Ethnology,*
[1949]    New York: E. P. Dutton. London: Methuen.

**Forero, J.**
2002     As Andean Glaciers Shrink, Water Worries Grow. Electronic document, http://www.nytimes.com, November 24.

**Fortes, M.**
1969     *Kinship and the Social Order: The Legacy of Lewis Henry Morgan.* Chicago: Aldine.

**Frownfelter, D. A.**
2001     Groundwater Withdrawal Permit Program Edwards Aquifer Authority. Paper presented at the symposium "The Changing Face of Water Rights in Texas 2001," The State Bar of Texas, San Antonio.

**Fulford, A. J. C., J. H. Ouma, H. C. Kariuki, F. W. Thiongo, R. Klumpp, H. Kloos, R. F. Sturrock, and A. E. Butterworth**
1996     Water Contact Observations in Kenyan Communities Endemic for Schistosomiasis: Methodology and Patterns of Behaviour. Parasitology 113:223–241.

**Ghersi, E.**
1997     The Informal Economy in Latin America. *The Cato Journal* 17(1). Electronic document, http://www.cato.org/pubs/journal/cj17n1-8.html.

**Gianella, J.**
1970     *Marginalidad en Lima Metropolitana.* Lima: Cuadernos DESCO A8.

**Giddens, A.**
1999    *How Globalization Is Shaping Our Lives: Runaway World.* London: Routledge.

**Gillette, E. A, M. M. Meza, M. G. Aguilar, A. D. Soto, and I. E. Garicial**
1998    An Anthropological Approach to the Evaluation of Preschool Children Exposed to Pesticides in Mexico. *Environmental Health Perspectives* 106(6):4–28.

**Gleick, P. H.**
1999    The Human Right to Water. *Water Policy* 1(5):487–503.
2004    The Myth and Reality of Bottled Water. In *The World's Water 2004–2005: The Biennial Report on Freshwater Resources,* edited by P. Gleick, pp. 17–43. Washington, DC: Island Press.

**Gleick, P. H., ed.**
1993    *Water in Crisis—A Guide to the World's Fresh Water Resources.* New York: Oxford University Press.

**Gleick, P. H., with W. C. G. Burns, E. L. Chalecki, M. Cohen, K. K. Cushing, A. S. Mann, R. Reyes, G. H. Wolff, and A. K. Wong**
2002    *The World's Water 2002–2003: The Biennial Report on Freshwater Resources.* Washington, DC: Island Press.

**Gleick, P., G. Wolff, E. Chalecki, and R. Reyes**
2002    The Privatization of Water and Water Systems. In *The World's Water 2002–2003: The Biennial Report on Freshwater Resources,* edited by P. Gleick, pp. 57–86. Washington, DC: Island Press.

**Glennon, R. J.**
2002    *Water Follies: Ground Water Pumping and the Fate of America's Fresh Waters.* Washington, DC: Island Press.

**Glick, T. F.**
1970    *Irrigation and Society in Medieval Valencia.* Cambridge, MA: Harvard University Press.
1979    *Islamic and Christian Spain in the Early Middle Ages.* Princeton, NJ: Princeton University Press.

**Global Water Partnership**
2000    *Water Dialogue* 1(1):1. Harare, Zimbabwe.

**Gohdes, D. M., and N. Acton**
2000    Diabetes Mellitus and Its Complications. In *American Indian Health: Innovations in Health Care, Promotion, and Policy,* edited by E. R. Rhoades, pp. 221–243. Baltimore: Johns Hopkins University Press.

**Goldman, M.**
2004    How Water for All! Policy Became Hegemonic: The Power of the World Bank and Its Transnational Policy Networks. Paper presented at the Troubled Waters Conference, University of Illinois, Urbana-Champaign.

# References

**Gootenberg, P. E.**
1989 *Between Silver and Guano: Commercial Policy and the State in Postindependence Peru.* Princeton, NJ: Princeton University Press.

**Government of Malawi (GOM)**
1999a *Draft Water Act. Water Resources Development Policy and Strategies.* Annex B, May 1999 Resubmission. Lilongwe, Malawi: Ministry of Water Development.
1999b *Community-Based Rural Water Supply, Sanitation and Hygiene Education Implementation Manual.* Lilongwe, Malawi: Ministry of Water Development.
2000 *Water Resources Management Policy and Strategies.* Lilongwe, Malawi: Ministry of Water Development.
2001 *Joint Review of Malawi Water and Sanitation Sector. Issues and Priorities.* Lilongwe, Malawi: Ministry of Water Development.

**Government of Namibia**
2004 The Water Resources Management Bill. Windhoek, Nambia: Ministry of Agriculture, Water, and Rural Development.

**Government of South Africa**
1998 National Water Act, No. 36. Pretoria: Government Gazette.
2000 The Philosophy and Practice of Integrated Catchment Management: Implications for Water Resource Management in South Africa. Department of Water Affairs and Forestry, Water Research Commission.

**Government of Spain**
1994 *Boletín Oficial del Estado* no. 58, March 9.
1996 *Boletín Oficial del Estado* no. 192, August 9.

**Government of Zimbabwe**
1998a Water Act, No. 31/1998.
1998b Zimbabwe National Water Authority Act, No. 11/1998.
2000a Statutory Instrument 33. Water (Catchment Councils) Regulations.
2000b Statutory Instrument 47. Water (Subcatchment Councils) Regulations.
2000c Towards Integrated Water Resources Management: Water Resources Management Strategy for Zimbabwe. Harare.

**Greaves, T.**
1998 Water Rights in the Pacific Northwest. In *Water, Culture and Power*, edited by J. Donahue and B. Johnston, pp. 35–46. Washington, DC: Island Press.

**Green, C., and S. Baden**
1994 Water Resources Management: A Macro-Level Analysis from a Gender Perspective. Briefings on Development and Gender (BRIDGE), report no. 21. Sussex, UK: Institute of Development Studies.

# References

**Grewal, I., and C. Kaplan**
1994 Introduction: Transnational Feminist Practices and Questions of Postmodernity. In S*cattered Hegemonies*, edited by I. Grewal and C. Kaplan, pp.1–33. Minneapolis: University of Minnesota Press.

**Grusky, S.**
2001 Privatization Tidal Wave: IMF/World Bank Water Policies and the Price Paid by the Poor. *Multinational Monitor* (September).

**Gubler, D., with G. Kund**
1997 *Dengue and Dengue Hemorrhagic Fever*. New York: CAB International.

**Guillet, D.**
1992 *Covering Ground: Communal Water Management and the State in the Peruvian Highlands*. Ann Arbor: University of Michigan Press.
1997 The Politics of Sustainable Agriculture: The Case of Water Demand Management in Spain. *South European Society and Politics* 2(1):97–117.
1998 Rethinking Legal Pluralism: Local Law and State Law in the Evolution of Water Property Rights in Northwestern Spain. *Comparative Studies in Society and History* 40(1):42–70.
2000 State Intervention and Water Property Rights in the Margins of Europe: The Orbigo Valley of Northwestern Spain. In *Negotiating Water Rights*, edited by B. Bruns and R. Meinzen-Dick, pp. 222–244. New Delhi: Sage.
2002a Water Matters: The Formulation and Application of Sustainable Water Management Policy for the 21st Century. Paper presented at the conference "Environment, Resources and Sustainability: Policy Issues for the 21st Century," Athens, GA.
2002b Rethinking Irrigation Efficiency. Unpublished paper.

**Hall, D., and E. Lobina**
2002 *Water Privatization in Latin America*. London: Public Services International. Electronic document, www.woels-psi.org, accessed February 2, 2004.

**Hammar, A., B. Raftopoulos, and S. Jensen**
2003 *Zimbabwe's Unfinished Business. Rethinking Land, State and Nation in the Context of Crisis*. Harare, Zimbabwe: Weaver Press.

**Hazell, S.**
1991 Environmental Aspects of the Hydro-Development in the James Bay Region. *Northeast Indian Quarterly* (Winter):20–24.

**Hearne, R. R., and K. W. Easter**
1995 *Water Allocation and Water Markets*. Washington, DC: World Bank.

**Helling-Giese, G., E. F. Kjetland, S. G. Gundersen, G. Poggensee, J. Richter, I. Krantz, and H. Feldmeier**
1996 Schistosomiasis in Women: Manifestations in the Upper Reproductive Tract. *Acta Tropica* 62(4):225–238.

# References

**Helling-Giese, G., A. Sjaastad, G. Poggensee, E. F. Kjetland, J. Richter, L. Chitsulo, N. Kumwenda, P. Racz, B. Roald, S. G. Gundersen, I. Krantz, and H. Feldmeier**
1996 Female Genital Schistosomiasis (FGS): Relationship between Gynecological and Histopathological Findings. *Acta Tropica* 62(4):257–267.

**Hellum, A.**
2001 *Towards a Human Rights Based Development Approach: The Case of Women in the Water Reform Process in Zimbabwe.* Warwick, UK: Law, Social Justice and Global Development. Electronic document, http://elj.warwick.ac.uk/global/issue/2001-1/hellum.html.

**Hellum, A., and W. Derman**
2004 Land Reform and Human Rights in Contemporary Zimbabwe: Balancing Individual and Social Justice through an Integrated Human Rights Framework. *World Development* 32(10):1785–1805.

**Hirji, R., P. Johnson, P. Maro, and T. M. Chiuta, eds.**
2002 *Defining and Mainstreaming Environmental Sustainability in Water Resources Management in Southern Africa.* Maseru, South Africa, Harare, and Washington, DC: SADC (with IUCN, SARDC, World Bank, and Sida).

**Holt, G.**
2000 Tribe Gathers Historic Clam Harvest. *Seattle Post-Intelligencer.* 16 February. Electronic document, http://seattlepi.nwsource.com/local/, accessed October 19, 2004.

**Hong, E.**
2000 Globalisation and the Impact on Health: A Third World View. Paper presented at The Peoples' Health Assembly, Savar, Bangladesh.

**Hoops, T., and E. Ashur**
2004 *La Crisis del Agua en Salta: Entre la Sequía y la Inundación.* Salta, Argentina: Fundación CAPACITAR.

**Howard, M. O., R. D. Walker, P. S. Walker, and E. R. Rhoades**
2000 Alcoholism and Substance Abuse. In *American Indian Health: Innovations in Health Care, Promotion, and Policy,* edited by E. R. Rhoades, pp. 281–298. Baltimore, MD: Johns Hopkins University Press.

**Huang, Y., and L. Manderson**
1992 Schistosomiasis and the Social Patterning of Infection. *Acta Tropica* 51(2):175–194.
1999 Socioeconomic Factors and the Prevalence of Schistosomiasis japonica in Rural Areas of China. *Chinese Journal of Schistosomiasis Control* 11(3):137–142.
2003 Rural People's Perceptions of Schistosomiasis and Other Diseases. *Chinese Journal of Schistosomiasis Control* 15(2):108–115.

# REFERENCES

**Hyatt, B. S.**
2004     Water Is Life, Meters Out! Women's Grassroots Activism and the Privatization of Public Amenities. Paper prepared for the Globalization Research Center, University of South Florida, Tampa.

**Hydrogen and Fuel Cell Letter**
2002     Hydrogen Is Challenge for New Breed of Economists, WHEC-14 Attendees Are Told. Electronic document, http://www.hfcletter.com/letter/July02/features.html.

**Imhoff, A., S. Wong, and P. Bosshard**
2002     *Citizens' Guide to the World Commission on Dams*. Berkeley: International Rivers Network.

**Indian and Northern Affairs, Canada**
2002     Information, Frequently Asked Questions about Aboriginal Peoples. Electronic document, www.ainc-inac.gc.ca/pr/info/index_e.html.

*Indian Country Today*
2001     Animas-LaPlata Request Unjustified. 9 May: A3.
2002a     Shooting Raises Issue of Racism in Klamath Basin Water Wars. 23 January: A1.
2002b     Cree Vote Yes on Quebec Deal. 13 February: A1.
2002c     Maine River Indians Reject Settlement of Clean Water Dispute. 22 May: B1.
2002d     Groups to Appeal Decision on Makah Whale Hunts. 29 May: B1, B2.
2002e     Swinomish Win Largest EPA Research Grant. 19 June: A6.
2002f     Alaska Firm Wants Role in Pipeline Project. 14 August: C1.
2002g     Pojoaque Leader Says Pueblo Will Fight Water Lawsuit. 2 October: B1.
2002h     Tesuque Switches Sides in Water Lawsuit. 13 November: C1.
2002i     Alaskan Sovereign Village Takes Charge of Its Own Tourism Destiny. 20 November: B2.
2002j     Crow and Cheyenne Worry about Water Contamination. 20 November: B2.
2002k     Mi'kmaq Shubenacadie Band. 27 November: A2.
2002l     Environmentalists Decry Proposed Grand Canyon Pipeline. 4 December: C1.
2003a     Te-Moak Western Shoshone Tribe. 8 January: B4.
2003b     Nez Perce Files New Appeal of Restoration Project. 19 February: B4.
2003c     Animas-La Plata Project Waits for Funds. 19 February: B4.
2003d     Gila River Tribe Approves Water Settlement Proposal. 19 February: B4.
2004     Switching Tribes to Escape Poverty. 9 June: D1, D4.

**Instituto Nacional de Estadísta e Informática**
1994     Censos Nacionales de 1993. Lima, Peru.

# References

1998    Compendio Estadística Departmental Lima-Callao. Lima, Peru.

2002    Compendio Estadística Peru. Lima, Peru.

**International Consortium of Investigative Journalists (ICIJ)**
2003    Cholera and the Age of the Water Barons. Report published by the Center for Public Integrity. Electronic document, http:///icij.org/dtaweb/water/.

**International Union for the Conservation of Nature (IUCN)**
2000    Vision for Water and Nature: A World Strategy for Conservation and Sustainable Management of Water Resources in the 21st Century. Glans, Switzerland: IUCN.

**ITT Industries**
1998    *The New Economics of Water: Private Enterprise and Public Utilities. An ITT Industries Guidebook with Key Definitions, Industry Profiles and Technical Definitions.* White Plains, NY: ITT Industries, Inc.

**Iyngararasan, M., L. Tianchi, and S. Shrestha**
2002    The Challenges of Mountain Environments: Water, Natural Resources, Hazards, Desertification and the Implications of Climate Change. Briefing paper presented at the Bishkek Global Mountain Summit, Kyrgyzstan. Electronic document, http://www.mtnforum.org/bgms/papere1.htm.

**Jackson, C.**
1993    Doing What Comes Naturally? Women and Environment in Development. *World Development* 21(12):1947–1963.

**Jackson, S., and A. Sleigh**
2000    Resettlement for China's Three Gorges Dam: Socio-Economic Impact and Institutional Tensions. *Communist and Post-Communist Studies* 33(2):223–241.

**James, M.**
1993 [1948]    *Merchant Adventurer: The Story of W. R. Grace.* Wilmington, DE: Scholarly Resources.

**Janes, C.**
2004    Medical Anthropology and Global Health Advocacy. Remarks prepared for the March meeting of the Society of Applied Anthropology, Dallas.

**Jiang, Q. W., L. Y. Wang, J. G. Guo, M. G. Chen, X. N. Zhou, and D. Engels**
2002    Morbidity Control of Schistosomiasis in China. *Acta Tropica* 82(2):115–125.

**Jiliberto, R., and A. Merino**
1997    Sobre la situación de las comunidades de regantes. In *La gestión del agua de riego,* edited by J. López-Gálvez and J. M. Naredo, pp. 183–201. Madrid: Argentaria-Visor.

**Johnston, B. R.**
1994    *Who Pays the Price? The Sociocultural Context of Environmental Crisis.* Washington, DC: Island Press.

1997    Life and Death Matters at the End of the Millennium. In *Life and Death Matters: Human Rights and the Environment at the End of the Millennium*, edited by B. R. Johnston, pp. 9–20. Walnut Creek, CA: AltaMira Press.

1998    Culture, Power, and the Hydrological Cycle: Creating and Responding to Water Scarcity on St. Thomas, Virgin Islands. In *Water, Culture, & Power: Local Struggles in a Global Context*, edited by J. Donahue and B. R. Johnston, pp. 285–312. Washington, DC: Island Press.

2001    Reparations and the Right to Remedy. World Commission on Dams briefing paper (July 2000). Contributing Report, Thematic Review 1.3: Displacement, Resettlement, Reparations, and Development. Electronic document, http://www.damsreport.org/docs/kbase/contrib/soc221.pdf.

2002    Considering the Power and Potential of the Anthropology of Trouble. In *Ecology and the Sacred: Engaging the Anthropology of Roy A. Rappaport*, edited by E. Messer and M. Lambeck, pp. 99–121. Ann Arbor: University of Michigan Press.

2003a    The Political Ecology of Water: An Introduction. *Capitalism, Nature, Socialism* 14(3):73–90.

2003b    Notes from the Field: Guatemalan Community Struggles with Chixoy Dam Legacy of Violence, Forced Resettlement. In *The American Association for the Advancement of Science Report on Science and Human Rights*, (3): Electronic document, http://shr.aas.org/report/xxiii/chixoy_dam.htm.

**Johnston, B. R., and C. Garcia-Downing**
In press    The Pehuecnche: Human Rights, the Environment, and Hydro-development on the Biobio River, in Chile. In *Indigenous Peoples, Development and Environment*, edited by H. Feit and M. Blaser. London: Zed Books.

**Johnston, B. R., and T. Turner**
1998    Censorship, Denial of Informed Participation, and Human Rights Abuses Associated with Dam Development in Chile. Professional Ethics Report, vol. XI, no. 2. The AAAS Scientific Freedom, Responsibility and Law Program, in collaboration with the Committee on Scientific Freedom and Responsibility.

**Josephy, A. M., Jr.**
1982    *Now That the Buffalo's Gone*. Norman: University of Oklahoma Press.

**Jubilee 2000 UK**
2000    Peru. Electronic document, http://www.jubilee2000uk.org/databank/profiles/peru.htm, accessed August 28, 2004.

**Junta de Castilla y León**
1997    *Plan de regadíos*. Valladolid: Junta de Castilla y León.

**Kaluwa, P. W. R., F. M. Mtambo, and R. Fachi**
1997    *The Country Situation Report on Water Resources in Malawi*. Lilongwe, Malawi: United Nations Development Programme/Southern African Development Community Water Initiative.

# References

**Kawachi, I., and B. P. Kennedy**
2002 *The Health of Nations.* New York: The New Press.

**Kearney, M.**
1996 The Local and the Global: The Anthropology of Globalization and Transnationalism. *Annual Review of Anthropology* 24:547–565.

**Kemper, K. E., and D. Olson**
2000 Water Pricing: The Dynamics of Institutional Change in Mexico and Ceara. In *The Political Economy of Water Pricing Reforms*, edited by A. Dinar, pp. 339–357. Oxford: Oxford University Press.

**Kendall, C., and J. Gittelsohn**
1994 Reliability and Measures of Hygiene Behavior: A Case Study. In *Studying Hygiene Behaviors: Methods, Issues and Experiences*, edited by S. Cairncross and V. Kochar, pp. 85–101. London: Sage.

**Kim, J. Y., with J. Millen, A. Irwin, and J. Gershman**
2000 *Dying for Growth: Global Inequality and the Health of the Poor.* Monroe, Maine: Common Courage Press.

**Kjetland, E. F., G. Poggensee, G. HellingGiese, J. Richter, A. Sjaastad, L. Chitsulo, N. Kumwenda, S. G. Gundersen, I. Krantz, and H. Feldmeier**
1996 Female Genital Schistosomiasis Due to Schistosoma haematobium—Clinical and Parasitological Findings in Women in Rural Malawi. *Acta Tropica* 62(4):239–255.

**Klare, M. T.**
2003 *Resource Wars: The New Landscape of Global Conflict.* New York: Henry Holt and Company.

**Klaver, I., J. Keulaertz, B. Gremmen, and H. van der Belt**
2002 Born to Be Wild: A Pluralistic Ethic Concerning Introduced Large Herbivores. *Environmental Ethics* 24:3–21.

**Kleemeier, E.**
2000 The Impact of Participation on Sustainability: An Analysis of the Malawi Rural Piped Scheme Program. *World Development* 28(5):929–944.
2001 The Role of Government in Maintaining Rural Water Supplies: Caveats from Malawi's Gravity Schemes. *Public Administration and Development* 21:245–257.

**Krauss, C.**
2002 Will the Flood Wash Away the Crees' Birthright? *New York Times*, 27 February: A4.

**Lane, L.**
2003 Hazard Vulnerability in Socio-economic Context. M.A. thesis, Department of Geography, University of South Florida, Tampa.

**Lee, K.**
2000 Impact of Globalization on Public Health: Implications for the UK Faculty of Public Health Medicine. *Journal of Public Health Medicine* 22:253–262.

# REFERENCES

**Lee, L. J., C. Chung, Y. Ma, G. Wang, P. Chen, Y. Hwang, and J. Wang**
2003    Increased Mortality Odds Ratio of Male Liver Cancer in a Community Contaminated by Chlorinated Hydrocarbons in Groundwater. *Occupational and Environmental Medicine* (60):364–369.

**Leonardt, D.**
2003    Globalization Hits a Political Speed Bump. *New York Times*, 1 June: B1, B10.

**Leopold, A.**
1949    *A Sand County Almanac*. New York: Oxford University Press.

**Lerer, L. B., and T. Scudder**
1999    Health Impacts of Large Dams. *Environmental Impact Assessment Review* 19(2):113–123.

**Lerner, R. N.**
1987    Preserving Plants for Pomos. In *Anthropological Praxis*, edited by R. Wulff and S. Fiske, pp. 212–222. Boulder, CO: Westview Press.

**Li, Y. S., A. G. P. Ross, D. B. Yu, Y. Li, G. M. Williams, and D. P. McManus**
1997    An Evaluation of Schistosoma japonicum Infections in Three Villages in the Dongting Lake Region of China. 1. Prevalence, Intensity and Morbidity before the Implementation of Adequate Control Strategies. *Acta Tropica* 68(1):77–91.

**Li, Y. S., A. C. Sleigh, G. M. Williams, A. G. P. Ross, Y. Li, S. J. Forsyth, M. Tanner, and D. P. McManus**
2000    Measuring Exposure to Schistosoma japonicum in China. III. Activity Diaries, Snail and Human Infection, Transmission Ecology and Options for Control. *Acta Tropica* 75(3):279–289.

**Liu, Q. H., J. W. Zhang, B. Z. Liu, Z. L. Peng, H. J. Zhang, S. Y. Wang, D. L. Mei, and L. N. Hsu**
2000    Investigation of Association between Female Genital Tract Diseases and Schistosomiasis japonica Infection. *Acta Tropica* 77(2):179–183.

**Lloyd, P.**
1980    *The "Young Towns" of Lima: Aspects of Urbanization in Peru*. Cambridge: Cambridge University Press.

**Lobo, S.**
1981    *A House of My Own: Social Organization in the Squatter Settlements of Lima, Peru*. Tucson: University of Arizona Press.

**Lock, M., and N. Scheper-Hughes**
1996    A Critical-Interpretive Approach in Medical Anthropology: Ritual and Routines of Discipline and Dissent. In *Medical Anthropology: Contemporary Theory and Method*, edited by C. F. Sargent and T. M. Johnson, pp. 41–70. New York: Prager.

# References

**Loewenson, R., and A. Whiteside**
1997   Social and Economic Issues of HIV/AIDS in Southern Africa. Report prepared for SAfAIDS, Occasional Paper Series, no. 2. Harare, Zimbabwe: Southern Africa HIV and AIDS Information Dissemination Service.

**Lovett, L.**
1998   "Step Inside This House." Universal City, CA: MCA Records, Inc.

**Maas, A., and J. Anderson**
1978   ...And the Desert Shall Rejoice. Cambridge, MA: MIT Press.

**Maclay, R. W.**
1988   Stratigraphic Subdivisions, Fault Barriers, and Characteristics of the Edwards Aquifer, South Central Texas. In *Aquifer Resources Conference Proceedings: Geological and Managerial Considerations Relating to the Edwards Aquifer of South Central Texas*. San Antonio: Trinity University, Division of Science, Engineering, and Mathematics, and the South Texas Geological Society.

**Macroconsult**
1996   Organización, Regulación e Incentivos de los Sistemas de Agua Potable y Saneamiento en el Perú. Final draft of paper prepared for Inter American Development Bank, Washington, DC.

**Mafiana, C. F., U. F. Ekpo, and D. A. Ojo**
2003   Urinary Schistosomiasis in Preschool Children in Settlements around Oyan Reservoir in Ogun State, Nigeria: Implications for Control. *Tropical Medicine & International Health* 8(1):78–82.

**Malhotra, S. P.**
1982   *The Warabandi System and Its Infrastructure*. New Delhi: Central Board of Irrigation and Power.

**Mangin, W.**
1957   Latin American Squatter Settlements: A Problem and a Solution. *Latin American Research Review* 2:3.
1959   Squatter Settlements. *Scientific American* 217:4.

**Maro, P., and L. Thamae**
2002   Policy, Legislative and Institutional Framework. In *Defining and Mainstreaming Environmental Sustainability in Water Resources Management in Southern Africa*, edited by R. Hjiri, P. Johnson, P. Maro, and T. M. Chiuta, pp. 261–294. Maseru, South Africa, Harare, and Washington, DC: SADC (with IUCN, SARDC, World Bank, and Sida).

**Matos Mar, J.**
1961   The Barriadas of Lima: An Example of Integration into Urban Life. In *Urbanization in Latin America*, edited by P. M. Hauser, pp. 170–190. Paris: UNESCO.

## References

1966    *Estudios de las Barriadas Limeñas.* Lima: Instituto de Estudios Peruanos.

**May, J.**
2002    Klamath Chinook Suffer Massive Die-Off. *Indian Country Today,* 9 October: A1, A3.

**May, P. A.**
1999    The Epidemiology of Alcohol Abuse among Native Americans: The Mythical and Real Properties. In *Contemporary Native American Cultural Issues,* edited by D. Champagne, pp. 227–244. Walnut Creek, CA: AltaMira Press.

**Mayor's Citizens Committee on Water Policy**
1997    Framework for Progress: Recommended Water Policy Strategy for the San Antonio Area. Final Report of the Mayor's Citizens Committee on Water Policy, submitted to the San Antonio City Council, January 23.

**Mbaya, S.**
2002    HIV/AIDS and Its Impact on Land Issues in Malawi. Paper presented at the FAO/SARPN Workshop on HIV/AIDS and Land, Pretoria, South Africa.

**McCaffrey, S.**
1992    A Human Right to Water: Domestic and International Obligations. *Georgetown Environmental Law Review* 5:1–24.

**McCully, P.**
2001    *Silenced Rivers, The Ecology and Politics of Large Dams: Enlarged and Updated Edition.* London: Zed Books.
2002    Avoiding Solutions, Worsening Problems: Critique of the March 25, 2002, Draft of the World Bank's Water Resources Sector Strategy. International River Network. Electronic document, http://www.irn.org/index.asp?id=/new/020527.wbwater critique.html.

**McDowell, E.**
2001    Indian Reservations Join the Tourist Circuit. *New York Times,* 3 June: TR3.

**McGrath, K. D., and T. Greaves**
2000    Dams and Environmentalists in Indian Country. Paper presented at the 99th Annual Meeting, American Anthropological Association, San Francisco.

**McMillan, M. E.**
2003    *La Purificacion Tepetitla: Agua Potable y Cambio Social en el Somontano.* Mexico City: Universidad Iberoamericana.

**McMurray, C., and R. Smith**
2001    *Diseases of Globalization: Socioeconomic Transitions and Health.* London: Earthscan.

# References

**Mehanna, S., N. H. Rizkalla, H. F. Elsayed, and P. J. Winch**
1994     Social and Economic Conditions in 2 Newly Reclaimed Areas in Egypt—Implications for Schistosomiasis Control Strategies. *Journal of Tropical Medicine and Hygiene* 97(5):286–297.

**Melmer, D.**
1996     Chairmen Divided Over Docket 74-A. *Indian Country Today*, 18 June: A1, A2.
2000     Agreement Means Improved Water Rights. *Indian Country Today*, 16 September: D1.
2002a     Tribal Water Coalition Chides BIA. *Indian Country Today*, 12 January: http://www.indiancountry.com.
2002b     Judge Supports Yankton. *Indian Country Today*, 19 June, A1: A2.
2003     Cuts Threaten Education and Clean Water for S. D. Reservations. *Indian Country Today*, 19 February: B1.

**Miess, F.**
2002     Felton Fights Privatized Water: Residents, Activists and Decision Makers Battle German Conglomerate RWE-AG over Acquisition of Felton's Water Rights. *The Alarm!* 2(19):1, 18.

**Military Toxics Project**
2002     Communities in the Line of Fire: The Environmental, Cultural, and Human Health Impacts of Military Munitions and Firing Ranges. Report by Military Toxics Project. Electronic document, http://www.kahea.org/current_issues_pdf/Military_Toxics_Campaign_Rpt.pdf.

**Mills, A.**
2002     The Gitxsan and Witsuwit'en in British Columbia. In *Endangered Peoples of North America*, edited by T. Greaves, pp. 59–78. Westport, CT: Greenwood.

**Ministerio de Medio Ambiente**
1998     Libro Blanco de Agua en España. Madrid.

**Morsy, S.**
1996     Political Economy. In *Medical Anthroplogy: Contemporary Theory and Method*, edited by C. Sargent and T. M. Johnson, pp. 21–40. New York: Praeger Press.

**Mott, K. E., P. Desjeux, A. Moncayo, P. Ranque, and P. Deraadt**
1990     Parasitic Diseases and Urban Development. *Bulletin of the World Health Organization* 68(6):691–698.

**Murry, D.**
1994     *Cultivating Crisis: The Human Cost of Pesticide Use in Latin America*. Austin: University of Texas Press.

**N'Goran, E. K., S. Diabate, J. Utzinger, and B. Sellin**
1997     Changes in Human Schistosomiasis Levels after the Construction of Two Large Hydroelectric Dams in Central Cote d'Ivoire. *Bulletin of the World Health Organization* 75(6):541–545.

**Nadal Reimat, E.**
1993    *Introducción al análisis de la planificación hidrológica.* Madrid: Ministerio de Obras Públicas y Transportes, Dirección General de Obras Hidráulicas.

**Neruda, P.**
1950    Amor América. *Canto General.* Mexico: Ediciones Oceano.

**New York Times**
2003    US Withholds Approval for Nuclear Waste Storage on Indian Reservation, 11 March: A19.

**Nickum, J., and D. Greenstadt**
1998    The Lake Biwa Project in Japan. In *Water, Culture and Power: Local Struggles in a Global Context,* edited by J. M. Donahue and B. R. Johnston, pp. 141–161. Washington, DC: Island Press.

**Nitze, W.**
2002    Meeting the Water Needs of the Border Region: A Growing Challenge for the United States and Mexico. Policy paper on the Americas. CSIS Americas Program XII.

**Olsen, E.**
1997    Pure Water or Pure Hype? Natural Resource Defense Council. Electronic document, http://www.nrdc.org/water/drinking/nbw.asp.

**Omran, A. R.**
1977    A Century of Epidemiological Transition in the United States. *Preventive Medicine* 6:30–51.

**Ortner, S.**
1994    Theory in Anthropology since the Sixties. In *Culture/Power/History? A Reader in Contemporary Social Theory,* edited by N. B. Dirks, G. Eley, and S. B. Ortner, pp. 272–411. Princeton, NJ: Princeton University Press.

**Orwin, A.**
1999    The Privatization of Water and Wastewater Utilities: An International Survey. Electronic document, http://www.environmentprobe.org/enviroprobe/pubs/ev542.html#South%20America, accessed June 21, 2004.

**Ostrom, E.**
1990    *Governing the Commons: The Evolution of Institutions for Collective Action.* Cambridge, MA: Cambridge University Press.

**Ostrom, E., R. Gardner, and J. Walker**
1994    *Rules, Games and Common-Pool Resources.* Ann Arbor: University of Michigan Press.

**Owusu, K., and F. Ng'ambi**
2002    *Structural Damage: The Causes and Consequences of Malawi's Food Crisis.* London: World Development Movement.

# References

**Pan American Health Organization (PAHO)**
2002     Core Health Data Selected Indicators. Data updated to 2002. Electronic document, http://www.paho.org/English/DD/AIS/cp_604.htm, accessed June 21, 2004.

**Pearce, F.**
2001     Bangladesh's Arsenic Poisoning: Who Is to Blame? *The Courier*. Electronic document, http://www.unesco.org/courier/2001_01/uk/planet.htm.

**Peet, R., and M. Watts**
1996     Liberation Ecology: Development, Sustainability, and Environment in an Age of Market Triumphalism. In *Liberation Ecologies: Environment, Development, Social Movements*, edited by R. Peet and M. Watts, pp. 1–45. London and New York: Routledge.

**Perrottet, A.**
1993     *Ecuador: Insight Guides*. APA Publications (HK) LTD. Published and distributed in Ecuador by Ediciones Libri Mundi, Quito, Ecuador.

**Perry, C. J.**
1995     *Alternative Approaches to Cost Sharing for Water Service to Agriculture in Egypt*. Research Report 2. Colombo, Sri Lanka: International Water Management Institute.
2001     *Charging for Irrigation Water: The Issues and Options, with a Case Study from Iran*. Research Report 52. Colombo, Sri Lanka: International Water Management Institute.

**Perry, C. J., M. Rock, and D. Seckler**
1997     Water as an Economic Good: A Solution or a Problem? Research Report No. 14. Colombo, Sri Lanka: Integrated Irrigation Management Institute.

**Peterson, I.**
2004     State, U.S. and Tribal Hurdles Stall New York Casino Deals. *New York Times*, 20 January: A18.

**Pevar, S. L.**
2002     *The Rights of Indians and Tribes*. Carbondale: Southern Illinois University Press.

**Picard, A.**
1990     James Bay: A Power Play. *The Globe and Mail*, 16 April. Electronic document, http://www.andrepicard.com/jamesbay.html.

**Plotkin, S.**
1987     *Keep Out: The Struggle for Land Use Control*. Berkeley: University of California Press.

**Poggensee, G., S. Sahebali, E. Van Marck, B. Swai, I. Krantz, and H. Feldmeier**
2001     Diagnosis of Genital Cervical Schistosomiasis: Comparison of Cytological, Histopathological and Parasitological Examinations. *American Journal of Tropical Medicine and Hygiene* 65(3):233–236.

# REFERENCES

**Postel, S.**
1992    *Last Oasis: Facing Water Scarcity.* New York: W. W. Norton & Company.

**Promotion of the Role of Women in Water and Environmental Sanitation Services/United Nations Development Program (PROWWESS/UNDP)**
1991    *A Forward-Looking Assessment of PROWWESS: Report of an Independent Team.* New York: PROWWESS/UNDP.

**Puckett, J., L. Byster, S. Westervelt, R. Gutierrez, S. Davis, A. Hussain, and M. Dutta**
2002    Exporting Harm: The High-Tech Trashing of Asia. The Basel Action Network (BAN) and the Silicon Valley Toxics Coalition (SVTC) with contributions by Toxics Link India, SCOPE (Pakistan), and Greenpeace China. Report published by Silicon Valley Toxics Coalition. Electronic document, http://www.svtc.org/cleancc/pubs/technotrash.pdf, accessed February 25.

**Rapport, D., R. Costanza, P. Stein, C. Guadet, and R. Levins, eds.**
1998    *Ecosystem Health.* London: Blackwell Science.

**Ravenga, C., J. Brunner, N. Henninger, K. Kassem, and R. Payne**
2000    *Pilot Analysis of Global Ecosystems: Freshwater Systems.* Washington, DC: World Resource Institute.

**Reardon, T., J. Codron, L. Bush, J. Bingen, and C. Harris**
2002    Global Change in Agrifood Grades and Standards: Agribusiness Strategic Responses in Developing Countries. *International Food and Agribusiness Management Review* 2(3):1–25.

**Reid, M.**
1985    *Peru: Paths to Poverty.* London: Latin American Bureau/Third World Publications.

**Reid, R.**
1998    Status of Water Disinfection in Latin America and the Caribbean. Electronic document, http://www.cepis.ops-oms.org/eswww/caliagua/simposio/enwww/ponencia/ponen1.doc, accessed March 2003.

**Reisner, M.**
1986    *Cadillac Desert: The American West and Its Disappearing Water.* New York: Viking.

**Relea Fernández, C. E., J. C. Ríos Pacho, and A. Panigua Mazorra**
1994    Tradición, estructura e implicaciones socioespaciales del movimiento ecologista en la provincia de León. *Polígonos* 4:115–125.

**Remoue, F., D. T. Van, A. M. Schacht, M. Picquet, O. Garraud, J. Vercruysse, and A. Ly**
2001    Gender-Dependent Specific Immune Response during Chronic Human Schistosomiasis haematobia. *Clinical and Experimental Immunology* 124(1):62–68.

**Robles, E., P. Ramírez, E. González, M. G. Saiz, B. Martínez, Á. Duran, and E. Martinez**
1999    Bottled-Water Quality in Metropolitan Mexico City Water. *Air and Soil Pollution* 113(2):217–226.

**Rojas, R., G. Howard, and J. Bastram**
1994    Groundwater Quality and Water Supply in Lima, Peru. In *Groundwater Quality*, edited by H. Nash and G. J. H. McCall, pp. 159–167. London: Chapman and Hall.

**Root, C., D. Wiley, and S. Peek**
2000    The Impacts of Globalization and Environmental Struggles in a South African City. In *Rethinking Globalization(s): From Corporate Transnationalism to Local Interventions*, edited by P. Aulakh and M. Schechter, pp. 198–217. Wilshire, UK: St. Martin's Press.

**Rosegrant, M., and H. Binswanger**
1994    Markets in Tradable Water Rights: Potential for Efficiency Gains in Developing Country Water Resource Allocation. *World Development* 22(11):1613–1625.

**Rosegrant, M., X. Cai, and S. Cline**
2002a    Global Water Outlook to 2025: Averting an Impending Crisis. International Food Policy Research Institute and International Water Management Institute presentation, Washington, DC, Colombo, Sri Lanka.
2002b    World Water and Food to 2025: Dealing with Scarcity. International Food Policy Research Institute and International Water Management Institute presentation, Washington, DC. Electronic document, http://www/worldfood prize.org/symposium/2002 symposium, accessed November 24.

**Russo, K.**
2002    The Lummi in Washington State. In *Endangered Peoples of North America*, edited by T. Greaves, pp. 97–116. Westport, CT: Greenwood.

**Rynard, P.**
2000    Welcome In, but Check Your Rights at the Door: The James Bay and Nisga'a Agreements in Canada. *Canadian Journal of Political Science* 32(3):211–244.

**Saleth, M. R., and A. Dinar**
1999    Water Challenge and Institutional Response: A Cross-Country Perspective. Policy Research Working Paper 2045. World Bank Development Research Group on Rural Development.

**Saliba, B. C., and D. B. Bush**
1987    *Water Markets in Theory and Practice: Market Transfers, Water Values, and Public Policy*. Boulder, CO: Westview Press.

# REFERENCES

**Sama, M. T., and R. C. Ratard**
1994      Water Contact and Schistosomiasis Infection in Kumba, South-Western Cameroon. *Annals of Tropical Medicine and Parasitology* 88(6):629–634.

**Schoenberger, K.**
2002      Silicon Valley's Dark Side: A Mercury News Special Report. *San Jose Mercury News*, 24 November: 1A, 16–18A.

**Schroeder, L.**
2000      Social Funds and Local Government: The Case of Malawi. *Public Administration and Development* (20):423–438.

**Seldon, R.**
2002      Fort Belknap Tribes Sue Mining Company. *Indian Country Today*, 4 September, A1, A2.
2003a     Positive Sign for Flathead Water. *Indian Country Today*, 19 February: B1.
2003b     Montana Water Bill Concerns Trickle In. *Indian Country Today*, 5 March: B1.

**Shah, M. K., N. Osborne, T. Mbilizi, and G. Vilili**
2002      *Impact of HIV/AIDS on Agricultural Productivity and Rural Livelihoods in the Central Region of Malawi.* Lilongwe, Malawi: CARE International.

**Shiva, V.**
2001      World Bank, WTO and Corporate Control over Water. *International Socialist Review* (August/September). Electronic document, www.thirdworldtraveler.com/Water/Corp_Water_Vshiva.html.
2002      *Water Wars: Privatization, Pollution and Profit.* Toronto: Between the Lines Press.

**Shively, L. A.**
2002      Zuni Salt Lake Mining Okayed. *Indian Country Today*, 17 July: A1, A3.

**Silicon Valley Toxics Coalition**
2004      Sustainable Water Page. Electronic document, http://svtc.igc.org/sust_water/.

**Sleigh, A., S. Jackson, X. Li, and K. Huang**
1998      Eradication of Schistosomiasis in Guangxi, China. Part 2: Political Economy, Management Strategy and Costs, 1953–92. *Bulletin of the World Health Organization* 76(5):497–508.

**Sleigh, A., X. M. Li, S. Jackson, and K. L. Huang**
1998      Eradication of Schistosomiasis in Guangxi, China. Part 1: Setting, Strategies, Operations, and Outcomes, 1953–92. *Bulletin of the World Health Organization* 76(4):361–372.

**Snow, J.**
1855      *On the Mode of Communication of Cholera.* Reprint, London: Churchill. Reproduced in *Community Health: An Epidemiological Approach* by B. C. Smith. New York: Macmillan Publishing Company, 1979.

# References

**Solo, T. M.**
2003 Independent Water Entrepreneurs in Latin America: The Other Private Sector in Water Services. World Bank References Report, pp. 1–12.

**Song, H.**
1999 The Impact of De-collectivisation on Women in Rural China. *Yunnan Geographic Environment Research* 11(supplement):138–150.

**Southgate, V. R.**
1997 Schistosomiasis in the Senegal River Basin: Before and after the Construction of the Dams at Diama, Senegal and Manantali, Mali and Future Prospects. *Journal of Helminthology* 71(2):125–132.

**Southgate, V. R., L. A. T. Tchuente, M. Sene, D. De Clercq, A. Theron, J. Jourdane, B. L. Webster, D. Rollinson, B. Gryseels, and J. Vercruysse**
2001 Studies on the Biology of Schistosomiasis with Emphasis on the Senegal River Basin. *Memorias Do Instituto Oswaldo Cruz* 96:75–78.

**Sow, S., S. J. de Vlas, D. Engels, and B. Gryseels**
2002 Water-Related Disease Patterns before and after the Construction of the Diama Dam in Northern Senegal. *Annals of Tropical Medicine and Parasitology* 96(6):575–586.

**Sparks, S.**
1988 Pesticides in Mexico. *Multinational Monitor* 9(10):1–3.

**Sparr, P., ed.**
1994 *Mortgaging Women's Lives.* London: Zed Books.

**Spronk, S.**
2004 The Perils of Privatization in Third World Cities and Its Alternatives: Case Studies from Bolivia. Paper presented at the Latin American Studies Association, Las Vegas, November.

**Star, S. L., and J. R. Griesemer**
1989 Institutional Ecology, Translations and Boundary Objects: Amateurs and Professionals in Berkeley's Museum of Vertebrate Zoology. *Social Studies of Science* 19:387–420.

**Starr, E. R.**
1996 Health Care Systems in Indian Country. In *Health of Native People of North America,* edited by S. R. Gray, pp. 7–39. Lanham, MD: Scarecrow Press.

**Statistics Canada**
2003 1996 Census: Nation Tables—Aboriginal (20% Sample Data). Electronic document, www.statcan.ca/english/census96/jan13/nalis9.htm.

**Steingraber, S.**
1998 *Living Downstream: A Scientist's Personal Investigation of Cancer and Environment.* New York: Vintage Books.

# REFERENCES

**Stephenson, J.**
2002    Bangladesh Arsenic Water Crisis. *Journal of the American Medical Association* 288:1708.

**Stott, P., and S. Sullivan**
2000    Introduction in *Political Ecology: Science, Myth and Power*, edited by P. Stott and S. Sullivan, pp. 1–14. London: Arnold.

**Sullivan, R.**
2000    *A Whale Hunt.* New York: Scribner.

**Swyngedouv, E., B. Page, and M. Kaika**
2002    Sustainability and Policy Innovation in a Multi-level Context: Crosscutting Issues in the Water Sector. Electronic document, http://www.geog.oz.ac.uk/bgage.files.Final Report (Water).

**Taliman, V.**
2002    Globalism Violates Human Rights. *Indian Country Today*, 8 May: A1, A3.

**Tax, S.**
1963 [1953]    *Penny Capitalism: A Guatemalan Indian Economy.* Chicago: University of Chicago Press.

**Torres, V.**
2003    Shifts in Paradigm: Health and the Environment. Paper presented at the Meeting of the American Anthropological Association, Chicago.
n.d.    The Cybor Political Ecology of Disease. Unpublished paper.

**Trostle, J.**
2000    International Health Research: The Rules of the Game. In *Global Health Policies, Local Realities*, edited by L. M. Whiteford and L. Manderson, pp. 291–311. Boulder, CO: Lynn Reiner Press.

**Tsur, Y., and A. Dinar**
1995    Efficiency and Equity Consideration in Pricing and Allocating Irrigation Water. Policy Research Working Paper 1460. Washington, DC: The World Bank.

**Tsybine, A.**
2001    Water Privatization: A Broken Promise. Report published by Public Citizen's Critical Mass Energy and Environment Program. Washington, DC: Public Citizen. Electronic document, http://www.citizenorg/cmep.

**United Nations Children's Fund (UNICEF)**
2004    Trends over the Decade. Electronic document, http://www/childinfor.org/eddb/water/trends.htm, accessed August 27.

**United Nations Conference on Environment and Development**
1992    Report of the United Nations Conference on Environment and Development, UN Doc A/CONF 151/26.

# References

**United Nations Educational, Scientific and Cultural Organization (UNESCO)**
2002 Substantive Issues Arising in the Implementation of the International Covenant on Economic, Social and Cultural Rights. Articles 11 and 12 of *The Right to Water.*
2003a Electronic document, www.unesco.org/water/wwap/wwdr/index.shtml, accessed March 9.
2003b *Water for People, Water for Life.* Barcelona: Berghahan Publishers.

**United Nations Environment Programme (UNEP)**
1997 Global Environment Outlook-1: The Global State of the Environment Report. Electronic document, http://www.grida.no/geo1/ch/toc.htm#exsum, accessed March 2003.
1999a World Day for Water, 22 March 1999. Joint statement of UNEP and United Nations University. Electronic document, http://www.worldwaterday.org/1999/press.html, accessed June 20, 2004.
1999b Global Environment Outlook 2. Nairobi, Kenya. Electronic document, http://www.unep.org/geo2000, accessed August 30, 2004.
2002 *Children in the New Millennium: Environmental Impacts on Health.* New York: UNEP, UNICEF, and WHO.

**United Nations HIV/AIDS Programme (UNAIDS)**
2000 Report on the Global HIV/AIDS Epidemic. AIDS Epidemic Update Report, June.

**United Nations Population Division (UNPD)**
2000 Department of Economic and Social Affairs, Commission on Population and Development, Population Division 37th Session. Electronic document, http://www.un.org/esa/population/unpop.htm, accessed June 20, 2004.

**United Nations Population Fund (UNFPA)**
1993 State of World Population. New York.

**United Nations World Water Assessment Programme (Wateryear 2003)**
2003 Facts and Figures: Did You Know…? International Year of Freshwater 2003. People and the Planet: World Water Assessment Programme, UNESCO Publishing. Electronic document, http://www.wateryear2003.org.

**United Nations World Water Development Report (UN WWDR)**
2003 Water for People, Water for Life: UN World Water Development Report. UNESCO Publishing. New York: Berghahn Books.

**Vlassoff, C., and L. Manderson**
1998 Incorporating Gender in the Anthropology of Infectious Diseases. *Tropical Medicine & International Health* 3(12):1011–1019.

**Walker, C.**
2001 *Agrarian Change, Gender and Land Reform: A South African Case Study.* UNRISD Social Policy and Development Program Paper, no. 10. Geneva: United Nations Research Institute for Social Development.

# References

**Walpole Island, First Nation, Canada**
2003    Reserve website, Electronic document, http://www.iisd1.iisd.ca/
        50comm/commdb/desc/d09.htm, accessed March 6.

**Wang, J.**
2000    An Investigation of De-agriculturalization and Changes in the Position of
        Rural Women in Family—The Example of Zhejiang Province. *Social Sciences
        in China* (Summer):89–98.

**Waters, W.**
2001    Globalization, Socioeconomic Restructuring, and Community Health.
        *Journal of Community Health* 26(2):79–92.

**Watts, S., K. Khallaayoune, R. Bensefia, H. Laamrani, and B. Gryseels**
1998    The Study of Human Behavior and Schistosomiasis Transmission in an
        Irrigated Area in Morocco. *Social Science & Medicine* 46(6):755–765.

**Welch, J., with P. Stekler**
1994    *Killing Custer, The Battle of the Little Bighorn and the Fate of the Plains Indians.*
        New York: Penguin Books.

**Whiteford, L. M.**
1997    The Ethnoecology of Dengue Fever. *Medical Anthropology Quarterly* 1(2):202.
1998    Children's Health as Accumulated Capital: Structural Adjustment in the
        Dominican Republic and Cuba. In *Small Wars: The Cultural Politics of
        Childhood*, edited by N. Scheper-Hughes and C. Sargent, pp. 186–201.
        Berkeley: University of California Press.
2000    Idioms of Hope and Despair: Local Identity, Globalization and Health in
        Cuba and the Dominican Republic. In *Global Health Policy/Local Realities: The
        Fallacy of the Level Playing Field*, edited by L. M. Whiteford and L. Manderson,
        pp. 57–78. Boulder, CO: Lynn Rienner Press.

**Whiteford, L., with A. Arata, M. Torres, D. Montano, N. Suarez, E. Creel, and K. Ramsey**
1999    Diarrheal Disease Prevention through Community-Based Participation
        Interventions. Activity Report No. 61. Arlington, VA: Environmental Health
        Project.

**Whiteford, L., with C. Laspina and M. Torres**
1996    Cholera Prevention in Ecuador: Community-Based Approaches for Behavior
        Change. Activity Report No.19. Arlington, VA: Environmental Health
        Project.

**Whiteford, S., and F. Bernal**
1996    Campesinos, Water and the State: Different Views. In *Reforming Mexico's
        Agrarian Reform*, edited by L. Randall, pp. 215–222. New York: Sharpe.

**Whiteford, S. and A Cortez-Lara**
1996    Conflictos urbano/rurales sobre el agua del río Colorado en el ámbito inter-
        nacional. In *Agua: Desafios y oportunidades para el siglo XXI*, edited by Claudio
        Vargas and Joajuín Sosa Ramírez, chapter 10. Aguascalientes: Gobierno del
        Estado de Aguascalientes.

# References

**Whiteford, S., and R. Melville, eds.**
2002 *Protecting a Sacred Gift: Water and Social Change in Mexico.* La Jolla: Center for U.S./Mexico Studies, University of California, San Diego.
2003 *Protecting the Sacred Gift: Power and Water in Mexico.* Berkeley: University of California Press.

**Wiarda, H. J.**
2001 *The Soul of Latin America: The Cultural and Political Tradition.* New Haven, CT: Yale University Press.

**Williams, T.**
2003 Salmon Stakes. *Audubon* 3. Electronic document, http://magazine.audubon.org/incite/incite0303.html.

**Winpenny, J.**
1994 *Managing Water as an Economic Resource.* London: Routledge.

**Witter, S., and S. Whiteford**
1999 Water Security: The Issues and Policy Challenges. *International Review of Comparative Public Policy* 11:1–25.

**World Bank**
1993 Water Resources Management: A World Bank Policy Paper. Washington, DC.
1994 World Development Report. Washington, DC.
1999a Intensifying Action against HIV/AIDS in Africa: Responding to a Development Crisis. Washington, DC.
1999b Malawi: A Safety Net Strategy for the Poorest. Washington, DC.
2002a Water, Sanitation and Hygiene. Electronic document, http://wbln0018.worldbank.org/HDNet/hddocs.nsf, accessed March 2003.
2002b Bridging Troubled Waters. Washington, DC: Operations Evaluation Department.
2004 Water Resources Sector Strategy. Washington, DC: World Bank. Electronic document, http://lnweb18.worldbank.org/ESSD/ardext.nsf/18ByDocName/Strategy.

**World Commission on Dams (WCD)**
2000 Dams and Development: A New Framework for Decision Making. Final report of the WCD. Electronic document, http://www.wcd.org.

**World Commission on Health and the Environment**
1992 Our Planet, Our Health. Report of the WHO Commission on Health and the Environment. Geneva: World Health Organization.

***World Gazetteer***
2004 World Gazetteer Peru 2004. Electronic document, http://www.gazetteer.de and http://www.gazetteer.de/t/t_pe.htm, accessed October 23.

# REFERENCES

**World Health Organization (WHO)**
1998      The World Health Report 1998: Message from the Director-General. Electronic document, http://www.who.int/whr2001/2001/archives/1998/message.htm, accessed March 2003.
2000      Global Water Supply and Sanitation Assessment 2000 Report. Electronic document, http://www.who.int/water_sanitation_health/Globassessment/Foreword1.htm, accessed March 2003 and http://www.who.int/docstore/water_sanitation _health/Globassessment/Global1.htm, accessed June 20, 2004.

**WHO World Water Day Report**
2001      Electronic document, http://www.worldwaterday.org/2001/report/index.html, accessed February 13, 2003.

**World Water Council**
2000      Water Secure World: Vision for Water, Life and the Environment. World Water Vision Commission Report. Montpellier, France: World Water Council.

**World Water Forum**
2000      The Africa Water Vision for 2025: Equitable and Sustainable Use of Water for Socioeconomic Development. The Hague: World Water Forum.

**Yokwe Online**
2002      Kwajalein at Risk—Environmental Impact due to Toxin Perchlorate. Marshall Islands Message Board. Electronic document, http://www.yokwe.net/phpBB2/viewtopic.php?t=565.

**Yuan, H. C., J. G. Guo, R. Bergquist, M. Tanner, X. Y. Chen, and H. Z. Wang**
2000      The 1992–1999 World Bank Schistosomiasis Research Initiative in China: Outcome and Perspectives. *Parasitology International* 49(3):195–207.

**Zheng, J., X. G. Gu, Z. L. Qiu, and Z. H. Hua**
1997      Transmission Factors of Schistosomiasis japonica in the Mountainous Regions with Type of Plateau Canyon and Plateau Basin. *Chinese Medical Journal* 110(2):86–89.

**Zwarteveen, M. Z.**
1997      Water: From Basic Need to Commodity: A Discussion on Gender and Water Rights in the Context of Irrigation. *World Development* 25(8):1335–1349.

# Index

9/11 disaster, 245, 260

Aboriginals, 180n1. *See also* indigenous people
access to health care. *See* health care
access to information, 242
access to water and resources: demand management and, 186–87; disparities in, 4, 260; in Ecuador, 32; equity in policies, 48; health and, 19–23; privatization and, 189; safe water statistics, 9; in Southern Africa, 227; water scarcity and, 135–36; in Zimbabwe, 223–25
Acequia Real del Júcar, 199
Achuar people, 31
acre-feet measurements, 126n4
activism: collectivism, 92; Mexico's farmers and, 261; middle classes and, 205; political activism, 174; Spain's water policy and, 202–3; technology and, 235; transcending borders, 234
Africa, 90. *See also* Southern Africa; *names of specific nations*
age, disease and, 52, 73–74, 75
Agreement on Technical Barriers to Trade (TBT), 36, 42
Agreement on the Application of Sanitary and Phytosanitary Measures (SPS), 42
Agreement on Trade-Related Aspects of Intellectual Property (TRIPS), 36, 42
Agricultural Chemicals Group, 244
agriculture. *See* farming
Aguas del Rtunari, 149
Alaska Native Claims Settlement Act, 180n8
Alaskan native corporations, 173, 180n8
ALCOA company, 120
alcoholism, 176, 178
Aleuts, 180n1
All-American Canal, 242
Allan, T., 214, 229n10
Alma Ata Declaration, 41
American Anthropological Association, 7
American Indians: casinos. *See* casinos; colonizers and, 153–54; cultural impacts on, 169–70, 174–75; economic impacts on, 171–74; environmental impacts on, 175–76; globalization and, 169–78; health impacts on, 176–78; legal issues, 167–69; multitribal coalitions, 170, 171; Native Alaskans, 157, 173, 180n8; off-reservation claims, 162–65, 167–69; political impacts on, 170–71; populations, 156–58; research scope, 159–60; sovereignty, 156, 161; terminology, 179–80n1; tourism, 172–74; water disputes and, 142, 158–65; water-linked food resources, 165–67
American Water Company, 144–45
American Water Works, 191

Amnesty International, 170, 230n23
Andean climate change, 136
Andean Development Corporation, 40
Anhui province, China, 75
animals, 95–96, 102–3
Animas-La Plata Project, 163
anthropogenic factors in water scarcity, 141–46
anthropology: global ethnography, 86; policy issues and, 7–8; scope of inquiry, 262. *See also* research
anti-schistosomiasis workers, 82
anti-terror measures, 178
Appadurai, A., 154
appropriation of water, 188. *See also* partitioning water
aquaculture, 171
aquifers and groundwater: American Indian rights to, 163; as commons or property, 118, 121; contamination of, 122–23, 132, 134, 242–46; Edwards Aquifer. *See* Edwards Aquifer; in irrigation, 187–88; lack of information on quality, 247–49; Lima's situation, 94; in Mexicali Valley, 238, 239, 242–43; as Mexican state-owned, 248; perception of, 243; permits for, 118; recharge areas, 112, 117–18, 119, 243; rights and, 188; salinity, 93; saltwater intrusions, 91, 93, 136; testing, 253n5; in Virgin Islands, 133–34; water insecurity, 261–62; water laws and, 109

303

# INDEX

Aragón, Spain, 199
Armelagos, G., 11
arsenic, 130, 138, 139, 151
ascariasis, 77
Asia, 90. *See also names of specific countries*
Assiniboine tribe, 162, 163
Aswan dam, 71
"augmenting supply," 185
Austin, Texas, 120
automobile manufacturing, 113
avian flu, 178
Azurix company, 191, 194

Bacterial diseases, 27
Baer, H. A., 252n3
Bangladesh, 138, 151
Barlow, M., 26
Barrios de Luna dam, 197
Barrios de Luna syndicate, 201
Basel Convention, 140
BASF pesticides, 244
BASIS program, 64n1, 66n8
Bayer de Mexico, 244
Bechtel Corporation, 149, 194
behavior: disease-related, 12, 27, 33–34, 35, 89; water insecurity and, 14
belief systems: cholera-related, 33–34; development formulas as, 235
Belloni, R., 166
Bexar County, Texas, 107, 115, 119, 122–23
bilharziasis. *See* schistosomiasis
Bill and Melinda Gates Foundation, 14
birth control, China, 79–80
birth defects, 139
Black Hills, South Dakota, 168–69
Blackstone, W., 188
black waters, 10
Boldt decision, 167
Bolivia, 38, 39, 136, 149, 194
Border Environmental Cooperation Commission, 240
borders: food inspections, 241; Mexican assembly plants, 240; between Mexico and U.S., 232, 241–42; political coalitions transcending, 234; security, 260
boreholes, 57, 58–59, 65n6
bottled water: companies, 237, 248, 249, 254n9; costs of, 40; designer water, 144; quality of, 251; testing, 249; U.S. sales, 254n9
boundary objects: negotiation and, 116–18; water management and, 124–25; water politics and, 108–10
Brazil, 71, 189
breast milk, 41, 42
Brennan, T., 177
Broadening Access and Strengthening Input Market Systems (BASIS), 64n1, 66n8
bureaucracy, 120, 123
Bureau of Indian Affairs, 170–71
Buroway, M., 21–22, 85–88

Cai, X., 215
California-American Water Company, 143–44
California Public Utilities Commission, 144
Cameroon, 72
campesino communities, 190
*Campylobacter jejuni*, 96
Canada: Hydro-Quebec projects, 147, 158–59, 172; Indian reserves, 156–58
canal irrigation, 188, 196, 239, 242
cancer, 139, 141
Canto Grande, Peru, 89, 93, 97–101
capital in globalization, 154
cardiovascular problems, 245
caregiving, HIV/AIDS and, 53
Caribbean region, 39–40, 90. *See also names of specific countries*
car manufacturing, 113
Carrizo-Wilcox Aquifer, 120
cash crops, 112
cash economy, 77–78, 82, 155
cash resources, 77, 80, 81, 82, 83
casinos: competition for, 172–73, 182n21; disputes over, 168; effects of, 174; health care and, 178; Pojoaque Pueblo, 162, 165; Swinomish tribe, 162
Catchment Councils, Zimbabwe, 224
Cato Institute, 105
Celilo Falls, Columbia River, 158
Center for International Community-Based Health Research, 89
Center for Policy Analysis on Trade and Health (CPATH), 26
Central America, 251n1. *See also names of specific countries*
Central Irrigation Syndicate, Barrios de Luna, 197
Centro Nacional de Sindacatos, Spain, 199
*cercariae*, 69–70, 73
CGIAR (Consultative Group on International Agricultural Research), 218, 229n12
Chachis people, 31
Chavula, G., 64n1
checkerboard reservations, 160
chemotherapy, 75
children: China's birth control program and, 79–80; Convention on the Rights of the Child, 219; diarrheal diseases in, 95; educational and domestic demands on, 82; health focus of organizations, 260; mortality rates, 9, 25, 39–40; orphans, 53; reducing mortality, 259–60; schistosomiasis and, 73
Chilima, G., 65n1
Chilton, J., 91
China: birth control in, 79–80; dams, 68–69, 84; educational system, 79–80, 81, 82; health care resources, 82–83; lake pollution, 137; male work-

# INDEX

force, 81–82; market economy and, 82; schistosomiasis in, 74–83; uneven development patterns, 83
chlorination, 34, 94
cholera: in Ecuador, 30–35; incidence of, 27; increasing after privatization, 146; in Lima, 91; in London, 12–13; in Malawi, 55, 61, 62; reintroduction of, 35; in South America, 28, 151–52; in Southern Africa, 222; transmission of, 31–32; as waterborne disease, 9
chromium, 130, 140, 151
chronic diseases, 12
churches, 51, 59, 61, 88. *See also* religion
Citizens Utilities, 143
Clarke, R., 26, 91
Clean Water Act, 142
climate change, 90, 136, 137
Cline, S., 215
clinic fees, 36, 38
Clorpiriphos pesticide, 244–45
CNA (Comisión Nacional del Agua), 245, 250–51
Coca Cola, 237, 249, 254n9
Cochabamba, Bolivia, 194, 207
Cohesion Fund, E.U., 204
El Colegio de la Frontera Norte, 253n5
collaboration and cooperative behaviors: boundary objects and, 108–10; de-collectivization, 82; in Dublin Principles, 212; irrigators and, 206–8; labor movements, 199; lack of, 102-103, 100; Malawi water reforms and, 59–60; multi-tribal coalitions, 170, 171; participatory project management, 259; promotion of, 92; in *pueblos jovenes*, 100, 102–3; research participation, 6; in rural water programs, 59; in Spain's water policy, 202–3; trade unions, 200; transcending borders, 234; working

water-use arrangements, 197
Collaborative Research Support Program (CRSP), 64n1
collectivism, 92
Colombia, 36–37
colonialism, 31, 155, 221
Colorado River, 123, 234, 238, 239, 243
Colorado River Compact, 238
Columbia River, 158, 166
Comal County, Texas, 111–12, 115
Comisión Nacional del Agua (CNA), 239, 245, 250–51
commercial fishing, 165–67
commercial water, 223
Committee on International Agreements on Trade in Endangered Species, 228n2
commodities: drinking water as, 231, 237; groundwater as, 116–17; health care as, 38; human rights and, 152; loan structures and, 149–50; natural resources and, 26; rights and, 26, 50, 126; water's value as, 68–69, 120, 129–30, 133–35
"the commons" (public property): access to, 23; aquifers as, 109, 116, 121, 123–25; canal irrigation and, 196; ecosystem health and, 125; groundwater as, 116–17; negotiation and, 116–18; tragedy of, 26; water as, 119
communication technologies, 234, 241–42
community: activism. *See* activism; Alaskan Native villages, 157; defined in policies, 56; health care and, 82–83; local identities, 88; local processes, 6; Malawi's water policies and, 57, 61; male dominance in governance, 81; migrants returning to, 35; neighbors, 100; *pueblos jovenes*, 89, 94, 97,

98–101; research participation, 6; trade organizations' impact on, 28; *vs.* user groups, 60; village priorities, 81. *See also names of specific communities*
Community-Based Participatory Intervention (CPI), 33
*Community Based Rural Water Supply, Sanitation and Hygiene Education Implementation Manual*, 65n4
Conferación Hidrológica del Duero, 201
confusion about water programs, 59
conjunctivitis, 10, 55
connections between sites: global connections, 88; in globalization studies, 86–88; in *pueblos jovenes*, 97–98, 104; water problems and, 89–92
Consejería del Medio Ambiente y Ordenación del Territorio, 202
conservation easements, 117–18, 119
conservation of water. *See* water conservation
Consultative Group on International Agricultural Research (CGIAR), 218, 229n12
consumers. *See* customers
consumption, patterns of, 264
consumption-based water fees, 192–93
consumptive water uses, 190, 192–93
contamination of water, 13, 34, 247. *See also* pollution; toxic wastes
continuous water delivery, 190
contractual mechanisms, 88. *See also* international trade organizations
contrived scarcity. *See* manufactured scarcity
Convention on the Elimination of All Forms of

305

# Index

Discrimination against Women, 50
Convention on the Rights of the Child, 219
cooperation. *See* collaboration and cooperative behaviors
La Coordinadora, 194
Coordinadora Ecologista de Castilla y León, 202
coordination. *See* collaboration and cooperative behaviors
copyrights, 42–43
corporate farming, 234, 241
corporations: Alaskan Native, 173, 180n8; bottled water and, 237; corporate farming, 234, 241; development corporations, 40, 122–23; energy scarcity and, 147; in globalization, 5, 154, 234; pesticide companies, 244–45; privatization and, 149, 191, 194, 232, 252n4; water as commodity and, 117, 133–35; water taken by force and, 26
Cortez-Lara, A., 19, 130, 132, 231–54
cost recovery in water systems: Bolivian riots and, 149; cholera and, 151–52; in Felton, California, 145; Malawi water policies, 55, 56; pricing water, 191–93; rates increases and, 146; San Antonio Water System, 120; as top-down mechanism, 148; volumetric pricing and, 186
costs: groundwater-based irrigation, 187–88; health care, 36–37, 38; mismanagement of resources, 265; water measurement devices, 193
Cote d'Ivoire, 71
cotton, 239
CPATH (Center for Policy Analysis on Trade and Health), 26
Cree tribe, 159, 172, 180–81n9

crimes against water users, 3, 265
critical medical anthropology, 43, 233–34, 236, 263, 264–65
Crow tribe, 163
cryptosporidiosis, 27
cultural impacts of globalization: culture as charter, 85; economic development vs. cultural rights, 142–43; fishing and, 174; on indigenous peoples, 169–70, 174–75; lifestyle diseases, 12; power and water scarcity, 141–46; "project" culture, 120; water shortages and, 185
currency, devaluation of, 37, 40
customers: definition of water quality, 236; indigenous peoples as, 155; patterns of consumption, 264

Dalles Dam, The, 158
dams: American Indians and, 158–59; in China, 68–69, 84; displacement effects of, 69, 257, 260; impacts on populations and ecology, 137; manufactured scarcity and, 146–50; in Mexico, 252n1; pricing of water and, 225; problems with, 259; schistosomiasis and, 71; Southern Africa's colonial era, 221; World Bank's projects, 257; in Zimbabwe, 230n22
Dawes Severalty Act, 160
DDT pesticide, 246
de-agriculturalization, 82
death. *See* mortality
debt crisis of 1980s, 96
debt servicing. *See* loan structures
decentralization of services: in Ecuador, 28; gender and, 49; government policy partnerships and, 108; in Malawi, 56, 58–62; neoliberal reforms and, 258–59; public health infrastructure breakdown, 36–41; in

Southern Africa, 50; trends towards, 47–48; World Bank loans and, 241, 258
de-collectivization, 82
deforestation, 136
dehydration, 95, 96
deindustrialization, 87
deinstitutionalization, 87
delivered water: fixed delivery of water, 190; in Latin America, 236–37; in Lima, 94; in *pueblos jovenes*, 100–101
demand for water: daily needs, 13–14; in Europe, 95; industrialization and, 138–39; in Lima, 94, 95; quarrels over water, 80; reducing by per-unit fees, 192; water scarcity and, 135–36. *See also* water conservation
demand management-based strategies: in Malawi, 56, 57; multinational organizations and, 45–46; per-unit fees and, 191–92; privatization as, 186–87, 189–91; resistance to, 194–95, 206–8; river basin management and, 48; World Bank and, 48
Democratic Republic of Congo, 229n9
demographics and diseases, 68
dengue, 10, 40, 84n1
deregulation, 26, 27, 237
Derman, W., 130–31, 209–30, 252n3
desalinization plants, 143–44
De Soto, H., 100, 103–4, 105
devaluation of currency, 37, 40
developed nation disease rates, 27–28
Devereux, S., 51–52
diabetes, 176
Diama Dam, Senegal, 71
diarrheal diseases: child mortality and, 39–40; in China, 77; in Lima, 86, 95; mortality and, 12, 39–40, 91, 138; pesticides and, 244; prevention of, 27; risk behav-

306

# INDEX

iors for, 89; in Southern Africa, 222; water shortages and, 95; world statistics, 9, 30. *See also* cholera
diffusion, 88
dirtiness, concepts of, 101
Disability Adjusted Life Years (DALYS), 36
disadvantaged. *See* poverty and the poor
discourses, 214; scale and, 131; scarcity frameworks, 214–17; water-as-economic-good framework, 217–18; water-as-human-right framework, 218–19; water-health interface, 255; water-in-environment framework, 220–21; water policy frameworks, 212–14
discretionary income, 77, 80, 81, 82, 83
diseases: American Indian statistics, 167, 176–78; annual rates of, 27; contaminated water and, 136; economic effects of, 36; epidemiological transitions, 11–13, 28–29; leading causes of death, 12; prevention, 27, 33; Southern African reforms and, 211; types of, 9–10; vectorborne, 67–69. *See also names of specific diseases*
disenfranchisement: disparities in access to resources, 4, 260; economic priorities and, 142–43; mechanisms of, 8; structural violence and, 262; in U.S. Virgin Islands, 134; user groups *vs.* communities, 60–61. *See also* access to water and resources
displacement: dams and, 69, 257, 260; indigenous peoples and, 155; schistosomiasis and, 71
division of labor, 78–79
domestic animals, 95–96, 102–3
domestic water use: in Malawi, 56–57, 58; in Mexicali Valley, 239; schistosomiasis and, 73; women's role in, 49. *See also* drinking water
domestic work, 79, 80, 102
Dominican Republic, 37, 38
Donahue, J., 22, 107–26, 126n1, 253n6
Dongting Lake region, China, 75
Douglas, O., 170
Dow Elanco, 244
Drexel Chemical Company, 245
drinking water: Colorado River as, 234; contaminants in, 138; costs of, 39; deaths related to, 9; de-emphasis in policies, 64; epidemiological transitions and, 11; lack of access to, 251n1; in Malawi, 54–58, 64; mitigation of illness and, 57; piped water supplies, 34; pollution and, 91; privatization of, 236–37; public health efforts and, 138; quality issues, 231–33; in San Antonio, 123; in Southern Africa, 211; in Zimbabwe, 225–26
droughts: in Southern Africa, 211; in Spain, 198; in St. Thomas, 133–34; in Texas Hill Country, 114; water use restrictions, 116
drugs, 178
Dublin Principles, 212; in Southern Africa water reform, 222; water-as-economic-good framework, 217–18; water management and, 46
Dupont company, 244
dysentery, 27, 55, 61, 222

*E. coli*, 95
Eastern Cree tribe, 159, 172, 180–81n9
Ebro River basin, Spain, 203
ecofeminist literature, 48–49
ecological anthropology, 4
Ecologistas en Acción, 204
ecology. *See* ecosystem health; environment
economic anthropology, 263
economics and economic development: American Indians and, 171–74; Dublin Principles values, 212; economic effects of illness, 36; economic pressures on populations, 155, 171–74; *vs.* environmental and cultural rights, 142–43; favoring over pollution, 123; global agreements, 132; global forces in, 88; health's political economy, 43; health's relationship to, 14–15, 20, 26, 36, 43; impact on wetlands and lakes, 137; indigenous peoples and, 155, 171–74; Lima's growth and, 94; loss of control in globalization, 155; Malawi's impoverishment and, 50–54; manufactured scarcity and, 150–52; moral economy. *See* moral economy; neoliberal. *See* neoliberal economic policies; penny consumerism, 100, 102–3, 104; prioritization in water management, 142–43; *vs.* public health water issues, 64; Spain's reforms and, 195–96; water-as-economic-good framework, 217–18; water scarcity and, 150–52
ecopolitics, 143
ecosystem health: prioritizing ecology, 151; privatization and, 117; public health and, 122–23; public property concept and, 125; San Antonio's water plan and, 118–20; vectorborne diseases and, 68; water-in-the-environment framework, 220–21; in water policies, 126n9
Ecuador: cholera outbreak, 30–35; currency devaluation and loss, 37, 40; loan restructuring, 40–41; map, 29; privatization and decentralization in, 28
education in China, 79–80, 81, 82

307

# Index

Edwards Aquifer: administration and rights, 114–16; as boundary object, 108–10, 124–25; discharge, 126n5; hydrology and movement, 110–14; size, 126n4
Edwards Aquifer Authority, 109, 114–16, 119, 121
Edwards Underground Water District, 115
Egypt, 71, 192
E-H2 corporation, 147
*ejidatarios*, 239
elected officials, 124–25, 198
electronics companies, 139–40
elephant products, 228n2
elite classes, 227, 258
eminent domain, 144
empowerment: equitable participation in management, 148; of local agencies, 257–58; in Malawi's policies, 57–58, 63; World Health Organization disempowerment, 41, 43. *See also* power
enclosure, 46, 62
endangered species, 114, 142, 171, 228n2
Endangered Species Act, 114, 142
Endosulfan Sulfate, 244
energy crises, 147
enforcement, 148. *See also* regulations and laws
English riparian water law, 118
Enron Corporation, 191, 194
enteritis, 12
enteropathogens, 95
environment: American Indian preservation efforts, 164; changes in, 68, 90, 136, 233; climate changes, 90, 136, 137; costs of protecting, 140; ecosystem framework, 220–21; global freshwater water stress, 90; greenhouse gases, 137; indigenous peoples and, 164, 175–76; Malawi's policies and, 57; political ecology and, 212; populations and, 90; redefining nature, 249; regulations as ideological globalization, 235; rights to water, 48, 216; San Antonio's issues, 122–23; sustainability and, 220–21; vectorborne diseases and, 68; water-as-economic-good framework and, 217–18
environmental activism, 202–3, 205, 242
environmental anthropology, 264
environmental changes, 68, 90, 136, 233
Environmental Health Project, 33
Environmental Protection Agency, 242, 245
Environmental Rights Action, 170
EPA (Environmental Protection Agency), 242, 245
epidemics: cholera. *See* cholera; epidemiological transitions, 11–13, 28–29; epidemiology, 11; HIV/AIDS. *See* HIV/AIDs epidemics; schistosomiasis, 74–83
equality: exposure to health risks, 234; health and, 4; in land distribution, 189; participation in management, 148; patterns of disease and poverty, 32; unequal power relationships, 234; in water access policies, 48
Eskimo peoples, 157, 180n1
ethnoscapes, 154
Euro-Mediterranean Irrigators Community, 205
European Regional Development Fund, 204
European Union: demand management policies, 207; Water Framework Directive, 205; water policy, 201
Euro-Quebec Hydrogen Pilot Projects, 147
eviction, water bills and, 146
exploitation, globalization and, 87
export markets: hydrogen, 147; Malawi products, 51; Mexican products, 240; power and utilities market, 172; World Bank encouragement of, 37–38
external forces, 86–92, 96–97, 104
external risk, 233

Facilities: breakdown of, 59. *See also* public health infrastructure; sanitation systems; water supply
Fairchild Semiconductor, 139
famine, 52
Farmer, P., 7, 8, 43–44
farmer-managed irrigation systems (FMIS), 187, 195–204, 207
farming: appropriation of land, 230n20; Chinese village agriculture, 78, 82; corporate farming, 234, 241; dam construction and, 137; de-agriculturalization, 82; demand management strategies and, 186–87, 192, 206; Edwards Aquifer and, 111; Klamath River water rights and, 142; Malawi agriculture, 50–51, 58; Mexicali Valley agriculture, 238–40, 241; NAFTA's effect on, 240; pesticides and chemicals in, 241; schistosomiasis and, 75; Southern African reforms and, 211; standards and, 241; subsidies for, 221; Texan cash crops, 112; water pricing structures, 191–93; water security and insecurity, 261–62; women's role in, 49. *See also* farmer-managed irrigation systems
fecal coliform, 61, 66n8
feces and fecal contamination: in aquifers, 94; cholera transmission and, 31–32, 33; Lima's water tests, 95; *pueblos jovenes* adaptations, 102–3; schistosomiasis and, 75

# INDEX

Federacíon Ecologista de Castilla y León, 202
fees. *See* clinic fees; user fees; water fees
Felton, California, 143–44
feminism: ecofeminist literature, 48–49; traveling theories of, 87
Ferguson, A., 20–21, 45–66, 252n3
filariasis, 10, 83, 84n1
financescapes, 154
First Nations, 180n1
fish: American Indian preservation efforts, 172; cultural roots and, 174; dams and, 137, 158; "fish-ins," 166; globalization's impacts on indigenous peoples and, 171; hatcheries, 165, 171; salmon fishing, 166, 167; salmon kills, 142–43, 164; salmon runs, 158
fisher folk: "fish-ins," 166; marine resources, 165–67; salmon fishing, 166, 167; salmon kills, 142–43, 164; schistosomiasis and, 75
fixed delivery of water, 190
fixed flow dividers, 208n3
fixed water providers, 236
Flathead Reservation, 161
flooding, 211
FMC Corporation, 244
FMIS (farmer-managed irrigation systems), 187, 195–204, 207
FNCR (National Federation of Irrigation Communities), 199, 200, 205
food: cholera and, 33; fecal contamination and, 95; food riots, 37; genetically-modified foods, 178–79; water-linked food resources, 165–67
*forasteros*, 197, 208n4
Forde, C. D., 85
Fort Peck reservation, Montana, 162
Fraser River, Canada, 167
free market/privatization incentives: managing water as economic good, 217–18; multilateral agreements and, 149–50; Spain's water reforms, 203; water conservation and, 262
free riding water use, 208n4
Free Trade Area of the Americas (FTAA), 26, 27
freshwater: crisis in, 90, 185; dams and, 137; in Dublin Principles, 212; irrigation's demand on, 135
friendships, 88
Frownfelter, D., 121
FTAA (Free Trade Area of the Americas), 26, 27
Fukumoto, M., 89

Garci Crespo, 237
Gates Foundation, 14
GATS (General Agreement on Trade in Services), 36
GATT (General Agreement on Tariffs and Trade), 145, 240, 250, 260
GBM pesticides, 244
gender: cholera and, 13; disease exposure and, 78–79, 80; health care and, 83; Malawi's policies and, 59, 62, 63; schistosomiasis infection and, 72–74, 75, 83; scope of research, 46; water management roles, 48–49, 65n4; in World Bank policies, 228n6
General Agreement on Tariffs and Trade (GATT), 145, 240, 250, 260
General Agreement on Trade in Services (GATS), 36
General Allotment Act, U.S., 160
genetically-modified foods, 178–79
genital schistosomiasis, 73
Ghana, 194
Giago, T., 181n10
giardiasis, 9, 55
Giddens, A., 233
Gila River, Arizona, 163
Gleick, P. H., 49–50, 217, 254n9
global connection. *See* connections between sites
global ethnography, 86
global forces (external forces), 86–92, 96–97, 104
global imagination, 88; cleanliness and disease, 101–2; expectations and, 105n1; in globalization studies, 86–88; in *pueblos jovenes*, 104
globalization, 5, 28; Buroway's three axes, 86–88; casualties of, 25–30; constraining forces on, 178–79; cultural impacts. *See* cultural impacts of globalization; domains of impact on lifeways, 169–70; economic impacts of, 171–74; environmental effects of, 175–76, 213; forces in, 88; government policy partnerships and, 108; grounded globalization, 85–88, 89–92, 104–5; impact on indigenous peoples, 154–56, 170–71, 175–76; *vs.* modernization, 154; NGOs and, 5, 59, 214, 235, 261; political effects of, 170–71; processes in, 234–36; public health infrastructure and, 35–41; time-sensitivity of issues, 265; water-health interface in, 14–15, 43–44, 255; water's commodity value and, 68–69; of water supplies and water control, 151
global warming, 90, 136, 137
global water apartheid, 45
Global Water Corporation, 26
Global Water Partnership, 211, 261
gold discoveries, 169
golf courses, 122–23
Goshute tribe, 175
Gover, K., 170
Gowan, T., 86
gray water, 10
Greaves, T., 130, 153–83
greenhouse gases, 137
Greenpeace, 204
Gros Ventre tribe, 163

309

# Index

grounded globalization, 85–92, 104–5
groundwater. *See* aquifers and groundwater
Groundwater Conservation Districts, Texas, 121
group taps, in Lima, 94
growth retardation, 77
Guadalupe-Blanco River Authority, 114
Guadalupe River, Texas, 123
Guanxi, China, 74
Guayaquil, Ecuador, 32
Guillet, D., 130–31, 185–208
guinea pigs, 96
Guiyu, China, 140

Hacienda system, 190
hand washing, 101
Harare, Zimbabwe, 226
Hawaiian peoples, 180n5
Hays County, Texas, 107, 111–12, 115
Hazardous Materials Storage Ordinance, 139–40
hazardous wastes. *See* toxic wastes
health: American Indians, 176–78; behaviors, 14, 33–34, 35, 89; casualties of globalization, 25–30; decentralization of, 258; economic development and, 14–15; ecosystems, 220–21; equity and, 4; farmer-managed irrigation systems and, 187; global disparities in, 4; high-tech industry waste and, 139, 140–41; loss of self-sufficiency and, 155; Millennium Challenge, 256, 259–60; moral economy and, 30, 41–44; native medicine and healing, 177; pesticides and, 244–45, 253n7; as private good, 38; as private responsibility, 121–22; privatization and, 117; rights model, 14–15, 43–44; Southern African reforms and, 211; trade organizations and, 28; unequal exposure to health risks, 234; water access and, 19–23; water-health interface in globalization, 255; water scarcity and, 136–41. *See also* health care
Health Behavior Interventions to Reduce the Incidence of Diarrhea in Lima, Peru (HBIRID), 88–89
health care: Chinese villages, 74, 82–83; free health care, 36; native medicine and healing, 177; privatization of, 258
heavy metals, 140
Hellum, A., 50
hemorrhagic fever, 77
hepatitis, 9, 76, 222
herbicides, 243–46
Hermandades Sindicales Agrarias, 199–200
hermeneutic society, 86
Hexaclorinebencene, 246
high-tech industry, 139–40, 141
Hill Country, Texas, 107
Hirji, R., 217, 219
history: context for water and health policies, 256; erasing, 7
HIV/AIDs epidemics: American Indian rates, 176; coexisting disease issues, 55; in Malawi, 52–54, 58–62; middle and upper class incidence of, 65n2; privatization's effects on, 146; in Southern Africa, 52–53, 222; structural violence and, 63
homicide rates, 176
Hong, E., 35–36
hookworm, 77
Hoopa tribe, 164
Hopi Pueblos, 163
housing in *pueblos jovenes*, 98–101
Huang, Y., 21, 67–84, 76
human rights: commodities and, 152; environmental sustainability and, 220–21; sanitation systems and, 43; vaccines and, 43; water as, 43, 45–46, 49–50, 218–19; in Zimbabwe, 230n23
Human Rights Watch, 230n23
hydrogen exports, 147
Hydro-Quebec projects, 147, 158–59, 172
hygiene: cash resources and, 81; cholera and, 32, 33–34, 35; diarrheal diseases and, 89; schistosomiasis and, 72–74; water insecurity and, 14

Ideological globalization, 235, 240
ideoscapes, 154
illiteracy in China, 80
illness. *See* diseases
images, adoption of, 88
imaginations from daily life. *See* global imagination
IMF. *See* International Monetary Fund (IMF)
immune system, 55
immunizations, 12, 36, 43
Imperial Irrigation District, 242
Imperial Valley, California, 238
*Indian Country Today*, 159–60, 181n10
Indian Trust Fund scandal, 168
India's irrigation charges, 192
indigenous people: American Indians. *See* American Indians; cultural impacts on, 169–70, 174–75; dams and, 137–38; economic impacts on, 171–74; in Ecuador, 31; environmental impacts on, 175–76; globalization's impacts on, 154–56, 169–70; Native Alaskans, 157, 173, 180n8; patterns of disease, 32; political impacts on, 170–71; sovereignty, 156, 161; terminology, 180n1
individualism, 102
industrialization: Chinese manufacturing, 82; deindustrialization, 87;

## INDEX

Edwards Aquifer and, 111; high-tech waste, 139, 140–41; Lima's water supply and, 94; Mexican manufacturing, 240; pollution and, 94, 112–13, 138–39; protecting environment and, 140; Texan rivers and, 112–13; water demands and, 138–39

inequities: exposure to health risks, 234; land distribution, 189; patterns of disease, 32; unequal power relationships, 234. *See also* equality

inflation, 40

informal adjustments to water reforms, 197

infrastructure: facilities, breakdown of, 59; public health. *See* public health infrastructure; sanitation systems. *See* sanitation systems; water supply. *See* water supply

input water pricing, 192

insecticides, 243–46

insects, 10, 84

Institute of Nutrition Research, 95

institutional project culture, 120

Instituto de Investigación Nacional, Peru, 89

Integrated Rural Water Supply and Sanitation program, Zimbabwe, 225

intellectual property, 42–43

Inter-American Development Bank, 232

International Boundary and Water Commission, 238

International Center for the Settlement of Investment Disputes, 149

International Code of Marketing Breast Milk Substitute, 41, 42

International Conference on Water and the Environment, 228n5

international corporations. *See* transnational corporations

International Covenant on Economic, Social and Cultural Rights, 46, 219

International Crisis Committee, 230n23

International Drinking Water Supply and Sanitation Decade, 25, 260

International Fund for Agricultural Development, 229n12

international law, 235. *See also* regulations and laws

international lending organizations, 214. *See also* International Monetary Fund; loan structures; World Bank

International Monetary Fund (IMF): cost recovery policies, 146; Ecuador's loans, 40; Malawi debts, 51; poverty and, 216; water scarcity report, 147

international trade organizations: community health and, 28; endangered species and, 228n2; health *vs.* economic growth formulas, 26; Hong's work on, 36; intellectual property and, 42; labeling agreements, 42; lack of rights-based approaches, 152; municipal water supplies and, 143–44; public health deregulation and, 26, 27; public health infrastructure tradeoffs, 35; research on global trade, 19. *See also* General Agreement on Tariffs and Trade; North America Free Trade Agreement; World Trade Organization

International Union for the Conservation of Nature, 214, 216

International Water Limited, 194

International Water Management Institute, 192, 218, 229n7, 261

intestinal schistosomiasis, 69, 70, 71

intestinal worms, 27

Inuit peoples, 157, 180n1

invasions (aquifer saltwater intrusions), 91, 93, 136

invasions (urban settlements), 93, 97, 98–101

irrigation: in China, 80; collaboration in, 206–8; dams and, 137; Euro-Mediterranean Irrigators Community, 205; farmer-managed. *See* farmer-managed irrigation systems; freshwater demand of, 135; health of irrigators and, 131; in Hill Country, Texas, 112; landscape watering, 111; Leon Irrigators Council, 201–4; in Malawi, 58; in Mexicali Valley, 239; in Orbigo Valley, 195–201; pesticides and, 233; pollution resulting from, 94, 135; property rights and, 187–89; rationing water and per-unit fees, 192; regulatory frameworks for, 200–201; subsidies for, 221; upstream users, 190; water security and insecurity, 261–62

irrigation communities, 131, 200–204, 205

isolation, 154

IUCN (International Union for the Conservation of Nature), 216

James Bay Hydroelectric Projects, Canada, 146–47, 158–59, 172

Janes, C., 14

Johannesburg summit, 45, 46, 92, 218

Johns Hopkins University, 89

Johnston, B. R., 129, 130, 133–52, 252n2

Josephy, A. M., 159

junior and senior water rights, 115

Junta de Castilla y León, 202, 203

Junta de Explotación, 197

311

# Index

Kambewa, D., 65n1
Kato-Katz technique, 76
Kendall, C., 21–22, 85–105
Kennewick Man, 168
Kerr, J., 65n1
Khaila, S., 64n1
kidney disease, 244
Kinney County, Texas, 112, 115
kinship, 88
Kinzua dam, 158, 174–75
Klamath River, California, 142–43, 163
Klaver, I., 22, 107–26, 125n1
knowledge-based property, 42–43
Koch, R., 13
Kootenai tribe, 161, 163
Kwajalein, Marshall Islands, 141

Labor movements in Spain, 199
lakes, 75, 137, 164–65
land: American Indian reservations, 156–58, 167–69; in China, 77–78, 82; inequities in distribution, 189; loss of, 54, 65n3; in Malawi, 54, 63; non-Indian leaseholders, 161, 181n12; Southern African redistribution, 221; water property rights and, 188–89, 206, 224
landscape watering, 111
large-scale water projects. *See* "mega" projects
Latin America: child mortality in, 39–40; drinking water privatization and, 236–37; hacienda system, 190; rapid urban growth in, 90. *See also names of individual countries*
latrines, 98, 103
lawns, 111
laws. *See* regulations and laws
lead poisoning, 140
leaking chemical tanks, 139
leasing native lands, 161, 181n12
legal systems and challenges. *See* regulations and laws
Leon Irrigators Council, Spain, 201–4
Leopold, A., 125
Lerer, L. B., 71
levies. *See* tariffs and levies
Ley de Modificación de Aguas, Spain, 204–5
lifestyles. *See* behavior; cultural impacts of globalization
lifeways. *See* cultural impacts of globalization
Likangala River district, Malawi, 58
Lima, Peru: cholera in, 91; diarrhea prevention in, 88–89; European water use compared to, 95; penny consumerism, 100; privatization in, 92; *pueblos jovenes*, 89, 94, 97–101; seismically active areas, 99; urban growth in, 94; water scarcity in, 85–86, 93–96; water supply and contamination, 92–96; water vendors, 94
literacy in China, 80
liver disease, 176, 244
loan structures: commodities and, 149–50; contractual relationships and, 149; decentralization of services and, 241, 258; demand management-based water strategies and, 48; in Ecuador, 40–41; effects on health, 25; health care as part of, 43; as implementing belief systems, 235; lack of rights-based approaches in, 152; in Malawi, 51–52; in Mexicali Valley, 239; middle classes and, 40–41; in Peru, 96; policy changes and, 213; restructuring, 40–41; for schistosomiasis control, 75, 84; structural adjustment policies, 37, 40, 50; water resource management and, 46–50; World Bank requirements for, 241. *See also* international lending organizations; International Monetary Fund; World Bank
lobster harvesting, 165, 166
local agencies: decentralization and, 38; desires for local control, 259; empowerment of, 257–58; financial support for policies, 64; in Malawi, 51–52, 57, 58–62; negotiations in policy making, 108; public health infrastructure breakdown, 36–41; responsibility for infrastructure, 35; village priorities in China, 80–81; water disinfection and, 34; water rights and, 227. *See also* collaboration and cooperative behaviors; community
Local Government Act, Malawi, 60
local identities, 88
local processes, 6
logging protests, 168, 175
London cholera outbreak, 12–13
Lovett, L., 107, 125
low-cost health care, 36
Lower Brule tribe, 164, 171
Lumberman's Investment Corporation, 122–23
Lummi tribe, 162–63, 164, 165, 174

Maintenance of water supply, 57, 59, 60, 193
Makah tribe, 167, 171
malaria, 10, 30, 40, 55, 83, 84n1
Malathion, 244–45
Malawi: HIV/AIDs epidemic, 52–54; impoverishment and economics, 50–54; map, 47; Ministry of Water Development, 57, 60; National Water Development Project, 55; rural health and gender water issues, 58–62; water policies, 54–58
Malawi Social Action Fund, 59
males: dominance in governance, 81; health care access, 83; loss of land, 65n3; migration of work-

312

## INDEX

force, 81–82; schistosomiasis and, 73, 83; workload, 80. *See also* gender; women
Manderson, L., 21, 67–84
manufactured risk, 233, 250
manufactured scarcity (contrived scarcity), 233; economic agendas and, 150–52; manipulation of water and public opinion, 129, 262; *vs.* natural scarcity, 252n2; privatization and large scale projects, 146–50; St. Thomas, U.S. Virgin Islands, 134
manufacturing. *See* industrialization
maquiladoras, 240
marine resources, 165–67, 182n17
market economy. *See* cash economy; free market/privatization incentives
Marshall Islands, 141
Mashantucket Pequot tribe, 182n22
Massachusetts Military Reservation, 141
matrilineal/matrilocal societies, 65n3
Mauritania, 71
Mbaya, S., 54
Mbeki, T., 45
McCaleb, N., 170
measles, 37
measuring water, 188, 191–93, 196
mediascapes, 154
mediators in globalization, 88
medical anthropology, 4, 43, 46, 233–36, 252n3, 263–65
Medina County, Texas, 112, 115
"mega" projects: "augmenting supply" and, 185; cost recovery and, 148; manufactured scarcity and, 146–50; recommended bans on, 148; World Bank and, 150, 257
memes, 88
mercantilism, 155
mercury, 243
methane wells, 163, 182n14

Mexicali-Mesa de Andrade aquifer, 238, 242–43, 244, 247–49
Mexicali Valley, Mexico: agriculture and water quality, 238–40; bottled water sources, 249, 254n9; globalization's impacts on, 242, 249–51; pesticides and, 239, 243–46; trusting drinking water, 248–49; water table, 247; World Bank loans, 239
Mexico: borders, 232, 241–42; bottled water in, 237; lack of groundwater quality information, 247–49; Mexicali Valley. *See* Mexicali Valley, Mexico; NAFTA participation, 240; pesticides and, 243–46; structural myopia, 250; water conflicts with U.S., 238, 250; water insecurity, 251n1; water management program, 239; withholding pesticide information, 245–46
middle classes, 28–29, 40–41, 65n2, 203, 205
migrants: in China, 81–82; cholera and, 33, 35; in Ecuador, 34–35; global connections and, 88; globalization and, 87; schistosomiasis and, 71–72
militarism, 141, 151
Millennium Challenge, 256, 259–60
Millennium Development Goals, 257
mining, water issues and, 163–64
Ministry of the Environment, Spain, 201
Ministry of Water Development, Malawi, 57, 60
miracidium, 70
miscarriages, 139
missile defense tests, 141
mixed uses of water, 190
Mni Sose Intertribal Water Rights Coalition, 171
Mni Wiconi Project, 164, 171
mobile water providers, 236

mobility restrictions, in China, 79
mobilization. *See* activism
modernization, 154
Mohawk tribe, 168
mollusciding, 74–75, 76
monitoring systems: cholera prevention and, 33; difficulties in multilateral developments, 148; for Edwards Aquifer, 115–16; in Malawi, 58, 61, 64; in Southern Africa, 222
Monsanto pesticides, 244
moral economy: cholera and, 30–35; *vs.* demand management-based strategies, 45–46; disease patterns and, 32; globalization and, 30; health perspectives, 41–44; Malawi policies and, 62; public health infrastructure and trade, 35
morbidity. *See* diseases
Morocco, 73
mortality: American Indians, 176–78; Caribbean children, 39–40; children, 9, 25, 39–40, 259–60; cholera, 13, 31, 146; diarrheal diseases, 91, 96; Ecuador's cholera outbreak, 31; HIV/AIDS, 52, 65n2; Latin America children, 39–40; London's cholera outbreak, 13; reducing for children, 259–60; schistosomiasis, 70; tropical diseases, 68; U.S. leading causes of, 12; water-related diseases, 136, 251n1; WHO statistics, 30
multidisciplinary teams, 4, 32–33, 263–64
multilateral organizations, 213–14. *See also* International Monetary Fund; loan structures; World Bank
multinational corporations. *See* transnational corporations
multitribal coalitions, 170, 171

313

# Index

Mulwafu, W. O., 64n1
municipal water supplies: irrigation distribution in Spain, 197; Lima, Peru; Mexicali. *See* Mexicali Valley, Mexico; privatization, 117; San Antonio, 110–11, 113, 118–20, 122–23; trade agreements and, 143–44; Yingjiang Village, China, 75–81. *See also names of specific cities and villages*
munitions, 141

Nader, L., 236
NAFTA. *See* North America Free Trade Agreement (NAFTA)
Namibia: colonial water projects, 221; history, 230n15; rights to water, 227; water problems, 221; water scarcity, 217; water supply investments, 229n9
narrative analogy in frameworks, 212–14
National Action Council, Zimbabwe, 226
National Cap of Water, Ghana, 194
National Federation of Irrigation Communities (FNCR), 199, 200, 205
National Indian Gaming Regulatory Act, United States, 182–83n23
National Water Council, Spain, 198
National Water Development Project, Malawi, 55
nation-states: decline of, 213; developed nation disease rates, 27–28; impacts of water and health policies, 260–61; indigenous peoples in, 156; NAFTA legal challenges and, 26–27; porous borders and, 234, 250; social contracts and, 59; water ownership, 223; welfare obligations of, 258. *See also names of specific countries*

Native Alaskans, 157, 173, 180n8
Native Americans. *See* American Indians; indigenous people
Native Hawaiians, 180n5
native medicine and healing, 177
native peoples. *See* indigenous people
natural scarcity, 252n2
nature. *See* environment
Nature Conservancy, 261
Navajo Nation, 163
negotiation: mediators in globalization, 88; public property concepts and, 116–18; Spain's irrigation systems and, 198; United States and Mexico's water disputes, 250; water politics and boundary objects, 108–10
neighbors, 100
neoliberal economic policies: decentralization in, 258–59; Ecuador's adoption of, 34; in globalization, 5; in Malawi, 51–52; public health impacts, 28, 35–41; structural violence and, 25, 63
Nestle Corporation, 237, 249, 254n9
net fishing, 166
Nez Perce tribe, 164, 174
NGOs. *See* nongovernmental organizations (NGOs)
Niger, 72
Nigeria, 73–74
Nisqually tribe, 164
Nkhoma, B., 65n1
non-consumptive water uses, 190
nongovernmental organizations (NGOs): in globalization, 5; human rights and torture reporting, 230n23; importance of, 261; Malawi water programs and, 59; technology and, 235; World Bank policy critiques, 214
non-Indian leaseholders, 161, 181n12

North America Free Trade Agreement (NAFTA): binational agreements and, 250; challenges to local laws, 26–27; Mexico's participation in, 240; policy impacts on health, 26; water as commodity, 145
North American Commission for Environmental Cooperation, 240
North American Development Bank, 240
Northern Cheyenne tribe, 163
nuclear fuel, 175
NUKEM Nuclear Ltd., 144

Ogallala aquifer, 191
Oglala tribe, 164, 171
Oka golf course conflict, 168
Omaña Dam, Spain, 202
Omran, A. R., 11
onchocerciasis, 10, 84n1
Oneida Nation, 181n
Orbigo Valley, Spain: irrigation systems, 187; Leon Irrigators Council, 201–4; Ley de Modificación de Aguas, 204–5; water management history, 195–201
Organic Law on Trade Union Freedom, Spain, 200
organization. *See* activism; collaboration and cooperative behaviors
organochlorines, 246
Ó Riain, S., 86
orphans, HIV/AIDS and, 53
output water pricing, 192

Pacific islands, 136
parasites, 10, 27, 84n1
participatory management and behavior. *See* collaboration and cooperative behaviors
participatory research, 6
Partido Popular, Spain, 203
partitioning water, 188, 191–93, 208n3
Passamaquoddy tribe, 162

## Index

passions, in water issues, 3, 265
patents, 42–43
pathogens, 95
Patriotic Health Campaign, China, 74
patron-client relationships, 88
Peabody Energy Company, 163
Pedersen, D., 89
peers, global connections and, 88
Peet, R., 212
penny consumerism, 100, 102–3, 104
Penobscot tribe, 162
Pepsi Cola, 237, 249, 254n9
*pequeños propietarios*, 239
Pequot tribe, 182n22
perception: of groundwater, 243; of manufactured scarcity, 129, 146, 262; of water quality, 247
perchlorate, 130, 141, 151
permits, water, 118, 194, 223–24
pernicious moral relativism, 43–44
Perry, C. J., 192
personal computers, 140
Peru: Canto Grande, 89, 93, 97–101; loan structures, 96; map, 87; surface water supply, 93; underinvestment and underdevelopment, 96–97. *See also* Lima, Peru
per-unit water fees, 191–92, 197, 198, 206–7
pesticides, 233, 239, 241, 243–46, 253n5
Peters, P., 65n1
PHC (primary health care), 41
Pickens, T. B., 191
pinworm, 10
piped water, 34, 93–94
pipelines, 123
Plan Hidrológico Nacional, Spain, 203
Plan Nacional de Regadíos, Spain, 201, 203
pneumonia, 12, 222
Pojoaque Pueblo, 162, 165

policy issues: anthropology and, 7–8; cost recovery policies, 146; critique of policies, 214; decentralization and, 108; definitions of community and, 56; deregulation and health impacts, 26; discourses and, 212–14; ecosystem health and, 126n9; equitable access to water and resources, 48; historical context for, 256; impacts of water and health policies, 260–61; international lending organizations and, 214; lack of financial support for, 64; loan structures and, 213; negotiations in policy making, 108; neoliberal economics. *See* neoliberal economic policies; privatization and, 108; rights in water policies, 63; structural adjustment policies, 37, 40, 50; sustainable use policies, 216–17; water-borne diseases and, 263; water-related diseases and, 262
political activism. *See* activism
political anthropology, 263
political ecology: approaches in, 252n3, 263, 264–65; boundaries of, 46; environmental discourses and, 212; global forces in, 88; pollutants and, 233–34; "studying up" methodology, 236
political economy of health, 43
politics: casinos and, 173; indigenous people and, 170–71; manipulating public opinion, 262–63; manufactured scarcity and, 150–52; removing from water, 218
polluter pay systems, 222, 225
pollution: American Indian water supplies, 162; China's lakes, 137; Colorado River, 243; drinking water and, 91; escalation of, 265; exposure research, 233–34; favoring economic development over pollution, 123; as health issue, 122–23; high-tech industry and, 139–40; industrialization and, 94, 112–13, 138–39; irrigation and, 94, 135; in Malawi, 61, 62; militarism and, 141; poisoning water supply, 130; political ecology and, 233–34; regulations and laws, 62; rivers, 61, 62, 91, 243; sanitation systems and, 61; spread of, 91; strip mining and, 163; withholding information, 245–46
poor. *See* poverty and the poor
population growth, 90, 91, 92, 94, 108, 215
populations: American Indians, 156–58, 180n2; environmental change and, 90; freshwater estimates, 90; HIV/AIDS in, 52; impacts of dams on, 137; lacking sanitation systems, 90; lacking water supplies, 39, 90; local control and, 259; schistosomiasis in, 73–74, 75; terrorism and, 94; urban poverty, 90
porous boundaries of states, 250
Portugal, 185
potable water. *See* drinking water
poultry, 95–96
poverty and the poor: cholera and, 30–35; in Ecuador, 34–35; global trade and, 34–35; HIV/AIDS and, 52; intergenerational, 53; land redistribution and, 221; in Malawi, 51–54, 58–62; patterns of disease, 32; primary water and, 219; privatization and, 215–16, 232; *pueblos jovenes*, 97; selling water rights and, 190; in Southern Africa, 221;

315

# INDEX

urban populations and, 90; vectorborne diseases and, 68; water policies and, 58–62; water reforms and, 211
power: gender and, 49; HIV/AIDS and, 53; intellectual property rights, 43; participation in management, 148; unequal relationships, 234; water scarcity and, 141–46. *See also* empowerment
praziquantel treatment, 70, 76
*presas*, 196, 197
prevention of diseases, 12, 14, 27, 33–34, 35, 89
pricing water: commercial water in Zimbabwe, 225; cost recovery, 186, 191–93; dams and, 225; Dublin principles and, 215; European Union directive, 205; input and output pricing, 192; measuring water, 191–93; reducing water demand, 192; structures for, 191–93; volumetric pricing, 186, 191–93, 206–7
primary health care (PHC), 36, 41
primary water, 219, 223, 224
private drilling companies, 59
private property. *See* property rights
privatization: Bolivian riots and, 149; bottled water, 132, 249; demand-based strategies, 186–87; in Ecuador, 28; under FTAA rules, 27; government partnerships and, 108; of health care, 258; in Latin America, 236–37; in Lima, 92, 102–3; in Malawi, 56, 57; municipal water systems and, 117; public health infrastructure breakdown, 36–41; *vs.* public/private partnerships, 148–49; public utilities and, 150; resistance to,

149, 194–95, 253n4; in South Africa, 145–46; Spain's water laws and, 204–5; success of, 124; United States' promotion of, 92; water rights and, 189–91; water scarcity and, 146–50, 215–16; World Bank's backing of, 235, 256–59
Professional Golf Association, 122–23
project culture, 120
"projectization," 51–52
property rights: groundwater and, 116–17; irrigation and, 187–89; knowledge-based property, 42–43; land and water rights, 187–89, 206, 224; privatizing water and, 189–91; "pro-poor" companies, 232
protectionism, 179, 235
public good: centralized water management and, 258; drinking water as, 231; health as private good, 38; selling water rights and, 189
public health infrastructure: in China, 83; drinking water supplies and, 138; *vs.* economic market interests, 26; in Ecuador, 35; epidemiological transitions and, 11, 28–29; evisceration of, 35–41; globalization's consequences, 28; lack of funding for, 83; rapid urban growth and, 90; regulation and deregulation, 26; sanitation and water as rights, 12; schistosomiasis and, 74–75
public opinion, manipulating, 129, 262–63
public/private partnerships, 148–49
public property. *See* commons
public-right-to-know legislation, 140
public utilities, 143, 144, 150, 172
pueblos jovenes, 89, 94, 97,

98–101
Puerto Rico, 141
pumping caps, 119–20
pumps, municipal, 12–13
Puyallup tribe, 166, 174

Quality of water. *See* water quality
Quebec, Canada, 172
Quito, Ecuador, 32

Radioactive waste, 140
Rafeedie decision, 167
rationing water, 192
recharge areas for aquifers, 112, 117–18, 119, 243
recreational water use, 72, 73, 111, 172–74
reductions: in childhood mortality, 259–60; in farming subsidies, 259; in water demand, 192
reforms, water. *See* water reforms
regulations and laws: Canto Grande's legal challenges, 104; English riparian water law, 118; environmental regulations as ideological globalization, 235; global forces and legal mechanisms, 88; international water protection law, 235; Malawi water regulations, 58, 62; NAFTA legal challenges, 26–27; regarding aquifers and groundwater, 109; regarding surface water, 109; Spain's water laws, 196, 198, 200–201, 207; state level in water policies, 63–64; Zimbabwe's water law, 222–23
religion: church-based water programs, 51, 59, 61, 88; cleansing spiritual domains, 101; global imagination and, 88
relocation: dams and, 69, 257, 260; indigenous peoples and, 155; schistosomiasis and, 71. *See also* migrants
research: American Indian

# INDEX

water data, 159–60; assumptions and, 8; codes of ethics, 7; critical medical anthropology, 263, 264–65; ethnography and, 86; Kato-Katz technique, 76; local processes and, 6; methods used, 6; multidisciplinary teams, 4, 263–64; political ecology, 263, 264–65; scale and, 19; structural myopia, 254n8; study boundaries, 4–5

reservations and reserves: American Indian lands, 156–58; non-Indian leaseholders, 161, 181n12; off-reservation claims, 162–65, 167–69; on-reservation water issues, 160–62; populations on, 180n2; unemployment and income, 177–78

resistance and protests, 37, 122, 149, 194–95, 253n4

resource management: American Indian issues, 167–69; demand management *vs.* moral economy, 45–46; epidemiological transitions and, 11; globalization's preemption of, 155; health issues and, 4, 19; trends in, 46–50; water-linked food resources, 165–67. *See also* water management

Resources for the Future, 261

respiratory diseases, 12, 244–45

reused water, 100–101, 202

rice planting, 78–79

rights: American Indian water rights, 163, 181–82n13; appropriation of water and, 188; ceding rights, 202; *vs.* commodities, 26, 50, 152; drinking water as, 231; Edwards Aquifer usage, 115; fishing rights, 165–67; gender divisions and, 49–50; health as human right, 14, 46; local agencies and water rights, 227; Malawi's policies and, 57; moral economy and, 30, 43; property. *See* property rights; risks and, 42; sanitation as, 12; Spain's laws and, 196, 204–5; water as environment's right, 48, 216–17; water as human right, 12, 14, 45–46, 49–50, 218–19; in water policies, 63

Rio Summit Agenda 21, 46

riots and protests, 37, 149, 253n4

risk: behavior and disease, 89; manufactured risk, 233, 250; nondefinition of, 42; unequal exposure to, 234

river blindness (onchocerciasis), 10, 84n1

rivers: as boundaries, 67; pollution problems, 91; river basin management, 48. *See also names of specific rivers*

River Walk, San Antonio, 113

Rosebud Sioux tribe, 164, 171

Rosegrant, M., 215

RWE Aktiengesellschaft, 143, 191

Salinity, 93, 137, 143–44, 238, 243, 261

Salish tribe, 161, 163

salmon fishing, 158, 166, 167, 172, 174

salmon hatcheries, 165

salmon kills, 142–43, 164

saltwater invasions, 91, 93, 136

San Antonio, Texas, 110–11, 113, 118–20, 122–23

San Antonio Water System, 118–20

sanctions on water use, 198

Sandia Pueblo, 175

San Diego Water Authority, 242

sanitation systems: cash resources and, 81; in China, 77, 80–81; cholera and, 30–35; epidemiological transitions and, 11–13, 28–29; human rights to, 43; in Latin America, 237; in Malawi, 54–58, 61, 64; populations lacking access, 90; public health infrastructure and, 11; in pueblos jovenes, 102–4; in Southern Africa, 211, 222; UNICEF program, 260; in water-related diseases, 10

San Juan de Lurigancho, Peru, 89

San Lorenzo Valley Water District, 144

San Marcos aquifer, 253n6

Santa Clara, California, 139–40

Santa Cruz County, California, 144

SAPs (structural adjustment policies), 37, 40, 50

SARS virus, 178

Satiacum, R., 166

scabies, 9, 55, 62

scale, issues of, 19

scarcity frameworks, 214–17. *See also* manufactured scarcity; water scarcity

schistosomiasis: in China, 74–83; dams and, 68–69; gender differences in infection, 72–74, 83; HIV/AIDS and, 55; incidence of, 27, 70; in Malawi, 55, 61; peak shedding, 73; prevention workers, 82; in Southern Africa, 222; symptoms, 77; vectors and transmission, 69–72; as water-based illness, 10

Scudder, T., 71

seawater intrusion, 91, 93, 136

seismic activity, 99

selected primary health care, 36, 41

self-sufficiency, 155

selling water rights, 116, 189, 204–5

Seneca tribe, 158, 174–75

Senegal, 71

senior and junior water rights, 115

SEO/Birdlife group, 204

settlements: Canto Grande, 97; housing in, 98–101; in

317

# Index

Southern Africa, 221; urban growth and, 93
sewage systems. *See* sanitation systems
Shah, M. K., 54
shellfish, 165, 166, 182n17
shigella, 96
Shiva, V., 15
Shuar people, 31
Sichuan province, China, 75
Sierra Club, 114
Silicon Valley, California, 139–40
Sindicato Central de Riegos del Embalse de Barrios de Luna, 197
Sioux tribes, 162, 164, 168–69, 171, 174
skin infections, 77, 101
skin sepsis, 10, 55
Skull Valley Band, 175
sleeping sickness, 84n1
smallholder agriculture, 186. *See also* farming
snail fever. *See* schistosomiasis
snails, 69, 74–75, 76. *See also* schistosomiasis
Snoqualmie tribe, 174
Snow, J., 13
social contracts, breakdown of, 59
Society for Applied Anthropology, 7
Sohappy, D., 166
Sohappy, R., 166
Solo, T. M., 236
Song, H., 82
South Africa: catchment plan, 218; cholera, 151–52; colonial water projects, 221; cost recovery and, 145–46; South African Bill of Rights, 219; South African Water Act, 219; water rights in, 227
South African Water Act, 219
Southern Africa: HIV/AIDS in, 52–53; map, 210; nations in, 228n1; Southern African Development Community, 228n1; structural adjustment policies and, 50; water access challenges, 227; waterborne diseases in, 222; water frameworks in, 226–28; water reforms in, 209–11, 221–25
Southern African Development Community (SADC), 228n1
Southern Utes, 163
sovereignty, 156, 161
Spain: dam projects, 185; Ministry of the Environment, 201; National Water Council, 198; national water plan, 203; occupation of Ecuador, 31; Orbigo Valley irrigation systems, 187, 195–201; Organic Law on Trade Union Freedom, 200; reforms and economic development, 195–96; water laws, 196, 198, 200–201, 207
spiritual domains, 88, 101
spousal abuse, 177
springs, 111–12, 144
St. Thomas, Virgin Islands, 133–34
stakeholders: lacking water quality information, 247; Southern African decentralization and, 50; water management and, 218; water quality perception, 247; World Bank participation policies, 241, 257; Zimbabwe water reforms, 224
standards: agrifood industry, 241; as ideological globalization, 235; state level water policies, 63–64; water measurements, 193; water quality, 242
standards of living, 91
standpipes, 94
Stott, P., 213
street vendors, 33, 94
strip mining pollution, 163
structural adjustment policies (SAPs), 37, 40, 50
structural myopia, 132, 245, 248, 250, 254n8
structural violence: cholera as, 30–35; as framework, 8–9; HIV/AIDS and, 63; in marginalized groups, 130; political processes and, 262; processes of, 256; water scarcity as, 102–3; World Bank policies and, 259
"studying up" methodology, 236
Subcatchment Councils, Zimbabwe, 230n21
subsidies, 37, 47, 51, 259
Suez/ONDEO water company, 117, 191, 237, 252n4
suicide rates, 176
Sullivan, S., 213
supply-side dynamics, 48, 135
surface water: consumptive and non-consumptive uses, 190; Peru's supply, 93; rights to, in Texas, 118; testing, 253n5; water laws and, 109
sustainability, 216–17, 219–20
Sustainable Development Conference, 218
Swinomish tribe, 162

Tariffs and levies: commercial water in Zimbabwe, 225; economic nationalism and, 179; Ecuadorian system, 34; neoliberal reforms and, 234; Spain's water usage tariffs, 197; water pricing, 192
TBT (Agreement on Technical Barriers to Trade), 42
technology: activists' use of, 235; communication technologies, 234, 241–42; in globalization, 154; high-tech industry waste, 139, 140–41
technoscapes, 154
terraces, 196
terrorism, 94, 178
Texas: Commission on Environmental Quality, 118; Edwards Aquifer. *See* Edwards Aquifer; water laws in, 109
Thames Water Company, 144
The Dalles Dam, 158

## Index

"third space," 116–17
Thrasher Foundation, 89
Three Gorges Dam, China, 68–69, 84
tiered water pricing, 192
time-sensitivity of water and health issues, 265
tinea, 10
top-down management, 148
Torres, V., 252n3, 254n8
El Tor strain of cholera, 30
tourism, 113, 122–23, 134, 165, 172–74, 178
toxic wastes: Colorado River, 243; Hazardous Materials Storage Ordinance, 139–40; high-tech industry contamination, 139–40; industrial rates of creation, 138–39; militarism and, 141; water pollution. *See* pollution
trachoma, 10, 27
trade organizations. *See* international trade organizations
trade unions, 200
"tragedy of the commons," 26
transferring water rights, 116, 189, 204–5
transformative scale of globalization, 155
transnational corporations: bottled water and, 237; commodification of water and, 117, 133–35; in globalization, 5, 154, 234; pesticide companies, 244–45; privatization and, 149, 191, 194, 232, 252n4; water taken by force and, 26. *See also* corporations
transparency, 259
traveling theories of feminism, 87
treaties, 156, 167, 168–69, 180n4, 181–82n13, 238
treatment of schistosomiasis, 70, 75, 76
Treaty of Fort Laramie, 168–69
tribal sovereignty, 156, 161
trichloroethylene, 139
TRIPS (Agreement on Trade-Related Aspects of Intellectual Property), 42
trucking in water. *See* delivered water
trust, in drinking water safety, 236, 249
trypanasomiasis, 84n1
Tsimshian tribe, 173–74
tuberculosis, 12, 55, 77, 176, 222
two-part tariffs, 192
typhoid, 9, 27, 55, 61, 62, 243

Ulcers, 10, 55
Umatilla tribe, 166
underdevelopment, in Peru, 96–97
underinvestment, in Peru, 96–97
unemployment, 177
United Nations: Children's Fund, 260; Committee on Economic, Social and Cultural Rights, 219, 226; daily water needs statistics, 13–14; Development Program, 260; Environment Programme, 229n12; Food and Agriculture Organization, 229n12; "Global State of the Environment Report," 40; High Commission of Refugees (UNHCR), 13–14; International Covenant on Economic, Social and Cultural Rights, 46, 219; International Drinking Water Supply and Sanitation Decade, 25, 48; Millennium Challenge, 256, 259–60; Millennium Development Goals, 257; Permanent Forum on Indigenous Issues, 170; Population Fund, 90; rights-based approach of, 152; water scarcity report, 147; World Water Development Report, 147–48
United States: borders, 232, 241–42; bottled water sales, 254n9; negotiations for water disputes, 250; waterborne diseases, 27–28; water conflicts with Mexico, 238
United States government: Agency for International Development, 33; armed forces-generated toxic wastes, 141; Bureau of Indian Affairs, 170–71; Bureau of Land Management, 142; Environmental Protection Agency, 242, 245; National Indian Gaming Regulatory Act, 182–83n23
United Water company, 191
Upper Mekong/Lancang dam, China, 68
upstream users, 190
urban environments: Edwards Aquifer and, 111; effects of rapid urbanization, 91; housing in, 98–101; impact on wetlands and lakes, 137; indigenous peoples and, 155; Lima's environment, 92–96; *pueblos jovenes*, 97; schistosomiasis and, 71–72; urban growth worldwide, 90; water quality issues, 91; Zimbabwe water sales and, 226
urinary schistosomiasis, 69, 71
user fees: consumption-based, 192–93; cost recovery programs and, 146, 149; effects of, 206–7; Malawi water systems, 58; per-unit fees, 191–92, 197, 198, 206–7; polluter pay systems, 222, 225; riots and, 149; user pay policies, 224–25, 226
user groups: *vs.* community, 60; in Malawi, 63
user pay policies, 224–25, 226
USFilter, 191
Ute Mountain Utes, 163
Uvalde County, Texas, 112, 115

# Index

Vaccines, 12, 36, 43
Valencia, Spain, 199
values: Dublin Principles economic values, 212; global imagination and, 88; water as commodity, 68–69, 120, 129–30; water's value, 135
vecinos, 208n4
vectors: in disease transmission, 67–69; mortality rates of vectorborne diseases, 68; in schistosomiasis, 69–72; in water-related diseases, 10
vendor water, 33, 94. *See also* water companies
Vieques, Puerto Rico, 141
virtual water, 3, 215, 229n10
Vivendi Universal corporation, 117, 191, 237, 252n4
volumetric measuring and pricing, 186, 188, 191–93, 197, 202, 206–7

W. R. Grace corporation, 96
wage economy: China, 81–82; Ecuador, 34–35
Walpole Island Indian Community, 162
Wang, J., 82
warabandi irrigation system, 192
Washington Consensus, 51
wasting water. *See* water conservation
water: acre-feet, 126n4; boundary objects and, 108–10; as commodity, 68–69, 133–35; crises, 211–12; daily needs, 13–14; demand. *See* demand for water; freshwater estimates, 90; globalization of, 25–30; global water apartheid, 45; grounded globalization and, 89–92; human rights to, 45–46; management. *See* water management; markets, 186; moral economy of health and, 41–44; paradigm changes in rights model, 14–15, 43–44; as political resource, 67;

potable. *See* drinking water; pricing. *See* pricing water; rationing, 192; scarcity. *See* water scarcity; security. *See* water security and insecurity; use and demand statistics, 91; virtual water, 3, 215, 229n10; world statistics, 9, 90
Water Act of 1998, Zimbabwe, 222–23
Water Aid, 261
water banks, 204
water barrels, 98
water-based diseases, 10
waterborne diseases, 9; awareness of, 81; incidence of, 91; increases in after privatization, 146; in Malawi, 55; in Southern Africa, 222; transmission, 31–32; in United States, 27–28; water management policies and, 263
water companies: bottled water, 237; private water drilling companies, 59; utilities, 117, 143–45, 191, 237, 252n4
water conservation: conservation easements, 117–18, 119; free market incentives and, 262; privatization and, 215, 262; reused water, 100–101, 202; Southern African reforms and, 211
water fees and costs: Bolivian riots and, 149; effects of, 206–7; Orbigo Valley, Spain, 197; polluter pay systems, 222, 225; pricing structures, 191–93; *pueblos jovenes*, 100–101; South African cost recovery and, 146; urban areas, 91; user pay policy, 224–25, 226
water insecurity, 9–10, 14, 231–33, 251n1, 261–62
water-intensive cash crops, 112
Water Investment Act of 2002, United States, 145
waterlords, 189
water management: bound-

ary objects and, 108–10, 124–25; disease prevention efforts and, 83–84; economic prioritization in, 142–43; equitable participation in, 148; integrated approaches to, 48; Malawi water boards, 55; social structuring of, 130; trends in, 46–50; United Nations focus on, 257; water-related diseases and, 262; water scarcity and, 136, 148
water measurements, 188, 191–93, 196
water pricing. *See* pricing water
water projects: arsenic mitigation projects, 138; Colorado River rehabilitation project, 243; "mega" projects. *See* "mega" projects; Namibia colonial government, 221; participatory management in, 259; project culture and, 120; schistosomiasis and, 70, 71; small-scale localized projects, 148; Zimbabwe colonial government, 221
water quality: assessing, 231; bottled water, 251; community-based strategies in Malawi and, 61; crises in, 130; health issues and, 10; lack of information on, 247–49; in Mexicali Valley, 238–40; monitoring, 115–16; standards for, 220, 242; urban sewage problems, 91
water reforms: Bolivian resistance to, 149, 194; droughts and, 221; Dublin Principles and, 222; informal adjustments to, 197; Malawi water reforms, 58, 59–60; neoliberal reforms, 234, 259; poverty and, 211; resistance to demand management, 194–95; Southern African reforms, 222; Southern Africa reforms, 209–11, 221–25;

# INDEX

Spain's reforms, 195–96, 201, 203; water management and, 130, 132; Zimbabwe water reforms, 131, 210, 222–25, 223–25
water-related diseases, 9–10; factors in spread of cholera, 30–35; incidence, 91; mortality rates, 136, 251n1; vectorborne, 67–69; water management policies and, 262; world rates of, 30
water-related tourism, 172–74
Water Research Group, 215
water resource management. *See* water management
Water Resources Management Policy and Strategies, Malawi, 54
water-scarce diseases, 9, 55, 81, 85, 91
water scarcity: cultural and power dimensions in, 141–46; discourses about, 213–15; economic agendas and, 150–52; health and human consequences of, 136–41; in Lima, 93–96; local responses to, 85; manufactured scarcity, 129, 134, 146–50, 262–63; as relative construct, 135–36; scarcity frameworks, 214–17; in Texas, 109
water security and insecurity, 9–10, 14, 231–33, 251n1, 261–62
watersheds, 61, 108, 125, 142–43, 152, 203
water shortages. *See* water scarcity
Water Subcatchment Councils Regulations of 2000, 230n21
water supply: cholera and, 32; epidemiological transitions and, 11–13, 28–29; global threats to, 136; human rights to, 43; lack of records for, 60; Latin America systems, 236–37; Lima's issues, 92–96; Malawi systems, 54–58;

purchasing infrastructures, 252n4; Southern Africa systems, 50, 221; world's population without, 39, 90. *See also* drinking water
water-surplus and water-deficit watersheds, 203
water tables, 247
water taxes. *See* tariffs and levies
water use. *See* demand for water
water wars, 15, 109, 239
water-washed diseases (water-scarce diseases), 9, 55, 81, 85, 91
Watts, S., 212
WCD (World Commission on Dams), 148, 152
weapons testing, 141
wells, 93, 94, 161, 247. *See also* aquifers and groundwater
Western Shoshone tribe, 162
West Nile fever, 10
wetlands, 137, 164
whaling, 166, 167, 171
wheat, 239
Whiteford, L.: on future water and health challenges, 255–65; health and economics, 20; on health and water access, 19–23; on public health infrastructure's development, 150–51; research on global trade agreements, 19, 25–44; on water management, 129–32; on water paradigm change, 3–15
Whiteford, S.: on future water and health challenges, 255–65; on health and water access, 19–23; research on global trade agreements, 19; on U.S./Mexico border water issues, 231–54; on water management, 129–32; on water paradigm change, 3–15
WHO. *See* World Health Organization
widows, 54

Winters' Doctrine, 181–82n13
women: concern for water quality, 249; in Dublin principles, 212; exposure to disease, 78–79, 80; HIV/AIDS and, 53; in Malawi, 50–54, 56, 59, 62, 63; matrilineal/matrilocal societies, 65n3; mobility restrictions, in China, 79; role in water management, 48–49, 65n4; schistosomiasis and, 70, 72–74, 75, 83; sexual exploitation, 53; water policies and, 56, 59, 62, 63
women-in-development literature, 48–49
workforce: in China, 81–82; clean water supplies and, 11; in Ecuador, 34–35; public health and, 28–29
working arrangements in water use, 197
World Bank: arsenic mitigation projects, 138; Bolivian water system privatization, 194; CGIAR support, 229n12; Colorado River rehabilitation project, 243; contractual relationships and, 149; cost recovery policies, 145–46; demand-side orientation of, 48; escalation of poverty and, 216; ideology of, 5; loan requirements, 241; Malawi policies, 51, 55–56; "mega" project emphasis, 150; Mexicali irrigation and land loans, 239; new water policies, 217; nongovernmental organization critique of, 214; privatization emphasis of, 256–59; on "pro-poor" companies, 232; public health infrastructure breakdown and, 36–41; purchasing water infrastructures and, 252n4; schistosomiasis control and, 75, 84; Southern Africa focus, 222; structural adjustment policies. *See*

321

# Index

structural adjustment policies; Water Development Strategy, 257; Water Management Strategy, 228n6; Water Policy document, 257; water scarcity report, 147
World Commission on Dams (WCD), 134, 148, 152
World Health Organization (WHO): Action Programs on Essential Drugs, 41; children's health focus, 260; Commission on Macroeconomics and Health, 14; on daily water needs, 13; Diarrheal Diseases Control Program (CDD), 89; disempowerment of, 41, 43; ideology of, 5; International Code of Marketing Breast Milk Substitute, 41, 42; Lima diarrhea prevention project, 89; Medicinal Drug Promotion, 41; on mortality rates, 9, 30, 52; Special Program for Research and Training in Tropical Disease, 68; on trachoma cases, 27
World Resource Institute, 90
World Summit for Children and Water, 260
World Summit for Social Development, 26, 260
World Summit on Sustainable Development in Johannesburg, 45, 46, 92, 218
World Trade Organization (WTO): Agreement on Technical Barriers to Trade (TBT), 36, 42; constraints on trade and, 179; eliminating tariffs and barriers, 234; impact of trade on health, 28; public health infrastructure breakdown and, 36–41
World Vision, 261
World Water Forum, 117, 134, 147
worms, 27
WTO. *See* World Trade Organization (WTO)
WWF/ADENA group, 204, 208n6

Yakama tribe, 166, 174
Yangtze River, China, 69
Yankton Sioux tribe, 174
yellow fever, 10
Yingjiang Village, China, 75–81
Young, J., 166
young towns, 89, 94, 97, 98–101
Yunnan province, China, 75
Yurok tribe, 164

Zimbabwe: colonial water projects, 221; history, 230n15; Human Rights NGO Forum, 230n23; land and water reforms, 210; National Action Council, 226; National Water Authority, 225; National Water Authority Act, 222–23; primary water definition, 219; water reforms, 131, 222–25
zinc, 140
Zipingqu Dam, China, 68
Zomba district, Malawi, 58–62
Zuni Pueblo, 164–65
Zuni Salt Lake, 164–65

# School for Advanced Research Advanced Seminar Series

## PUBLISHED BY SAR PRESS

CHACO & HOHOKAM: PREHISTORIC REGIONAL SYSTEMS IN THE AMERICAN SOUTHWEST
*Patricia L. Crown & W. James Judge, eds.*

RECAPTURING ANTHROPOLOGY: WORKING IN THE PRESENT
*Richard G. Fox, ed.*

WAR IN THE TRIBAL ZONE: EXPANDING STATES AND INDIGENOUS WARFARE
*R. Brian Ferguson & Neil L. Whitehead, eds.*

IDEOLOGY AND PRE-COLUMBIAN CIVILIZATIONS
*Arthur A. Demarest & Geoffrey W. Conrad, eds.*

DREAMING: ANTHROPOLOGICAL AND PSYCHOLOGICAL INTERPRETATIONS
*Barbara Tedlock, ed.*

HISTORICAL ECOLOGY: CULTURAL KNOWLEDGE AND CHANGING LANDSCAPES
*Carole L. Crumley, ed.*

THEMES IN SOUTHWEST PREHISTORY
*George J. Gumerman, ed.*

MEMORY, HISTORY, AND OPPOSITION UNDER STATE SOCIALISM
*Rubie S. Watson, ed.*

OTHER INTENTIONS: CULTURAL CONTEXTS AND THE ATTRIBUTION OF INNER STATES
*Lawrence Rosen, ed.*

LAST HUNTERS–FIRST FARMERS: NEW PERSPECTIVES ON THE PREHISTORIC TRANSITION TO AGRICULTURE
*T. Douglas Price & Anne Birgitte Gebauer, eds.*

MAKING ALTERNATIVE HISTORIES: THE PRACTICE OF ARCHAEOLOGY AND HISTORY IN NON-WESTERN SETTINGS
*Peter R. Schmidt & Thomas C. Patterson, eds.*

CYBORGS & CITADELS: ANTHROPOLOGICAL INTERVENTIONS IN EMERGING SCIENCES AND TECHNOLOGIES
*Gary Lee Downey & Joseph Dumit, eds.*

SENSES OF PLACE
*Steven Feld & Keith H. Basso, eds.*

THE ORIGINS OF LANGUAGE: WHAT NONHUMAN PRIMATES CAN TELL US
*Barbara J. King, ed.*

CRITICAL ANTHROPOLOGY NOW: UNEXPECTED CONTEXTS, SHIFTING CONSTITUENCIES, CHANGING AGENDAS
*George E. Marcus, ed.*

ARCHAIC STATES
*Gary M. Feinman & Joyce Marcus, eds.*

REGIMES OF LANGUAGE: IDEOLOGIES, POLITIES, AND IDENTITIES
*Paul V. Kroskrity, ed.*

BIOLOGY, BRAINS, AND BEHAVIOR: THE EVOLUTION OF HUMAN DEVELOPMENT
*Sue Taylor Parker, Jonas Langer, & Michael L. McKinney, eds.*

WOMEN & MEN IN THE PREHISPANIC SOUTHWEST: LABOR, POWER, & PRESTIGE
*Patricia L. Crown, ed.*

HISTORY IN PERSON: ENDURING STRUGGLES, CONTENTIOUS PRACTICE, INTIMATE IDENTITIES
*Dorothy Holland & Jean Lave, eds.*

THE EMPIRE OF THINGS: REGIMES OF VALUE AND MATERIAL CULTURE
*Fred R. Myers, ed.*

CATASTROPHE & CULTURE: THE ANTHROPOLOGY OF DISASTER
*Susanna M. Hoffman & Anthony Oliver-Smith, eds.*

URUK MESOPOTAMIA & ITS NEIGHBORS: CROSS-CULTURAL INTERACTIONS IN THE ERA OF STATE FORMATION
*Mitchell S. Rothman, ed.*

REMAKING LIFE & DEATH: TOWARD AN ANTHROPOLOGY OF THE BIOSCIENCES
*Sarah Franklin & Margaret Lock, eds.*

TIKAL: DYNASTIES, FOREIGNERS, & AFFAIRS OF STATE: ADVANCING MAYA ARCHAEOLOGY
*Jeremy A. Sabloff, ed.*

## Published by SAR Press

Gray Areas: Ethnographic Encounters with Nursing Home Culture
*Philip B. Stafford, ed.*

Pluralizing Ethnography: Comparison and Representation in Maya Cultures, Histories, and Identities
*John M. Watanabe & Edward F. Fischer, eds.*

American Arrivals: Anthropology Engages the New Immigration
*Nancy Foner, ed.*

Violence
*Neil L. Whitehead, ed.*

Law & Empire in the Pacific: Fiji and Hawai'i
*Sally Engle Merry & Donald Brenneis, eds.*

Anthropology in the Margins of the State
*Veena Das & Deborah Poole, eds.*

The Archaeology of Colonial Encounters: Comparative Perspectives
*Gil J. Stein, ed.*

Globalization, Water, & Health: Resource Management in Times of Scarcity
*Linda Whiteford & Scott Whiteford, eds.*

A Catalyst for Ideas: Anthropological Archaeology and the Legacy of Douglas W. Schwartz
*Vernon L. Scarborough, ed.*

The Archaeology of Chaco Canyon: An Eleventh-Century Pueblo Regional Center
*Stephen H. Lekson, ed.*

Community Building in the Twenty-First Century
*Stanley E. Hyland, ed.*

Afro-Atlantic Dialogues: Anthropology in the Diaspora
*Kevin A. Yelvington, ed.*

Copán: The History of an Ancient Maya Kingdom
*E. Wyllys Andrews & William L. Fash, eds.*

The Evolution of Human Life History
*Kristen Hawkes & Richard R. Paine, eds.*

The Seductions of Community: Emancipations, Oppressions, Quandaries
*Gerald W. Creed, ed.*

The Gender of Globalization: Women Navigating Cultural and Economic Marginalities
*Nandini Gunewardena & Ann Kingsolver, eds.*

New Landscapes of Inequality: Neoliberalism and the Erosion of Democracy in America
*Jane L. Collins, Micaela di Leonardo, & Brett Williams, eds.*

Imperial Formations
*Ann Laura Stoler, Carole McGranahan, & Peter C. Perdue, eds.*

Opening Archaeology: Repatriation's Impact on Contemporary Research and Practice
*Thomas W. Killion, ed.*

Small Worlds: Method, Meaning, & Narrative in Microhistory
*James F. Brooks, Christopher R. N. DeCorse, & John Walton, eds.*

Memory Work: Archaeologies of Material Practices
*Barbara J. Mills & William H. Walker, eds.*

Figuring the Future: Globalization and the Temporalities of Children and Youth
*Jennifer Cole & Deborah Durham, eds.*

Timely Assets: The Politics of Resources and Their Temporalities
*Elizabeth Emma Ferry & Mandana E. Limbert, eds.*

Democracy: Anthropological Approaches
*Julia Paley, ed.*

Confronting Cancer: Metaphors, Inequality, and Advocacy
*Juliet McMullin & Diane Weiner, eds.*

## Published by SAR Press

DEVELOPMENT & DISPOSSESSION: THE CRISIS OF FORCED DISPLACEMENT AND RESETTLEMENT
*Anthony Oliver-Smith, ed.*

GLOBAL HEALTH IN TIMES OF VIOLENCE
*Barbara Rylko-Bauer, Linda Whiteford, & Paul Farmer, eds.*

THE EVOLUTION OF LEADERSHIP: TRANSITIONS IN DECISION MAKING FROM SMALL-SCALE TO MIDDLE-RANGE SOCIETIES
*Kevin J. Vaughn, Jelmer W. Eerkins, & John Kantner, eds.*

ARCHAEOLOGY & CULTURAL RESOURCE MANAGEMENT: VISIONS FOR THE FUTURE
*Lynne Sebastian & William D. Lipe, eds.*

ARCHAIC STATE INTERACTION: THE EASTERN MEDITERRANEAN IN THE BRONZE AGE
*William A. Parkinson & Michael L. Galaty, eds.*

INDIANS & ENERGY: EXPLOITATION AND OPPORTUNITY IN THE AMERICAN SOUTHWEST
*Sherry L. Smith & Brian Frehner, eds.*

ROOTS OF CONFLICT: SOILS, AGRICULTURE, AND SOCIOPOLITICAL COMPLEXITY IN ANCIENT HAWAI'I
*Patrick V. Kirch, ed.*

PHARMACEUTICAL SELF: THE GLOBAL SHAPING OF EXPERIENCE IN AN AGE OF PSYCHOPHARMACOLOGY
*Janis Jenkins, ed.*

FORCES OF COMPASSION: HUMANITARIANISM BETWEEN ETHICS AND POLITICS
*Erica Bornstein & Peter Redfield, eds.*

ENDURING CONQUESTS: RETHINKING THE ARCHAEOLOGY OF RESISTANCE TO SPANISH COLONIALISM IN THE AMERICAS
*Matthew Liebmann & Melissa S. Murphy, eds.*

## Now available from SAR Press

THE ARCHAEOLOGY OF LOWER CENTRAL AMERICA
*Frederick W. Lange & Doris Z. Stone, eds.*

CHAN CHAN: ANDEAN DESERT CITY
*Michael E. Moseley & Kent C. Day, eds.*

DEMOGRAPHIC ANTHROPOLOGY: QUANTITATIVE APPROACHES
*Ezra B. W. Zubrow, ed.*

THE DYING COMMUNITY
*Art Gallaher, Jr. & Harlan Padfield, eds.*

ELITES: ETHNOGRAPHIC ISSUES
*George E. Marcus, ed.*

ENTREPRENEURS IN CULTURAL CONTEXT
*Sidney M. Greenfield, Arnold Strickon, & Robert T. Aubey, eds.*

LOWLAND MAYA SETTLEMENT PATTERNS
*Wendy Ashmore, ed.*

METHODS AND THEORIES OF ANTHROPOLOGICAL GENETICS
*M. H. Crawford & P. L. Workman, eds.*

THE ORIGINS OF MAYA CIVILIZATION
*Richard E. W. Adams, ed.*

STRUCTURE AND PROCESS IN LATIN AMERICA
*Arnold Strickon & Sidney M. Greenfield, eds.*

## Published by Cambridge University Press

The Anasazi in a Changing Environment
*George J. Gumerman, ed.*

Regional Perspectives on the Olmec
*Robert J. Sharer & David C. Grove, eds.*

The Chemistry of Prehistoric Human Bone
*T. Douglas Price, ed.*

The Emergence of Modern Humans: Biocultural Adaptations in the Later Pleistocene
*Erik Trinkaus, ed.*

The Anthropology of War
*Jonathan Haas, ed.*

The Evolution of Political Systems
*Steadman Upham, ed.*

Classic Maya Political History: Hieroglyphic and Archaeological Evidence
*T. Patrick Culbert, ed.*

Turko-Persia in Historical Perspective
*Robert L. Canfield, ed.*

Chiefdoms: Power, Economy, and Ideology
*Timothy Earle, ed.*

Reconstructing Prehistoric Pueblo Societies
*William A. Longacre, ed.*

## Published by University of New Mexico Press

New Perspectives on the Pueblos
*Alfonso Ortiz, ed.*

The Classic Maya Collapse
*T. Patrick Culbert, ed.*

Sixteenth-Century Mexico: The Work of Sahagun
*Munro S. Edmonson, ed.*

Ancient Civilization and Trade
*Jeremy A. Sabloff &
C. C. Lamberg-Karlovsky, eds.*

Photography in Archaeological Research
*Elmer Harp, Jr., ed.*

The Valley of Mexico: Studies in Pre-Hispanic Ecology and Society
*Eric R. Wolf, ed.*

Explanation of Prehistoric Change
*James N. Hill, ed.*

Meaning in Anthropology
*Keith H. Basso & Henry A. Selby, eds.*

Explorations in Ethnoarchaeology
*Richard A. Gould, ed.*

Southwestern Indian Ritual Drama
*Charlotte J. Frisbie, ed.*

Simulations in Archaeology
*Jeremy A. Sabloff, ed.*

Shipwreck Anthropology
*Richard A. Gould, ed.*

Late Lowland Maya Civilization: Classic to Postclassic
*Jeremy A. Sabloff & E. Wyllys Andrews V, eds.*

## Published by University of California Press

Writing Culture: The Poetics and Politics of Ethnography
*James Clifford &
George E. Marcus, eds.*

## Published by University of Arizona Press

The Collapse of Ancient States and Civilizations
*Norman Yoffee &
George L. Cowgill, eds.*

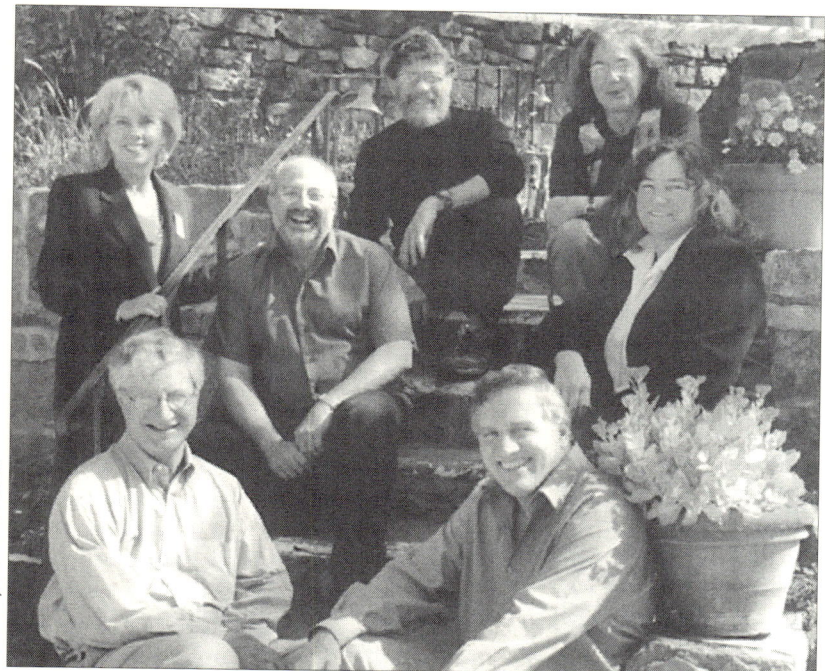

Photo by Katrina Lasko

Participants in the School of American Research contemporary issues seminar "Globalization, Water, and Health: Resource Management in Times of Scarcity," Santa Fe, New Mexico, October 8–9, 2002. Back from left: Linda Whiteford, Carl Kendall, William Derman, Anne Ferguson, Barbara Rose Johnston. Front from left: David Guillet, Scott Whitford.

Made in the USA
San Bernardino, CA
14 September 2013